The
Aromatherapy
Beauty Guide

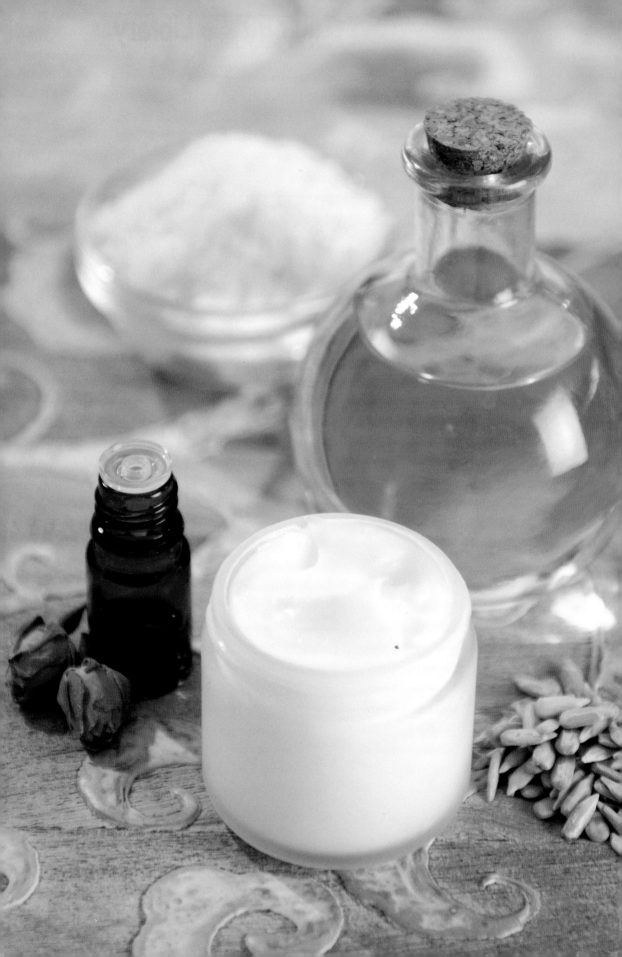

The Aromatherapy Beauty Guide

Using the Science of Carrier & Essential Oils to Create Natural Personal Care Products

Danielle Sade, BSc, CAHP

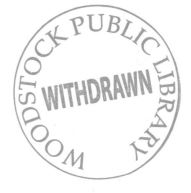

Robert
ROSE

For complete cataloguing information, see page 374.

Disclaimer

The author and the publisher are not responsible for any adverse effects or consequences resulting from the use of the information in this book. It is the responsibility of the reader to consult a physician or other qualified health-care professional regarding his or her personal care.

To the best of our knowledge, the recipes or formulas in this book are safe for ordinary use and users. For those people with allergies or health issues, please read the suggested contents of each recipe or formula carefully and determine whether or not they may create a problem for you. All recipes or formulas are used at the risk of the consumer.

We cannot be responsible for any hazards, loss or damage that may occur as a result of any recipe or formula use.

For those with special needs, allergies, requirements or health problems, in the event of any doubt, please contact your medical adviser prior to the use of any recipe or formula.

Design and production: Kevin Cockburn/PageWave Graphics Inc.
Senior editor: Judith Finlayson
Formulations editor: Tracy Bordian
Copyeditor/proofreader/indexer: Gillian Watts
Photography: Michael Tenaglia (except as noted below)
Formulation preparation: Danielle Sade

Additional images (pages 6, 8, 26, 35, 42, 74, 86, 94, 204, 224, 234, 250, 268, 284, 292, 302, 334, 356): © gettyimages.com

Illustration (page 278): © gettyimages.com

The publisher gratefully acknowledges the financial support of our publishing program by the Government of Canada through the Canada Book Fund.

Canada

Published by Robert Rose Inc.
120 Eglinton Avenue East, Suite 800, Toronto, Ontario, Canada M4P 1E2
Tel: (416) 322-6552 Fax: (416) 322-6936
www.robertrose.ca

Printed and bound in Canada

1 2 3 4 5 6 7 8 9 TCP 25 24 23 22 21 20 19 18 17

Contents

For my mother,
whose wisdom lives within me forever
and who is subtly woven into this book

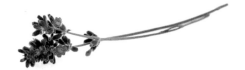

Acknowledgments

I feel blessed and honored to be the teacher from whom my students choose to learn aromatherapy. This book might not have been possible if it weren't for them, the people who inspired me to delve deeply into the unfamiliar scientific territory of aromatherapy to discover solid evidence of the effectiveness and healing potential of essential and carrier oils. Over the past two decades many of my students who have graduated and become professional aromatherapists have also become my colleagues and friends, and we have worked together to create standards of education in aromatherapy. As specialists in an uncommon subject, this has put us in a class of our own, pioneering the use of essential oils in natural skin care, health and well-being.

Many thanks to my colleagues who supported me and encouraged me to continuously share my experience and knowledge. These individuals have significant supporting roles in the writing of this book. Thanks to: Elaine Goodman, for your belief in me. Dr. Janice Goodman, for the confidence you gave me to present my work to a larger audience of professionals. Linda Prussick, Chantal Corriveau, Sue Todd and Chris Carrothers, for your support during times of uncertainty, providing me with the clarity to start a new page.

I am also blessed and filled with gratitude to Ken, my husband and best friend. His soft-spoken words continuously encourage me to believe in what I am doing. And, of course, thank you to my beautiful children, my supportive father and family, who have a fundamental role in whatever I do.

Thank you, also, to David Thomlinson and the Absolute Aroma team of chemists who throughout the years provided me with the gas chromatography tests that lie at the heart of understanding the essential oils I use daily in my work and my teaching.

A special thanks to the Robert Rose team. It is a rare occasion to be presented with an opportunity to write a book. When publisher Bob Dees asked me to write a book on natural skin care, I was unaware of what it took to make words into a manuscript, a manuscript into pages and pages into a book. When I was introduced to the brilliant Robert Rose publishing team, I recognized the significance of each person's role in the creation of this book. I would like to thank Judith Finlayson, Tracy Bordian, Joanna Lorenco and Gillian Watts for giving my words clarity. Thanks as well to Kevin Cockburn at PageWave Graphics for his book design and photo selection, and to Joseph Gisini for his art direction.

Finally, special thanks to you, the reader, who will give the formulations in this book a life of their own!

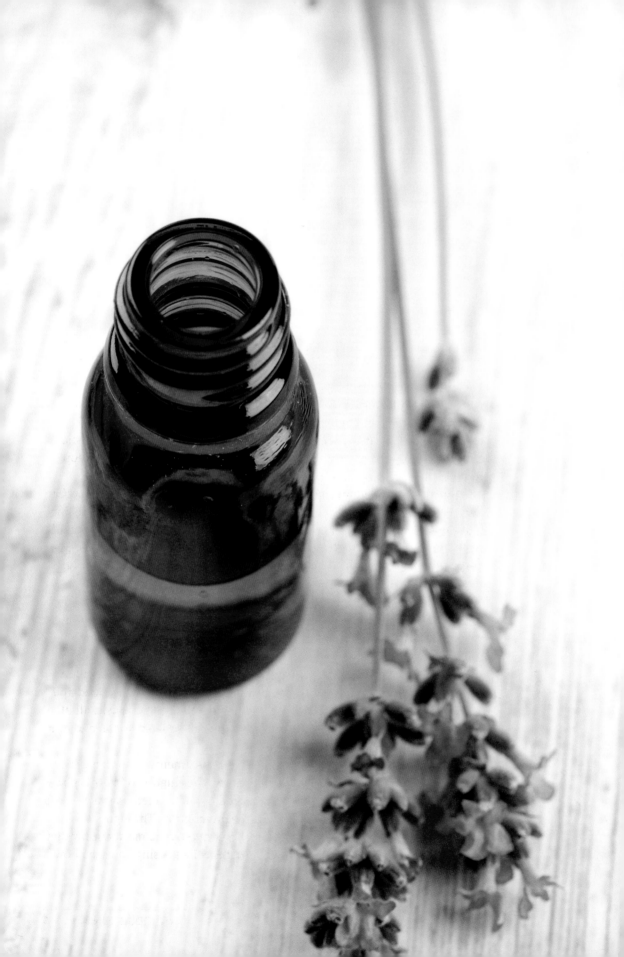

Introduction

The inspiration for this book began in the early 1970s. I have vivid recollections of being a young girl, walking past glitzy beauty counters in department stores and being fascinated by all the eye-catching personal care products. Like many teenage girls, I imagined that I too would be able to miraculously change my appearance and become as gorgeous as the top models whose photographs promoted them.

That illusion ended very quickly. At the age of 26, married and the mother of two boys ages three and six, I had my first outbreak of psoriasis, a baffling and unpredictable autoimmune disease that affects the skin. Within a month, over 80 percent of my body was covered with inflamed red lesions. They were both painful and itchy. It felt so disfiguring that I became withdrawn, in my close relationships as well as socially.

I recall asking one of the many dermatologists I visited, "When will this go away?" Her answer was, "You will have to live with this for the rest of your life." Without further explanation or guidance, she silently wrote a prescription for a stronger cortisone cream. What I perceived to be her indifference made me extremely emotional and probably overly compliant. I became vulnerable to accepting the treatments that doctors prescribed and didn't pay attention to potential risks. I visited many skin specialists, all of whom prescribed different treatments, from topical cortisone to tar, and even sunbathing at the Dead Sea.

With hindsight I can see that this cocktail of treatments was putting me at risk for skin cancer. Luckily, that didn't happen. The "highlight" of this phase came when one doctor prescribed a chemotherapy drug, methotrexate. That's when I drew the line — I refused to take the prescription. Throughout this entire experience, no medical professional ever questioned me about my diet or lifestyle, inquired about the skin-care products I was using, or asked how I was feeling emotionally.

I spent about three years in this troubling cycle, with no relief from my symptoms. Not surprisingly, I became very frustrated. The conventional approach to my illness wasn't getting me anywhere, so I began to research natural and holistic treatments. Little did I know this would lead me to where I am today!

The tipping point was my realization that my diet, lifestyle choices and emotional state played a huge role in my condition. I found this both comforting and empowering. It gave me an opportunity to be active and to take control of my health. I realized that I could cope. I could tame my psoriasis to the point where I could live with it.

In those days, information about plant-based medicine was not as available as it is today. The term *naturopath* seemed like a foreign word, and I associated aromatherapy with a relaxing massage and smelly candles. I was living in Israel at the time, and I went to see a naturalist in a small village. He told me to stop eating red meat, poultry, dairy products, wheat and sugar. I thought I would starve. He also told me to stop using all soap products, perfumes, cosmetics and detergents. At that point I was so desperate I would have done anything. I eliminated all foods that were not nurturing, began to substitute natural for synthetic products, and started investigating natural alternatives for personal care products. During this time I made my first homemade cream, and since then I have never purchased a commercially prepared moisturizing product.

I also started meditating and practicing relaxation techniques, using essential oils. Over time I became very conscious of how the external world influenced the way my mind and body felt. The process wasn't quick, but I can confirm that within myself I began to feel peaceful. I felt as if the struggles and frustrations were subsiding and harmony was taking over my whole being. Within six months, the angry red skin patches began to lighten and my skin returned to its normal state.

Occasionally I do have flare-ups. When that happens, I remind myself that my skin is a shield with a radar system. It is telling me that I need to take a deeper look at my lifestyle: nutrition, environment, the products I use, my stress levels. As soon as my skin comes into contact with an ingredient — natural or synthetic — that does not agree with my body, I experience a flare-up.

In the course of my recovery and my emerging understanding that diet and detoxification are crucial to healthy skin, I decided to further educate myself in the plant-based sciences. I went back to school and received a BSc in nutrition. In 1987 I read *Love, Medicine and Miracles*, by Bernie Segal. This book had a tremendous impact on me. It changed the way I thought about how to help myself — and, by extension, my clients — by directing me toward meditation and guided visualization practices. I'm a bit of a type A personality, so this was not an easy task. My mind wants to jump around, and it would not shut down. Coincidentally, at this time I was taking a class where a colleague introduced me to the scent of orange essential oil. I inhaled the aroma and then spontaneously exhaled the sound of *aahhhh* as my body released tension, shifting my nervous system into a parasympathetic state.

I began to experiment with essential oils and was absolutely amazed at how they could help my mind travel into peacefulness, no matter what was going on around me. Cross-linking nutritional medicine and aromatherapy soon moved to the forefront of my career. It made me realize that detoxifying the body is only one step; the mind also needs to be in a state of calm. Recognizing that essential oils are instrumental in mediating this task was a pivotal point in my studies and my practice.

I began to research the science behind aromatherapy. I was fascinated to learn how the scent from the aromatic volatile molecules of a plant has the power to shift the way you feel in an instant. At the same time, the essential oils from plants have therapeutic properties that can influence physical states. They have been shown to prevent and reduce inflammation, to have sedative properties, to assist with pain relief, and to prevent bacterial and fungal infections.

The dynamics of these therapeutic actions are crucial in my approach to skin care. Taking care of your skin should not be motivated purely by vanity. When you treat skin conditions with essential oils, you are also having an impact on your entire body. Skin care is much more than aesthetics; it is a complementary approach to healthy living. Because they have such a wide range of therapeutic benefits, using essential oils in personal care products allows you to establish a connection between inner well-being and external beauty.

Today I have more than 30 years of experience in teaching and practicing complementary health. My focus is on promoting health, nutrition and lifestyle awareness for my clients. I create educational certificate programs in aromatherapy and develop workshops for making naturally formulated products for personal and professional use. Interestingly, many of those who participate in the programs have one major thing in common: they are seeking sound knowledge that will lead them to a healthier lifestyle. This is not an easy feat, given the proliferation of misleading information available via the media, not to mention the skeptics who dismiss natural therapies out of hand. One of the reasons I wanted to write this book is that aromatherapy is a wild frontier. A great deal of misinformation is being disseminated. This needs to be corrected, and the sound scientific basis on which aromatherapy is built needs to be made available to both practitioners and the general public.

In this book I want to educate you, the consumer, by introducing you to evidence-based information about skin care and natural ingredients, in particular essential oils. It is a rational and realistic approach to creating natural products. Armed with the facts, you will be able to create signature products that will complement a natural lifestyle and meet all your skin-care needs.

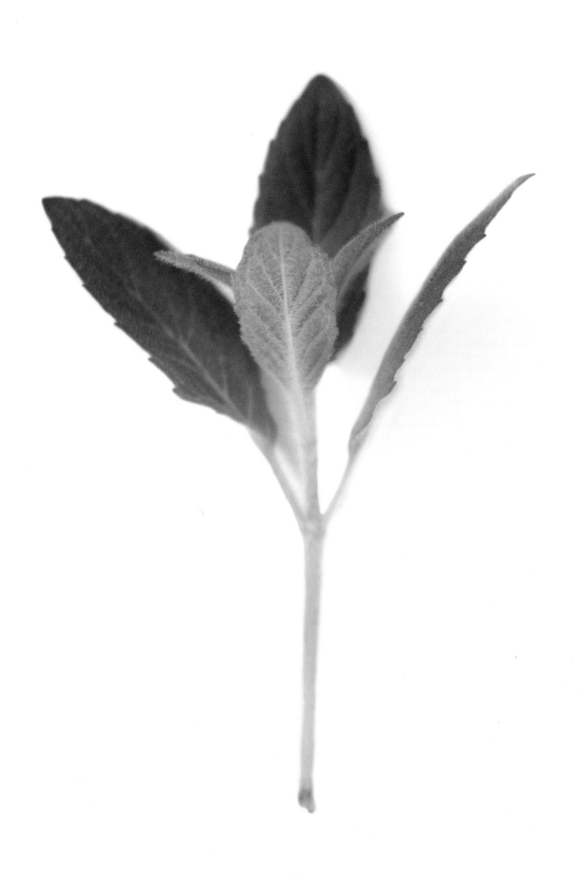

PART 1

The Foundations

The Skin

Skin is the living shield that protects
the body and radiates inner beauty.
— DANIELLE SADE

ANATOMY OF THE SKIN

Your skin is a complicated structure. It is continuously changing and responding to both internal and external changes. Physical and mental stress, poor nutrition and certain medications will alter its balance from the inside out. Exposure to chemicals, harsh water and extreme weather conditions are environmental stressors that can disrupt your skin from the outside. These imbalances show up in skin disorders, the major symptoms of which are inflammation, redness, swelling, burning, itching, dryness and congestion.

When creating personal care products, it's important to have a basic understanding of how your skin is structured and what it needs to stay healthy. This knowledge of its physiology will help you to target your formulations to achieve the desired benefits or to relieve particular skin concerns.

Let's start by exploring the three major layers of the skin: the epidermis, the dermis and the hypodermis.

The Epidermis

The epidermis is the outermost layer of the skin, and it plays a significant role in maintaining its health and beauty. It contains closely packed layers of tissue and is not directly connected to the body's blood supply. Most of the body's surfaces are covered by four layers of epidermis, while the palms of the hands and soles of the feet have five layers.

The innermost layer of the epidermis is called the stratum basale. In terms of skin care, this layer contains a type of cell that is particularly significant — melanocytes. These cells produce melanin, which provides skin with pigmentation and protects it from ultraviolet (UV) rays. Overexposure to UV affects melanocyte cells by causing them to produce excess melanin. This can create hyperpigmentation. Merkel is another type of cell found in the epidermis. These cells communicate the sense of touch to the brain, producing different sensations.

On top of the stratum basale is the stratum spinosum, the layer in which the major type of skin cells — keratinocytes — start to synthesize keratin. Keratin is the tough, fibrous insoluble protein that makes up skin, hair and nails. It also creates a waterproof barrier for the skin.

There is a lot of activity in the next layer, the stratum granulosum. This thicker layer is where keratin proteins and other waterproofing lipids are organized. Overexposure to soaps, detergents and some cosmetics can change your skin's pH and interfere with keratin production in this layer. This causes the skin to lose its strength and resiliency.

The stratum corneum is the outermost layer of the epidermis. It's composed of 15 to 30 layers of dry, dead cells called corneocytes, which protect the skin from microbial invasion and dehydration. In healthy skin, this layer is shed and completely replaced every 30 days. This rejuvenated state can be accelerated through exfoliation, which removes the dead skin and allows new cells to emerge on the surface.

Additionally, there's the stratum lucidum, a layer that is present only in thick skin such as the palms of the hands and the soles of the feet. The cells of the stratum lucidum are flattened and contain an oily substance that acts as a barrier and gives this layer waterproof properties.

The Dermis

The dermis is the middle layer of the skin, which contains nerve endings, sweat and sebaceous glands, hair follicles, muscle fibers and blood and lymph vessels. It is about $1/8$ inch (3 mm) thick.

The overall health of your skin relies on this intermediate barrier. The dermis is the body's reservoir of water and electrolytes, and the blood in this layer regulates blood temperature. The dermis's major function is to supply nourishment from the internal body to the skin's surface. In this way it acts as the link between nutrition and physical activity and the health of your skin.

The two layers of the dermis are the papillary and reticular layers. The papillary layer contains a thin arrangement of collagen fibers, while the reticular layer is made up of thicker collagen fibers. Collagen is found throughout the body, and its role is to provide strength and structure. Collagen is important for keeping skin looking youthful, as it helps to maintain its firmness and elasticity.

Collagen Production

As you age, the collagen in your skin is produced at a slower rate: it's estimated that your body loses at least 1 percent of its collagen every year. This contributes to the look of aging skin — think sagging, dryness, fine lines and wrinkles. Factors accelerating collagen decline include excessive sun exposure, cigarette smoke, environmental pollution, alcohol, stress and poor nutrition.

The Hypodermis

The hypodermis is the innermost layer of skin, also known as subcutaneous tissue. This layer contains fat cells and connective tissue that houses larger blood vessels and nerves. This is the thickest layer of skin. Its size varies throughout the body and from person to person.

HEALTHY LIFE, HEALTHY SKIN

Your lifestyle choices have a direct impact on your skin, and no amount of cream or lotion can totally repair the damage caused by unhealthy habits such as smoking or sunbathing. Here are the most important things you can do to get healthy, radiant skin.

ENJOY A HEALTHY DIET AND DON'T SMOKE

Glowing, radiant skin comes from eating foods with a good amount of essential fatty acids, which help create a natural oil barrier on the skin. This is so important to keeping skin hydrated and plump. Consuming protein is also key, as this macronutrient is broken down into the amino acids that go into making collagen. Steer clear of sugars, processed starches, coffee and alcohol, as these can aggravate skin conditions such as rosacea, acne, eczema and psoriasis. Cigarette smoke is particularly damaging; in addition to being harmful to your general health, it leads to dry skin and wrinkles, so don't smoke, and stay away from second-hand smoke.

KEEP HYDRATED

Skin cells are made up of water, so they cannot function properly if you are dehydrated. Lack of hydration results in skin that is dry and flaky and feels tight. Make sure to drink six to eight glasses of water every day. (Filtered water is best, because of its lower pH. For more on pH, see page 23) However, ingested water doesn't go straight to the skin, so make sure to keep hydrated in other ways too. Avoid over-consuming alcohol and caffeine, both of which can dehydrate you. And stay away from moisture-depleting environments, such as places with dry heat, and avoid taking long baths.

LIMIT SUN EXPOSURE

Too much sun exposure can damage skin in different ways. Excessive sun exposure in a short period of time can cause a sunburn, leading to red, itchy skin that feels hot to the touch. Sun exposure over time causes photo-aging of the skin, the effects of which can appear decades after exposure, in the form of wrinkles and brown spots. Be sun-smart — avoid being outside or, at the very least, stay in the shade between the hours of 10 a.m. and 3 p.m., when the sun is at its most powerful.

EXERCISE REGULARLY

Regular exercise promotes good circulation and helps the body to eliminate toxins. Also, a good, sweat-inducing workout boosts the amount of oxygenated blood going to the skin, which leaves you with a healthy glow.

THE NATURE OF SKIN TYPES

Classifying skin according to type can be complicated. In the early 1900s, Helena Rubenstein, a beauty entrepreneur, defined four different skin types: dry, oily, combination and sensitive. Since then we have recognized other factors that determine how skin is classified, such as age, sex, color, hydration and whether it is sensitive or resilient. Skin-care products should always be formulated to meet these specific needs.

Dry Skin

Dry skin has a dull, rough and leathery appearance. It's predisposed to feeling tight and developing fine lines. Sensitive dry skin is a subcategory of dry skin. It's cracked, flaky and inflamed and may occur alongside conditions such as eczema, psoriasis or various types of dermatitis.

What Causes Dry Skin?

Skin can be dry for many reasons. It may be because of a lack of fluids in the top layer, the stratum corneum. Another cause is poor cellular lipid synthesis, which means that your oil glands are not producing enough sebum — the body's natural oil — to keep your skin lubricated. There may also be a genetic predisposition; some populations, such as African Americans, seem to have a higher incidence of dry skin. Other factors include skin diseases such as eczema and dermatitis, which erode the skin barrier, and climate conditions such as extreme heat or cold or overexposure to UV rays. Cigarette smoke and alcohol are particularly damaging.

Recommended Treatments

Dry skin benefits from daily cleansing morning and night, with additional gentle exfoliation two to three times a week. If you have dry skin, massage your face nightly while applying serum. Dry skin also benefits from periodic aromatic steam treatments and moisturizing masks.

Recommended Oils for Dry Skin and Dry Sensitive Skin

	DRY SKIN		DRY SENSITIVE SKIN	
Carrier oils	• Argan • Avocado • Borage • Coconut	• Hempseed • Rosehip seed • Sweet almond	• Apricot kernel • Argan • Evening primrose	• Jojoba • Marula • Shea butter
Essential oils	• Frankincense • Geranium • Mandarin • Neroli	• Rose otto • Sandalwood (Australian) • Ylang-ylang	• Chamomile, German • Chamomile, Roman • Frankincense • Helichrysum	• Lavender • Neroli • Patchouli

Note: Oils that are ideal for these skin types are listed here. For a broader spectrum of oils and butters, you can investigate, see pages 57 to 76.

Oily Skin

Oily skin is shiny, looks greasy and is prone to acne. It is often characterized by large pores on the cheeks, nose, chin and forehead. Males are more likely to have oily skin than females.

What Causes Oily Skin?

Oily skin results from overactive sebaceous glands, which produce too much sebum. Sebum protects your skin from becoming dehydrated, but in excess it can lead to acne and seborrhea, a red, itchy skin rash that can affect the scalp, face, ears or torso. Diet matters too: junk food and processed food can cause oily skin.

Changing hormone levels at puberty or perimenopause, for example, can cause oily skin. That's why acne is common in teenagers; it's a time when the body produces more hormones that stimulate the oil glands to secrete more sebum.

Recommended Treatments

Oily and sensitive oily skin benefit from cleansing the skin and unclogging pores through gentle exfoliation. Oily skin also benefits from periodic aromatic steam treatments and clay masks.

Recommended Oils for Oily and Oily Sensitive Skin

	OILY SKIN	OILY SENSITIVE SKIN
Carrier oils	• Argan • Apricot kernel • Borage • Grapeseed • Jojoba	• Argan • Evening primrose • Grapeseed • Hempseed • Jojoba
Essential oils	• Clary sage • Geranium • Juniper berry • Lavender • Palmarosa • Tea tree	• Chamomile, German • Chamomile, Roman • Frankincense • Helichrysum • Neroli • Patchouli

Note: Oils that are ideal for these skin types are listed here. For a broader spectrum of oils, you can investigate, see page 57 to 73.

Combination Skin

Combination skin refers to skin that is both oily and dry. Combination skin coexists on different parts of the face as well as on the body. When it appears on the face, it is known as an oily T-zone: the forehead, nose and chin qualify as oily while the skin around the mouth, on the cheeks and around the eyes is dry. On the body it can affect areas such as the upper back and shoulders.

What Causes Combination Skin?

The reasons for combination skin can vary from genetics to hormone imbalances. The condition may be aggravated by the use of skin-care products that contain ingredients that irritate skin or that are harsh, causing some areas of the face to become dry, while other areas that may have been oily already are stimulated to produce more oil.

Recommended Treatments

It is crucial to vary the products used on combination skin and to adapt those products to the skin's different needs. Combination skin also benefits from regular facial massages.

Recommended Oils for Combination Skin

Carrier oils	• Argan
	• Apricot kernel
	• Evening primrose
	• Jojoba
	• Rosehip seed
Essential oils	• Chamomile, German
	• Helichrysum
	• Juniper berry
	• Patchouli
	• Sandalwood (Australian)

Note: Oils that are ideal for these skin types are listed here. For a broader spectrum of oils, you can investigate, see page 57 to 73.

Sensitive and Resilient Skin

Sensitive skin is skin that is easily irritated. It can appear on any part of the body and in people with any type of skin. Sensitive skin seems to "flare" — it looks red and is at times accompanied by a burning sensation.

Resilient skin can also occur with any skin type. It is balanced and is not prone to becoming inflamed when exposed to topical application of products or environmental stress. However, even the most resilient skin can react from overexposure to products to which it is allergic or sensitive.

Aging Skin

Even though the skin is a living system that undergoes continuous renewal, its functioning declines with the passage of time. So no matter what type of skin you have — oily, dry or combination — you will eventually be faced with aging skin. And at this stage in life, your lifestyle choices will have an even bigger impact on the appearance of your skin.

Why Does My Skin Look Older?

As you age, your cells don't regenerate as quickly as they once did. One result is that your skin appears thinner. Collagen and elastin production is less efficient, and as a result, your skin will tend to sag. Natural oils are less abundant as well. There's also a reduction in melanin production, which may lead to sporadic development of pigmented areas known as age spots.

Recommended Treatments

It's important to use oils that are high in essential fatty acids, such as borage or evening primrose. Products made with rich plant butters can also help dry aging skin.

Recommended Oils for Aging and Aging Sensitive Skin

	AGING SKIN	AGING SENSITIVE SKIN
Carrier oils	• Argan • Borage • Jojoba • Rosehip seed • Sesame seed • Sweet almond	• Apricot kernel • Camellia seed • Evening primrose • Hempseed • Jojoba
Essential oils	• Frankincense • Geranium • Mandarin • Neroli • Rose otto • Sandalwood (Australian) • Ylang-ylang	• Chamomile, German • Chamomile, Roman • Frankincense • Helichrysum • Lavender • Neroli • Patchouli

Note: Oils that are ideal for these skin types are listed here. For a broader spectrum of oils and butters, you can investigate, see pages 57 to 76.

THE ART OF SKIN CARE

Since the beginning of time, caring for the skin has been observed as a ritualistic practice. Today the experience of daily cleansing seems more like a necessity than a pleasurable experience, but our connection to cleansing and bathing goes beyond personal hygiene and repelling germs. It is an opportunity to clear your mind and a self-pampering experience that enhances your sense of well-being. Using natural ingredients in skin care creates a kaleidoscope of sensory experiences that support health and well-being and contribute to radiant beauty.

Cleansing

Your face needs to be cleansed twice a day — morning and night. Cleansing the skin removes dead skin cells, oil, dirt, makeup and other impurities. It can also help unclog pores. Ideally, your cleansing ritual will be a gentle, mindful experience that engages most of your senses.

Daily Morning Cleansing

After a good night's sleep, your skin has repaired and detoxified. This process pushes dead skin cells to the top layer of the skin, where they accumulate. Because this could lead to clogged pores and create conditions such as acne and dull skin, gentle cleansing is important; it prevents these cells from building up. Also, clean skin enables you to start your day refreshed. It is a lovely canvas on which to apply light, nourishing creams and cosmetics that enhance your appearance and sense of well-being.

Keep morning cleanses simple and use essential oils appropriate to your skin type (see page 17 to 20) in small amounts. Those that are grounding are preferable, such as sandalwood, patchouli, neroli, bergamot, cardamom, tea tree, mandarin, lemon or cajuput.

Daily Evening Cleansing

Choose a cleanser that supports your skin type, and include essential oils that promote rest, such as rose, frankincense, clary sage, lavender or Roman chamomile, all of which complement every skin type.

Exfoliate, Don't Scrub

Do not scrub — be gentle! When it comes to exfoliation, many people go to extremes, using harsh chemicals to remove unwanted skin cells. This is not a good idea. The skin is a living organ, and your body's first line of defense against invading substances such as bacteria. Excessive exfoliation tends to weaken this natural defense system.

Deep Cleansing with Exfoliation

Your skin sheds millions of dead cells on a daily basis. Exfoliation helps remove those useless cells from the upper surface of the skin, leaving behind a clean, polished surface with reduced fine lines. Exfoliation also stimulates the production of new skin cells. You should exfoliate twice a week and follow up with a nourishing mask or serum on your restored skin.

Deep Cleansing with Masks

A mask is a more intense method of detoxifying, nourishing and restoring skin. It is packed with clays, flours or powders — dry ingredients that become active when combined with liquids. Use an herbal-based mask once or twice a week, preferably during the latter part of the day, when your skin has a greater ability to absorb ingredients.

A mask should be a luxurious experience. Find a quiet space and apply on clean, exfoliated skin. It should feel soft and velvety and it should dry or set within 10 to 20 minutes. Remove with warm water and follow up with toner and moisturizer.

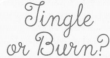

Tingle or Burn?

A mask can sometimes provoke a tingling feeling on the skin. This may indicate that its active components are penetrating the skin. However, if you experience a burning sensation, you are likely having a reaction to some of the ingredients. Your skin is being traumatized. If this happens, rinse off the mask as quickly as possible.

Toning

Toning is an essential step in skin care. A toner continues the cleansing process, removing any dirt or residue left behind. It also nourishes, hydrates and refreshes, restoring the skin's pH balance and creating a fresh canvas for moisturizing.

In general, two types of solutions are used for toning:

- TONERS: These are water-based and suitable for dry skin. A toner may or may not contain alcohol, and many contain glycerin. A hydrolat (see right) can be used on its own as a toner or as a component of a water-based toner.
- ASTRINGENTS: These solutions are a much stronger form of toner, and are suitable for oily or combination skin. They often contain alcohol, and possibly witch hazel or apple cider vinegar.

What Is a Hydrolat?

Hydrolats (also known as hydrosols or floral waters) are aromatic waters produced during the steam distillation process that creates essential oils. They can be used on their own as toners. They are alcohol-free. Some producers add alcohol to their formulations, which means they are not true hydrolats.

Morning Toning

After your cleansing, use a gentle morning toner that is suitable for your skin type. This will hydrate and protect your skin and balance your pH for the day.

Afternoon Toning or After Exercise

At midday, your skin is producing oil at maximum capacity. To control sebum buildup, mist your face with an astringent-based toner and pat dry. After exercising, spritz your skin with toner to refresh your face and prevent sweat from clogging your pores, which can lead to breakouts.

Toning Before Bed

During the evening, your skin is not producing as much oil as it did during the day. As a result, it is relatively dehydrated. You should avoid using strong, astringent-based toners and focus on water-based formulations. If your skin is particularly greasy, use an astringent-based toner with milder ingredients, such as alcohol-free witch hazel hydrolat.

Moisturizing

The final step in your regular skin-care routine is moisturizing. All skin types need to be kept moisturized, both during the day and at night. Moisturizing protects, tones and nourishes the skin. Selecting a moisturizer that suits your skin is crucial to keeping it balanced.

Moisturizers for normal, combination or oily skin should be based on gels or light carrier oils such as apricot, grapeseed or jojoba. Those for dry skin will rely on carrier oils with a higher percentage of saturated fats, such as sweet almond, avocado or coconut oil.

Daytime Moisturizing

After cleansing and toning, apply your daytime moisturizing cream. If you will be applying makeup, allow one to two minutes for the moisturizer to settle in before starting that step.

Evening Moisturizing

During the evening, your pores are much more dilated than they were in the morning, making it an ideal time to feed your skin with antioxidants and nutrient-rich products. After cleansing and toning, apply a nighttime serum and cream. No matter which type of skin you have, use lighter formulas. Stay away from heavy oils so that your skin can breathe during the night.

Your Skin's pH

The pH scale has a range from 1 to 14, with 1 being highly acidic, 7 neutral and 14 highly alkaline. Typical healthy skin has a pH level between 4.5 and 5.5, which means it is slightly more acidic than alkaline. This is a protective factor — your skin is working to prevent pathogens from entering your body. The pH of your skin varies for different areas of the body and at different times of the day. Other factors that affect the skin's pH are age and gender.

When preparing skin-care products, it's a good idea to measure the pH level of their components to ensure that your skin pH is not upset. (You can easily measure your formulations by using pH strips, which can be purchased at most health food stores.) This is especially important for products such as toners, since they are used to balance the skin. For oily or combination skin, you should use a toner that is slightly acidic, with a pH of 5. If necessary, add vinegar, which has a pH of 2.5 to 2.9, or witch hazel, a hydrolat that has a pH of 4.0 to 4.2. If you have dry skin, use a toner that has a pH of about 6. To increase the pH of a formulation, add aloe vera gel or glycerin.

SYNCHRONIZING YOUR SKIN WITH SKIN CARE

Have you ever stopped to think that your skin depends on you to make it look vibrant and healthy? Good skin-care products are just one piece of the puzzle. Another is synchronizing your skin-care program with your biological clock. Aligning your routine with your body's circadian rhythm will maximize the effectiveness of your personal care products.

Circadian Rhythms and Your Skin

The circadian rhythm is a 24-hour physiological cycle. An individual's biological clock is controlled by the part of the brain that responds to light and darkness, which receives signals sent through the optic nerve. When exposed to light, the hypothalamus — the part of the brain that controls the autonomic nervous system, among other functions — wakes up the body. It initiates hormonal secretions that regulate body temperature and circulation and prepares your body for physical activity. When your eyes are exposed to darkness, your brain understands that it should make you sleepy. At this stage it is preparing your body to repair and rejuvenate itself. Your skin works along with your biological rhythms, so synchronizing your personal products to work with these rhythms will enhance their effectiveness.

Your Skin-Care Schedule

Early Morning (4 a.m. to 8 a.m.)

YOUR SKIN: At this time of day, your skin is developing its natural protective barrier, so is not likely to absorb thick products or the active ingredients in those products. There's also a tendency during the early morning to have skin reactions.

SKIN-CARE RECOMMENDATIONS: Wash your face with a gentle cleanser and warm water. Your choice of essential oils for the cleansing process should be light, so choose ones like bergamot FCF, mandarin or lemon. Avoid using penetrating masks and serums.

Late Morning (8 a.m. to 12 p.m.)

YOUR SKIN: During the morning hours, your body is warming up and picking up the pace, which results in more blood flow to the surface of the skin. And remember, you are more likely to be sensitive to products or to have allergic reactions during the morning hours.

SKIN-CARE RECOMMENDATIONS: Your skin-care products should be light-textured, protective and moisturizing. Use essential oils moderately; some to try include rose otto, lime (distilled) or tea tree. Avoid using penetrating masks and serums.

Afternoon (12 p.m. to 5 p.m.)

YOUR SKIN: In the afternoon, there is a slow proliferation of new cell tissue and your body is secreting more sebum to the skin. People with oily or combination skin tend to take on a shiny appearance. Skin conditions such as psoriasis and eczema may look worse.

SKIN-CARE RECOMMENDATIONS: Freshen up with a spritz of a lovely gentle hydrolat. Make sure it's an alcohol-free formulation.

Evening (5 p.m. to 10 p.m.)

YOUR SKIN: Your skin's ability to absorb ingredients is much higher in the evening. This means it is more prone to respond to topical skin care.

SKIN-CARE RECOMMENDATIONS: This is the time to deep-cleanse the skin and to use exfoliants, facial masks, active serums and rich moisturizing oils. Choose essential oils that are calming and relaxing and support skin health, such as sandalwood, rose otto, neroli, patchouli, frankincense, Roman chamomile or German chamomile.

Night (9 p.m. to 4 a.m.)

YOUR SKIN: This is the time when the skin begins to repair itself by replacing old skin cells with new ones. It's producing less sebum and has a slightly lower pH, making it prone to dryness and itchiness.

Prepare for Bed and Getting a Good Sleep

Healthy skin relies on a good night's sleep. There are a number of things you can do to create an environment that invites a sound sleep. Do not go to bed on a full stomach or engage in stimulating exercise. Light stretching, however, is appropriate. Reduce exposure to electronics, such as television and computers and ensure that your bedroom is clean and pleasant, A good night's sleep is always important, but particularly if you are going through transitions in life, such as the various stages of menopause and menstrual cycles, as well as pregnancy.

Expert Tip

Consider diffusing essential oils into your environment an hour before bed to help calm your nervous system. Some good choices are lavender, bergamot, juniper berry and geranium.

Creating Your Own Skin-Care Products

SKIN CARE 101

Your skin is the largest organ of your body. It's affected by what you eat, how much physical activity you engage in, and the environment in which you live. Naturally, it will also react to the products you put on it and to the chemicals that make up the ingredients in those products.

Because you are taking steps toward making your own skin-care formulations, you owe it to yourself, as well as to anyone else who might be using them, to have a firm understanding of the ingredients they contain. You want your products to be as effective as possible and you also want to make sure they are safe to use. That means doing your best to avoid potential concerns such as skin irritation, sensitization and photosensitization. Arming yourself with this knowledge will give you the confidence and know-how to begin creating your own skin-care formulations using essential oils.

Responsibly creating products also means paying attention to their shelf life, and that means adding preservatives. Many preservatives used in commercial formulations can cause troubling side effects (I've included a rundown of the most problematic ones later in this chapter), which is why we recommend the use of synergies of essential oils containing anti-microbial properties to help prolong the shelf life of your products. These can be added to any formulation and will help keep your products safe from contamination.

Finally, this chapter concludes with an overview of the supplies and equipment you'll need to safely prepare, package and store your personal care products. By the end of this section you'll be well on your way to setting up your very own skin-care apothecary.

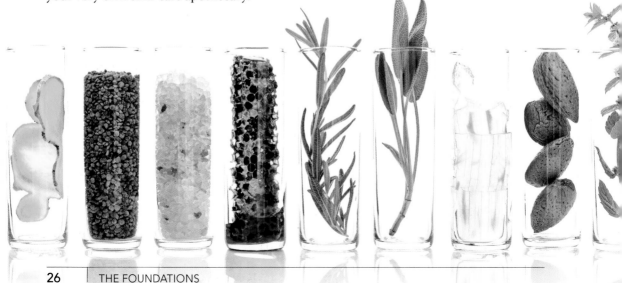

POTENTIAL REACTIONS TO NATURAL INGREDIENTS

Many plants, including those used as herbal remedies, may have adverse effects that can manifest in different ways. When applying essential oils, there are three main types of skin reactions that can occur: skin irritation, sensitization and photosensitization.

Skin Irritation

Most people have experienced skin irritation as a reaction to a particular ingredient. Skin irritation usually presents as a rash, appearing at the site of contact. Other symptoms include inflammation, itchiness, redness and hives. In very rare cases, there is even the risk that a serious reaction can cause anaphylactic shock.

It's difficult to predict if an individual will have a negative reaction to an essential oil. The good news is that, in most cases, the reactions are localized and short-lived. Still, before using any essential oil or blend of oils, it is a good idea to do a skin patch test. If you observe a reaction, that's a good indicator that you are sensitive or even allergic to that essential oil and should not use it on your skin. And if an essential oil comes with a caution that it is a potential irritant if you have sensitive skin, you should be careful about using products containing that oil.

Doing a Skin Patch Test

Mix a drop of essential oil into a small amount of carrier oil (such as coconut) and apply to a section of your inner arm. Over the next hour, check to see if there is a reaction. If your skin turns red or feels tingly, wash it with soap and water and avoid using that particular oil.

Sensitization

Some skin reactions are immediate; others can develop over time. Overexposure to any substance, natural or synthetic, can lead to a delayed response, which may even show up in different areas of your body.

Sensitization occurs when there is a gradual reaction of the immune system to any ingredient, synthetic or natural. Signs can include a rash; raised, itchy skin; or even eczema. Here's what happens: When an ingredient is absorbed into the skin, it interacts with the proteins in your skin. If those proteins are altered, they can become antigens — foreign substances that provoke an immune response. Your body considers the antigens to be invaders and will respond with inflammation and other allergic responses. The reaction may not be immediate; it can take a few days, weeks or even months of repeatedly using the ingredient.

Several factors can increase your risk of sensitization. Frequent use of the same ingredient is one. Some ingredients tend to be more sensitizing than others. In the case of essential oils, some contain constituents that are classified as sensitizers. Therefore, applying undiluted essential oils to the skin can also lead to sensitization, so always dilute your essential oil with a carrier oil or plant butter (see page 91).

How Do I Find Out Which Constituents Are in a Particular Oil?

If you are making natural personal care products, you should know what you are using. When it comes to essential oils, that means being aware of the chemical constituents of each oil you use. The pie chart that accompanies information on each essential oil listed in Part 3 provides a general picture of the oil's main chemical constituents. However, the percentages can vary from batch to batch. The best way to determine an essential oil's chemical constituents is by examining its gas chromatography analysis.

A gas chromatography (GC) test identifies the quantities of chemicals present in an essential oil. This analysis should be as recent as possible, because the amounts of individual constituents can change from year to year and from crop to crop. For instance, the percentage of benzyl benzoate found in jasmine essential oil can range from 10 to 22 percent, and carotol, a constituent unique to carrot seed essential oil, can range from 75 to 85 percent of the oil.

A reputable essential oil supplier should be able to provide you with GC test results; many suppliers now offer these on their website. You can also ask for the report at health food stores or other reputable retailers of essential oils. Don't be shy — ask for these tests at the counter.

Every year, billions of dollars are spent on personal care products. Ironically, a significant portion of that is spent on products to correct damage — either from overexposure to potentially harmful ingredients in those products or from their incorrect use.

Certain essential oils are known sensitizers. However, your skin can become sensitized to any essential oil, which is why it's a good idea not to overuse any particular skin-care product. Play it safe by regularly varying the oils you use in your formulations. And, contrary to popular belief, continued use of a sensitizing oil will not solve the problem. If you become sensitized to a particular oil, stop using it.

Alternating Essential Oils in Products

To avoid sensitization, do not exceed the recommended amounts of essential oil in a formulation (see page 91). Another technique I recommend is to create a two-phase line of products. For each phase, choose formulations that contain different essential oils. Alternate between the two phases every three months.

Photosensitization

Photosensitization is a skin reaction in the presence of ultraviolet (UV) rays. This reaction can occur when an essential oil is applied to skin that is exposed to direct sunlight or to UV radiation from a tanning bed. In other words, the oil becomes toxic when exposed to UV light. Reactions range from a blotchy red rash to dark pigmentation to a more serious burn. Several citrus essential oils, such as grapefruit and lime, can cause photosensitization.

NATURAL SUBSTANCES THAT CAN TRIGGER ADVERSE EFFECTS

It's a common assumption that products found in nature are safer than those created in a factory or lab. Unfortunately, that isn't always the case. Even natural ingredients can contain elements that cause sensitivity or irritation, and some may even be toxic. Just look at essential oils. These pure oils have wonderful therapeutic properties when applied to the skin or inhaled, but they should never be ingested, and they should always be used in the suggested quantities.

Below is a list of some of the chemicals in essential oils that can cause adverse reactions. (For more on the chemical constituents of individual oils, see Part 3.) Oils that contain these chemical constituents should be used with caution.

Benzyl Benzoate

Benzyl benzoate, found in many fragrant flowers, is what gives jasmine and ylang-ylang their distinctive sweet balsam scent. This chemical is classified as an allergen; when it makes up 27 percent of a formula, it is sensitizing. Benzyl benzoate is found in the following essential oils:

Benzoin 40–60%
Ylang-ylang 11–12%
Jasmine 10–22%

Citral (Geranial and Neral)

Geranial and neral are constituents that are usually found together as the chemical citral. Citral is highly irritating to the skin and has a high oxidation rate (see "Oxidation and Essential Oils," below). Citral is found in one essential oil featured in this book:

Lemongrass 75–80%

Oxidation and Essential Oils

The natural constituents of an essential oil begin to degrade when exposed to oxygen. This process, known as oxidation, can increase the risk of skin irritation and sensitization.

To avoid oxidation, always cap bottles of essential oil as soon as you have finished using them, and make sure not to leave bottles open for long periods of time. (It helps to decant larger quantities of oils into small bottles to prevent the remainder of the oil from being overexposed to oxygen.) Heat and light also damage essential oils, so be sure to store oils and natural skin-care products in sealed containers in a cool, dark environment.

Eugenol

Eugenol, which is often used in perfume for its spicy, aromatic fragrance, has a long history of use in dentistry for its analgesic and disinfecting properties. However, eugenol is a known sensitizer, so it should be used with caution; essential oils that contain a large amount of eugenol should be eliminated from daily use. Eugenol is found in the following essential oils featured in this book:

Sweet basil CT.. 10–30%
Jasmine.. 2–3%

Farnesol

Farnesol is known for its anti-inflammatory and antimicrobial properties. It's used extensively in anti-aging products, as well as in perfumes. This chemical constituent is found in trace amounts in many essential oils. Although it is generally non-irritating and is not found in high levels in any essential oil, if you are sensitive to it, it may create a reaction. People with sensitive skin should do a skin patch test (see page 27) before using the oils below. Farnesol is found in the following essential oils:

Australian sandalwood 8–10%
Lemongrass.. 5%
Neroli 2–3%
Rose otto... 2%

Geraniol

Geraniol has a rose-like scent. This chemical constituent is a skin irritant as well as a known sensitizer. Overexposure to geraniol can lead to an allergic reaction. People with sensitive skin should do a skin patch test (see page 27) before using the oils below. Geraniol is found in the following essential oils:

Palmarosa..................... 75–82%
Geranium...................... 20–35%
Rose otto...................... 20–25%
Citronella...................... 19–25%

Coumarins

Coumarins belong to a unique class of chemicals; they are organic compounds found in many plant species. Coumarins are present in essential oils such as bergamot (unless FCF), carrot seed, lemon and lime (unless distilled). These compounds become phototoxic when exposed to sunlight, so you should avoid using these essential oils on unprotected skin. Save them for night creams and for use in the winter, when you're likelier to spend less time outside.

Limonene

Used extensively in the food and fragrance industries, limonene is found in most citrus oils. It's what gives the fruits' peel its distinctive citrus scent. Exposing limonene to heat or air will gradually degrade it, which can lead to skin irritation. Essential oils with high levels of limonene should be stored in a cool location. Limonene is found in the following essential oils:

Mandarin 87–95%
Orange 84–95%
Grapefruit 84–95%
Lemon 55–70%
Lime 55–60%
Bergamot 2–35%

Linalool

Linalool is found in many essential oils, including lavender and rose. Synthetic linalool is a very common fragrance used in many mainstream products, such as detergents, fabric softeners, air fresheners and cosmetics. This chemical constituent has a tendency to oxidize quickly, leading to skin irritation. At high concentrations, oxidized linalool can cause an allergic reaction, so use these oils with caution. Linalool is found in high concentrations in the following oils:

Sweet basil linalool 55–70%
Lavender 25–30%

Allergies and Natural Ingredients

An allergy to a certain food or substance may be a precursor to an allergy or sensitivity to an essential oil or other natural substance. For example, if you are allergic to wheat, you should avoid wheat germ oil; if you are allergic to bee stings, do not use beeswax or honey in your skin-care products. Remember, essential oils are concentrated and therefore very powerful. Use common sense. If you are allergic to a particular substance, do not apply that substance to your skin in the form of an essential oil.

PRESERVATIVES

In the realm of personal care products, preservatives are used to extend what is described as "shelf life," the time frame during which the product remains effective and safe from bacterial contamination. Natural organic materials can be used as preservatives, but complex, synthetically produced chemicals may also be used.

Products that can sustain their appealing characteristics during a long shelf life are both convenient and economically attractive. But in the past two decades many preservatives have been linked to unpleasant reactions, as well as to more serious health risks. For example, some of the most common preservatives used in cosmetic formulations are known endocrine disruptors, meaning that they can interfere with your body's hormones and cause adverse health effects.

Health authorities have deemed chemicals such as parabens and formaldehyde to be safe in low concentrations. I might agree with this assessment if the average person used only one or two personal care products a day. But the reality is that we apply dozens of products to our bodies each and every day, and with each product we are adding to the levels of parabens, formaldehyde and other chemicals on our skin. Worse, studies show that health conditions may not be apparent after initial exposure to a chemical but may appear in later years.

Today there is much greater public awareness of these problematic synthetic preservatives and their effect on physical health than there was just a few years ago. This awareness is linked to the growing demographic of consumers who are educating themselves about the ingredients in their personal care products. The modern consumer is increasingly demanding safer alternatives to synthetic preservatives that can have major negative consequences.

What Affects a Product's Shelf Life?

There are many things that influence a product's shelf life. A big one is cross-contamination once the product has been opened — such as when you stick unwashed fingers in a pot of moisturizer. Here are some other factors that can cause a product to spoil quickly:

- Contaminated raw materials or water
- Unsanitary manufacturing conditions or packaging
- Not enough preservatives in product
- Poor storage of raw materials and finished products
- Cross contamination
- Exposure to heat
- Ingredients such as flour, wheat or water that encourage the growth of microorganisms

CHEMICALS YOU CAN LIVE WITHOUT

The demand for safer preservatives has pressured the cosmetic industry to respond, and to a large extent it has, by creating effective preservatives that will not cause harm. Many products on sale today have a shelf life of one to two years, using safe ingredients. However, there are concerns that many products still contain chemicals that have been linked to skin sensitivities and even disease. Here is an overview of the most problematic ones.

METHYLISOTHIAZOLINONE

Methylisothiazolinone (MIT or MI) is used as a preservative in lotions, cosmetics, shampoos and conditioners, liquid soaps and household cleaning products. It's used extensively, so it may lead to a wide range of skin reactions and sensitizations. Studies have shown that exposure to high levels of MIT can cause acute eye and skin irritation, and some research suggests it may even damage brain cells.

BHA AND BHT

BHA (butylated hydroxyanisole) and BHT (butylated hydroxytoluene) are common preservatives in cosmetics such as sunscreens, lipsticks and moisturizers. These chemicals can cause allergic reactions in the skin. What's more, numerous studies have classified BHA and BHT as endocrine disrupters, and there's also research showing that they may cause cancer. Some evidence indicates that these chemicals can mimic estrogen, so it is recommended that pregnant women steer clear of products containing them.

PARABENS

Parabens, which include methyl, butyl, propyl, isobutyl and ethyl paraben, are the most common preservatives used in toiletries. They are found in shampoos, conditioners, gels, moisturizers, lotions and various forms of makeup. Parabens are prolific, so even at low levels in individual products, their extensive use may result in overexposure. Research has shown that they can penetrate into the skin, blood and digestive system. Paraben accumulation has been linked with reduced sperm quality and breast and skin cancers, and accumulation of these substances in breast tissue has been found to be a result of topical application of creams, cosmetics and deodorants.

continued on next page

FORMALDEHYDE

Formaldehyde is used as a preservative and disinfectant in nail polish, nail glue, eyelash glue, hair gel, hair-smoothing products, baby shampoo, body soaps and washes and cosmetics. It has been identified by the U.S. National Toxicology Program as a potential human carcinogen and may also cause skin sensitivities resulting in dermatitis. As well, formaldehyde is classified as one of the top indoor pollutants.

POLYETHYLENE GLYCOL (PEG)

PEG is a petroleum-based compound used in many personal care products such as moisturizers, deodorants, makeup, soaps, toothpaste and hair removal products. It's used to help these products foam and to penetrate the skin. One problem with PEG is that it's likely to be contaminated by particular substances that have been identified as possible carcinogens. Even uncontaminated versions of PEG can lead to skin irritation and dermatitis.

Forget about Foaming

Who isn't familiar with the soft, silky texture of a foamy cleanser, body wash or shampoo? It might feel good, even necessary, but foaming has absolutely nothing to do with getting you clean. In fact, the ingredient typically used to get a product to foam — sodium lauryl sulfate (SLS) — can be quite harmful. A common ingredient in personal care products, SLS is a harsh chemical that can cause skin irritation. Steer clear of products that use it as a foaming agent.

USING ESSENTIAL OILS AS NATURAL PRESERVATIVES

As you can see, some preservatives in personal care products are potentially harmful chemicals. Still, a product is not likely to be safe without any preservatives to keep out germs and prevent bacterial overgrowth. And it certainly won't have a shelf life beyond a few months. So what can you turn to for preserving your natural skin-care products? To essential oils, of course!

Essential oils are prime candidates as natural preservatives. Many oils have strong antimicrobial activity, meaning that they kill or slow the spread of potentially harmful microorganisms such as bacteria, fungi and parasites. And you can boost an essential oil's antimicrobial power by adding certain raw ingredients. Honey and beeswax, for example, are well-known for their antibacterial properties. Finally, added ingredients that have preservative properties, such as sugar and alcohol glycerin, will combine to make potent natural preservatives.

Expert Tip

When creating products for your own use, I recommend that you make them in small batches. Most have a life expectancy of a maximum of three months and can be safely used for that period. However, adding a synergy may extend the shelf life beyond this time frame, as will keeping your products refrigerated.

The following synergies have been developed so that they can be used as natural preservatives in your personal care products. These natural blends, which I call Antimicrobial Synergies, were formulated based on evidence of their antimicrobial properties and may help to extend the shelf life of your products.

Creating Synergies

These synergies may be added to any products to extend their shelf life. Choose a synergy based on your preferred scent. Use a beaker and a glass stirring rod to mix the ingredients, then pour the final product into a glass dropper bottle (see page 41 for packaging materials). These synergies have a shelf life of one year, if you keep them refrigerated. I recommend making them in small batches for personal use.

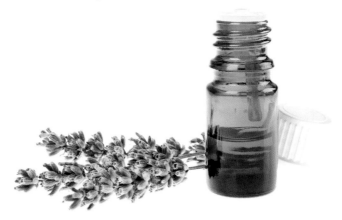

Rose-Scented Antimicrobial Synergy

Makes 5.5 mL

• **10 mL dropper bottle**

20 drops (1 mL)	palmarosa essential oil
20 drops (1 mL)	tea tree essential oil
10 drops (0.5 mL)	sweet basil (linalool) essential oil
20 drops (1 mL)	liquid vitamin E
40 drops (2 mL)	70% alcohol or glycerin

1. In beaker, combine palmarosa, tea tree and sweet basil essential oils. Add liquid vitamin E and alcohol or glycerin. Stir with glass rod. Pour into dropper bottle. Seal tightly and label. Shake well before using.

Citrus Antimicrobial Synergy

Makes 6 mL

Tip

Make sure to use bergamot FCF essential oil, particularly if you will be using your products while exposed to sun.

• **10 mL dropper bottle**

20 drops (1 mL)	lemongrass essential oil
20 drops (1 mL)	orange essential oil
10 drops (0.5 mL)	bergamot essential oil
20 drops (1 mL)	liquid vitamin E
50 drops (2.5 mL)	70% alcohol or glycerin

1. In beaker, combine lemongrass, orange and bergamot essential oils. Add liquid vitamin E. Add either alcohol or glycerin. Stir with glass rod and pour into a dropper bottle. Seal tightly and label. Shake well before using.

Minted Camphor Antimicrobial Synergy

Makes 6 mL

- **10 mL dropper bottle**

20 drops (1 mL)	rosemary essential oil
20 drops (1 mL)	sweet basil (linalool) essential oil
10 drops (0.5 mL)	peppermint essential oil
20 drops (1 mL)	liquid vitamin E
50 drops (2.5 mL)	70% alcohol or glycerin

1. In beaker, combine rosemary, sweet basil and peppermint essential oils. Add liquid vitamin E. Add either alcohol or glycerin. Stir with glass rod and pour into a dropper bottle. Seal tightly and label. Shake well before using.

Floral Antimicrobial Synergy

Makes 6 mL

- **10 mL dropper bottle**

20 drops (1 mL)	benzoin essential oil
20 drops (1 mL)	lavender essential oil
10 drops (0.5 mL)	clary sage essential oil
20 drops (1 mL)	liquid vitamin E
50 drops (2.5 mL)	70% alcohol or glycerin

1. In beaker, combine benzoin, lavender and clary sage essential oils. Add liquid vitamin E. Add either alcohol or glycerin. Stir with glass rod and pour into a dropper bottle. Seal tightly and label. Shake well before using.

Earthy Antimicrobial Synergy

Makes 6 mL

• **10 mL dropper bottle**

20 drops (1 mL)	patchouli essential oil
20 drops (1 mL)	clary sage essential oil
10 drops (0.5 mL)	geranium essential oil
20 drops (1 mL)	liquid vitamin E
50 drops (2.5 mL)	70% alcohol or glycerin

1. In beaker, combine patchouli, clary sage and geranium essential oils. Add liquid vitamin E. Add either alcohol or glycerin. Stir with glass rod and pour into a dropper bottle. Seal tightly and label. Shake well before using.

CREATING YOUR PERSONAL SKIN-CARE APOTHECARY

To begin creating your own personal care products, you need to set up a space in your home that will be used exclusively for this purpose. (Your work area should be kept free of pets, as their fur and dander can end up in products.) Here's what you need to set up your own personal apothecary.

Your Apothecary Checklist

Work Area and Storage Supplies

- WHEELED TROLLEY: This can be used as counter to make your products and to store your sealed ingredients. Some wheeled trolleys come with a handy cupboard or shelves underneath.
- PLASTIC BINS: These should have covers. I like to use medium-size bins, which measure 12 by 24 inches (30 by 60 cm).
- GLASS JARS: Store raw ingredients such as waxes, granules and herbs in various sizes of glass jars. I especially like Mason jars for storage.
- LABELS: used for identifying products.
- SMALL BAR FRIDGE: This isn't required but it really comes in handy for storing essential oils, raw ingredients and finished products.

Basic Equipment

- MEASURING CUPS: Sizes should range from $\frac{1}{4}$ cup to 1 cup (60 to 250 mL). These are used to measure liquid and dry ingredients.
- MEASURING SPOONS: used to measure liquid and dry ingredients.
- BEAKERS: Sizes should range from 25 to 500 mL. They are used to measure essential oils and carrier oils.
- DOUBLE BOILER: used to safely melt and heat emulsifying waxes and oils. The formulations in this book use a bowl-style double boiler, which is simply a heatproof glass bowl or measuring cup set over water simmering in a saucepan.
- GLASS BOWLS AND MEASURING CUPS: You should have various sizes of bowls and cups that can hold from 1 to 4 cups (250 mL to 1 L) of liquids.
- HOTPLATE: used to heat the water in the double boiler. An alternative to a hotplate is a rice cooker, in which you can place a glass bowl to heat the waxes. NOTE: A stovetop element can also be used to melt waxes, but I recommend using a hotplate or rice cooker instead. As much as possible, try to avoid making things in the kitchen; it's preferable to have a space dedicated to making your personal care products. This precaution will help you avoid contamination.
- THERMOMETER: used to check the temperature of your products as you are formulating them.
- ELECTRIC MIXER: used to mix formulations.
- COFFEE GRINDER: used to grind up dry ingredients.

Mixing and Pouring Utensils

- FUNNELS: used for pouring products into bottles.
- HEAT-RESISTANT SPATULAS: to ensure that no plastic leaks into a formulation.
- GLASS STIRRING SPOONS OR RODS: used for mixing essential oils, carrier oils and the final product.
- SQUEEZE BOTTLE: Use a wide-mouthed (2 to 3 inches/5 to 7.5 cm) condiment bottle to dispense thicker ingredients into smaller bottles.
- PLASTIC PIPETTE DROPPERS: used to drop small quantities into formulations.

Disinfecting and Sterilizing Tools

- FRAGRANCE-FREE DISHWASHING SOAP: used for initial washing of packaging materials.
- WHITE VINEGAR AND BICARBONATE OF SODA: used for soaking utensils.
- WASH BIN: Use one that fits in the sink to clean utensils and jars.
- SCRUB PADS: used to wash utensils and jars.
- CLEAN MICROFIBER CLOTHS: used to wipe the work surface before and after preparing formulations.
- PAPER TOWELS: used to disinfect packaging and utensils.
- 70% RUBBING ALCOHOL IN A SPRAY BOTTLE: used to wipe down counters, equipment and jars with paper towels before and after preparing formulations.
- RUBBER GLOVES: used to prevent cross-contamination from hands and nails.
- HEAD COVERING: used to keep hair out of products. A plastic shower cap can be used.
- PLASTIC CLING WRAP: used to wrap utensils while in storage and to cover the work surface if you do not have a dedicated trolley.

Keep Things Clean

Use a few drops of tea tree essential oil dissolved in alcohol to spray and wipe down counters, equipment and jars.

PACKAGING YOUR PRODUCTS

It is ideal to use glass bottles for packaging natural products, to help increase the longevity of the product. But if you are concerned about breakage, and for products such as cleansers and exfoliants, PET (polyethylene terephthalate) plastic packaging is a good alternative. The following list suggests some appropriate containers for the various products.

SYNERGIES
- Amber bottles with short dropper cap (5 and 10 mL)

CLEANSERS
- PET Boston round containers with pump, 100–500 mL
- PET Boston round containers with flip cap, 100–500 mL
- Glass Boston round containers with pump, 100–500 mL
- Glass jars, 80–250 mL

TONERS
- PET Boston round containers with flip cap, 100–500 mL
- PET Boston round containers with spray nozzle, 100–500 mL
- Glass Boston round containers with pump, 100–500 mL

SERUMS AND MOISTURIZERS
- Glass pump bottles, 30–100 mL
- Glass jars, 30–550 mL
- Glass bottles with glass dropper
- Black PET (PRC) straight-sided jars
- PET heavy-walled jars with wide mouth, 30–100 mL

MASKS AND EXFOLIANTS
- PET heavy-walled jars with wide mouth, 250 mL
- PET Boston round containers with flip cap, 250–500 mL

BODY OILS
- PET Boston round containers with flip cap, 250–500 mL
- PET Boston round containers with spray nozzle, 250–500 mL
- Glass Boston round containers with pump, 250–500 mL
- Glass Boston round containers with spray nozzle, 250–500 mL

SHAMPOOS
- PET Boston round containers with pump, 100–500 mL
- PET Boston round containers with flip cap, 100–500 mL

DEODORANTS
- Roll-on deodorant bottles, 50–75 mL
- Glass or PET jars, 30–60 mL

LIP BALMS
- Lip balm tubes, 10 mL
- PET clear jars, 10 mL

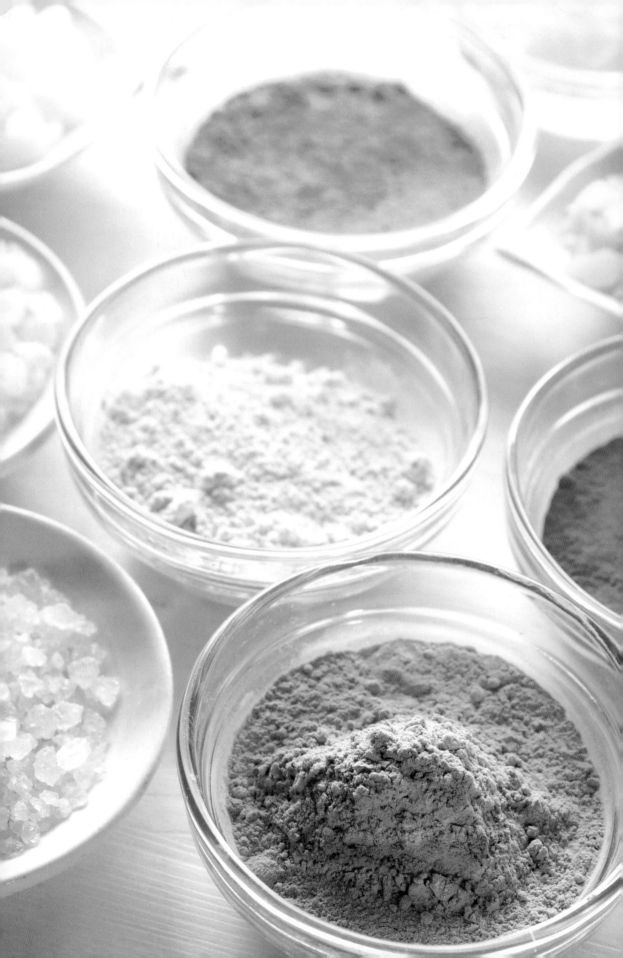

PART 2

Basic Ingredients

Natural Raw Ingredients

At their most basic, when creating the personal care products in this book, you'll start with a base — a carrier oil or plant butter — and then add one or more essential oils. But there are many other natural ingredients that can be added to formulations, from clays and flours to plant extracts, waxes and more. When it comes to creating your own skin-care products, the possibilities are endless. What you choose will depend on the function required of a product (thickening or emulsifying, for example) as well as the therapeutic properties with which you choose to enhance your formulation. Here are some of the different types of ingredients we'll explore in this chapter.

Clays, flours, grains and granules add texture to products and can thicken their consistency. Therapeutically, some can remove excess oil from the skin and slough away dead skin cells. Liquids and gels, on the other hand, are used as volumizers and for their wonderful skin-hydrating properties. Want to boost the therapeutic value of a formulation even more? Then consider adding an extract. There are various highly concentrated fruit, herb and seed extracts whose active ingredients have been shown to benefit the skin when topically applied.

Finally we come to one of the key elements in personal care products — the emulsifier. The ingredients in a formulation cannot combine properly or may separate later if you do not add an emulsifying agent. Waxes are the most commonly used emulsifiers, and there are a variety to choose from. The one you select will affect the texture and viscosity of your product (thicker in some cases, powdery in others) and may even provide highly desirable therapeutic benefits.

As you see, there are many options to choose from. Most of these ingredients can be found at health food stores or other supply stores. (If you don't have access to a reputable seller, consult my list of resources on page 371.) These raw ingredients are generally non-irritating, but, as always, if you have an allergy or sensitivity to a specific ingredient or ingredient family, avoid using it in your personal care products.

CLAYS

Since prehistoric times humans have used clay for therapeutic purposes, and its popularity continues. Today it's used in facial care as a component of masks and exfoliants, and as a poultice after cleansing.

Clays are widely used in personal care products because they are so highly absorbent. That means they're able to pull excess oils and other impurities out of the skin. They can also exfoliate dead cells, thereby cleansing and tightening the skin. Some clays have been found to have antibacterial properties as well. Clays are also rich in minerals, especially calcium, which is beneficial for inflammation. In terms of their function in skin-care formulations, clays are used as thickening agents. This makes them useful in facial masks, deodorants and creams.

Several clays are available for making personal care products, but the two that I personally recommend are kaolin (white) clay and French green clay.

Kaolin Clay

This whitish gray-brown clay is also called white clay, white cosmetic clay or china clay. Kaolin helps purify the skin by eliminating oils and other impurities. It also has antiviral properties, which means it can help the body to fight off viruses and treat infections.

French Green Clay

Light grayish green in color, French green clay is used as an astringent and an exfoliant and for removing oils and impurities. It has been found to have antibacterial properties and is highly beneficial for treating wounds, acne and oily skin.

FLOURS AND GRAINS

Like clays, flours and grains have a long history in therapeutic natural cosmetics. These ingredients act primarily as thickening agents in products such as facial masks and exfoliants. However, be aware that adding a flour or grain to a product will decrease its shelf life.

Arrowroot Powder

Sold in stores as arrowroot powder or starch, this ingredient is derived from the root of the arrowroot plant, *Maranta arundinacea*. In skin-care products it's usually added to body powders because it has a smooth, silky feel on the skin and helps to absorb moisture.

Chickpea Flour

Also called garbanzo bean, gram, besan or ceci bean flour, chickpea flour is traditionally used in cooking. It is an excellent cleanser and can help reduce oiliness, making it ideal for use as an ingredient in facial masks and scrubs.

Oats

Oats are considered to have hypoallergenic properties and are often used in products to treat skin conditions such as eczema. They contain phytochemicals (chemicals that occur naturally in plants) that can help reduce itching and irritation. Oats are very soothing and can be used in facial masks, scrubs and soaps. Ground oatmeal can also be added to bathwater to ease dry, itchy skin, burns and insect bites.

GRANULES

Granules are tiny particles with a coarse texture that makes them suitable for use in exfoliants. Some granules, such as sugar, salt and coffee, can dissolve to form a solution if enough water is added to them. Otherwise the granules remain solid and, when a small amount of water or oil is added, will form a moist paste.

Baking Soda

Chemically known as sodium bicarbonate, baking soda is a common household product that is highly alkaline, with a pH of 8 to 9. This high pH means that it may irritate the skin, making it unsuitable as a facial cleanser or exfoliant. It should instead be used in deodorants or mouthwashes. Fungus breaks down in highly alkaline environments, so another way to use baking soda is in antifungal dry shampoos to treat seborrheic dermatitis, a condition that affects the scalp and sometimes the upper parts of the body, such as face and neck.

Citrus Zest

The dehydrated zest of lemons, oranges and grapefruits makes an excellent natural exfoliant. You can easily dehydrate these fruits at home. If possible, use organic citrus, as they won't contain traces of pesticide residues.

To dehydrate the zest, air-dry the fruit's peel for several days, or speed up the drying process by using an oven. Once you've dehydrated the peel, place it in a clean coffee grinder and grind until you get granules. Store the dried zest in an airtight container in a cool, dry area. Add citrus zest to scrubs and other exfoliating formulations.

Cocoa Powder

The cacao tree produces pods whose seeds are used to make cocoa powder and chocolate. Cocoa powder is rich in antioxidants such as flavanols, which may help to repair damage to skin cells. Cocoa powder can also stimulate blood circulation, so it's wonderful for rejuvenating skin and creating a nice healthy glow. Keep in mind, however, that cocoa is a stimulant, and too much cocoa may be irritating to sensitive skin.

Cocoa powder added to a formulation gives it a rich, smooth texture. Use unsweetened cocoa powder in facial masks, lotions and exfoliants.

Ground Coffee

Coffee granules are ground coffee beans. Coffee is rich in antioxidants, which can help fight skin aging. It can also help brighten skin, making it a terrific addition to facial masks. And it's an excellent exfoliator — it can be a bit harsh for the face, but it's ideal for body scrubs. Because it is a stimulant, overexposure to coffee grounds may irritate sensitive skin.

Gum Arabic

The use of gum arabic (also known as acacia gum) dates back thousands of years. It has traditionally been used in cooking as a thickening agent for candies, gels, glazes and gum. In powdered form, gum arabic is used in facial masks to create a gel-like texture and appearance.

IRRITATION ALERT

In rare cases, gum arabic may cause allergic reactions on the skin.

Salt

Many varieties of sodium chloride can be used in skin-care formulations, from Dead Sea salt to Himalayan pink salt and more. Salt is used as a natural preservative, and its texture makes it ideal in body cleansers or exfoliants. Salt is also great sprinkled in bathwater, to detoxify the skin and promote relaxation, but overexposure may lead to irritation.

Sugar

Sucrose, more commonly known as sugar, has been used since the beginning of time as a natural skin whitener and exfoliant. It is widely used as both a natural preservative and a biodegradable cleansing agent. Use sugar in facial cleansers and exfoliants. Because it has a pH of 7 (meaning that it is neutral), it is adaptable to any skin type.

LIQUIDS AND GELS

The addition of liquids and gels will add volume as well as therapeutic properties to your natural care products. Some liquids and gels act as humectants, meaning that they can hydrate skin by pulling moisture from the environment.

IRRITATION ALERT

Aloe vera contains salicylic acid and steroids, both of which have anti-inflammatory properties. It also contains beneficial phenolic compounds that help fight off infection. However, some of these compounds may irritate hypersensitive skin. What's more, products containing salicylic acid may foster hyperpigmentation, so be cautious about using them on skin that will be exposed to the sun.

Aloe Vera Gel

The aloe vera plant produces a gel-like sap that is known for its ability to help heal wounds. Its first-aid power is one reason why many people keep a plant in their home. Breaking open a leaf yields the sap, which can be spread on minor cuts and burns. Aloe vera contains saponins, plant chemicals that contribute to the cleansing and antiseptic effects of the gel. That, combined with the nutrient-rich plant's antimicrobial properties, makes it ideal for applying topically to wounds, sunburn and mild abrasions.

Aloe vera can help reduce skin inflammation, and the salicylic acid in the gel can be used to treat acne and to prevent pores from clogging. It's also widely employed in skin-care treatments to tighten and firm skin. Use it in masks, exfoliants, deodorants, lotions and creams.

Alcohol

Ethyl alcohol (ethanol) is produced by the fermentation of sugar, starch and other forms of carbohydrate. This clear, colorless liquid is widely used in the cosmetic industry because it is a natural preservative. It is generally found in perfumes, colognes and aftershaves and as a cooling agent in after-sun skin-care products. It is known for drying the skin.

IRRITATION ALERT

Alcohol can dehydrate the skin and may disrupt its protective barrier, so people with sensitive skin should avoid using it topically.

Glycerin

This gel-like compound is a natural humectant, making it ideal for use in wash-off products that moisturize the skin. Glycerin is also a mild emulsifying agent that can be used to add stability to products. It has preservative properties similar to sugar and a pH of 7, which is neutral (neither acid or alkaline), making it very adaptable for skin-care products.

Natural glycerin can be derived from animal sources or from plant-based oils such as coconut oil or palm kernel oil. It can be mixed directly into almost any skin-care product. It can also be infused with various herbs, spices or flowers to create herbal infusions, which make wonderful skin-nourishing additions to oil-based formulations such as creams, lotions, serums and balms (see page 83).

Squalene

Squalene occurs naturally in our own bodies, where it acts as a protective barrier on the skin. Squalene is an effective moisturizer because it's wonderful for repairing damaged and dehydrated skin. Unfortunately it also oxidizes very quickly (see page 29). The squalene used in personal care products is usually harvested from the livers of sharks, many species of which are nearing extinction. So, for practical and environmental purposes, the hydrogenated version known as squalane is usually used in cosmetics.

Squalane, obtained from plant sources such as argan oil and sunflower seed oil, is much less likely than squalene to oxidize. Thus it is more stable. It is also a much more sustainable option. When applied topically, squalane is a non-greasy emollient that helps other topical agents to penetrate the skin. When applied to damaged and dehydrated skin and hair, it is very healing and quickly restores moisture levels. It also has UV-absorption properties, helping to protect skin from the sun. Use it in moisturizing masks, face creams and body lotions.

EXTRACTS

Extracts are obtained from various natural sources such as fruits, herbs and seeds. Adding extracts to personal care products boosts their therapeutic effects. They contain highly concentrated active ingredients, however, so you should use them with moderation in skin-care products in order to avoid irritation.

Extracts can be purchased in liquid or powdered form. Here are several commonly used ones.

Bamboo

This extract comes from the leaves and stalks of the bamboo plant. It is best known for its high silica content. Silica plays a role in keeping skin, nails and hair healthy, so it's used in products to smooth and strengthen skin and hair. It can also prevent a buildup of greasy film and ensures that products spread smoothly. Use bamboo extract in hair masks, shampoos, conditioners and skin cleansers.

Grapeseed

Grapeseed extract is derived from the ground-up seeds of red grapes. Grape seeds contain significant amounts of polyphenols. These plant-based molecules have very strong antioxidant properties that help to destroy free radicals and prevent aging, specifically wrinkles and dryness. Grapeseed extract may also facilitate the healing of cuts, scrapes and burns, making it ideal for using in poultices and after-sun skin-care products.

Pomegranate

This extract is typically made from the peel of the pomegranate fruit. Adding pomegranate extract to a product will increase its ability to tighten and firm skin. The extract has also been shown to reduce the effects of sun damage, because of a phenol compound called catechin. This makes it particularly valuable in anti-aging products. Use this extract in masks, exfoliants, body washes, lotions and creams.

ALLERGY ALERT

Salicylates are chemicals found in certain vegetables, fruits, herbs and nuts. While the salicylate content of foods depends on many factors — it can vary from crop to crop or depend on ripeness, for example — some generally have a high content, such as grapes, almonds and honey. People with a salicylate sensitivity or intolerance should avoid products made with high-salicylate foods.

Rosemary

This extract is obtained by soaking rosemary leaves in a liquid such as alcohol. The active ingredients are extracted and then added to either alcohol or water to make a concentrated product that is very high in antioxidants. These antioxidants help protect against free-radical damage, as well as environmental stressors, making this extract ideal for use in anti-aging skin-care products such as cleansers, moisturizers, masks and exfoliants. Rosemary extract is also used as a preservative in natural personal care products. It is widely used in hair treatments, from shampoos and cleansers to scalp tonics.

Vitamin E

Vitamin E is found naturally in many plant-based oils and butters, such as argan oil and shea butter. It is a powerful antioxidant that aids in fighting off the free radicals that age the skin. It helps your skin retain its natural moisture, and strong photo-protective properties help guard against UV damage, making it well suited for after-sun products. It's also highly beneficial in formulations for healing cuts, burns and scrapes, because its anti-inflammatory properties calm and hydrate skin. Use vitamin E in masks, exfoliants, deodorants, body washes, lotions and creams.

Witch Hazel

Also called witch hazel hydrolat, this extract is distilled from the dried leaves and bark of the witch hazel shrub. Its astringent properties help cleanse pores, making it a very effective acne treatment. It's also an analgesic, so it can help relieve itchy skin, minor burns and other skin irritations. In addition, it's been shown to reduce erythema, or patches of red skin.

Witch hazel is acidic, but when diluted in water, the pH is increased to 5, similar to that of the skin. This makes it ideal for using in toners. Other uses include masks, exfoliants, deodorants, body washes, lotions and creams.

IRRITATION ALERT

Most witch hazel extracts that you find in stores contain a high percentage of alcohol. Look for alcohol-free witch hazel hydrolat, especially if you have sensitive skin.

EMULSIFIERS

One of the most important ingredients in a skin-care product is the emulsifier. Emulsifiers are substances that have the capacity to blend water and lipids (fats). When you are formulating personal care products, you are combining incompatible oil- and water-based ingredients. Think of an emulsifier as the glue that holds these ingredients together.

I like to use waxes as the emulsifying agent in my personal care products. There are many types of waxes to choose from, and the type you use will have a large impact on the texture and stability of your product. For example, some waxes thicken formulations while others add an almost powdery texture. Here are some of the most commonly used emulsifying agents.

Beeswax

ORIGIN: secreted by female honeybees.

USES: emollient; thickener.

BENEFITS: soothes and softens skin; protects from dehydration; has antibacterial properties.

CAUTION: may be irritating to skin.

USED IN: lip balms; creams; lotions; salves.

ALLERGY ALERT

If you are allergic to pollen or honey, avoid skin-care products that contain beeswax. When creating formulations, you may replace beeswax with candelilla or carnauba wax, but keep in mind that these waxes produce a much thicker consistency.

Candelilla Wax

ORIGIN: derived from the leaves of the candelilla shrub, which is native to Mexico.

USE: stiffening agent.

BENEFITS: protects creams from moisture loss; hardens other waxes.

CAUTIONS: none; generally recognized as safe to use in skin-care formulations.

USED IN: lip balms; body butters; lotions; hair products; perfumed balms.

Carnauba Wax

ORIGIN: derived from the leaves of the carnaúba palm tree, which is native to Brazil.

USE: stiffening agent.

BENEFITS: hardens other waxes; gives products a glossy finish.

CAUTIONS: none; generally recognized as safe to use in skin-care formulations.

USED IN: lip balms; body butters; perfumed balms.

If the term "carnauba wax" seems familiar, it's because it is a major component of the waxes used to polish cars and floors.

Emulsifying Wax NF

ORIGIN: manufactured by National Formulary from a combination of ingredients that include cetearyl alcohol, a mixture of fatty alcohols derived from coconut oil, which is used widely used in cosmetics; polysorbate-60; PEG-150 stearate; and steareth-20. The solid flakes are white and waxy.

USE: stabilizer.

BENEFIT: relatively inexpensive.

CAUTIONS: This wax is safe when used in recommended concentrations. The Cosmetic Ingredient Review, an independent safety review program for cosmetic ingredients, has concluded that this wax does not cause skin sensitization, although some highly sensitive people may react to some of the ingredients.

USED IN: creams; lotions; moisturizers.

Stearic Acid

ORIGIN: waxy solid fatty acid obtained from sources such as animal tallow and vegetable fats.
USE: stabilizer.
BENEFIT: promotes wound healing.
CAUTIONS: Stearic acid is classified as safe when used in recommended concentrations. Overexposure may lead to irritation.
USED IN: creams; lotions; moisturizers.

Emulsimulse

ORIGINS: a blend of cetearyl alcohol, glyceryl stearate and sodium stearoyl lactylate. The solid flakes are off-white in color.
USE: stabilizer.
BENEFITS: Creams and lotions made with EmulsiMulse leave the skin feeling soft and silky.
CAUTIONS: no known toxicity.
USED IN: creams; lotions; moisturizers.

Floral Waxes

ORIGINS: solid, creamy aromatic waxes derived from the petals of certain aromatic floral plants, including rose, jasmine, tuberose and mimosa. Carefully selected flower heads are placed in a solvent, then in alcohol; finally the solid plant wax is filtered out of the resulting solution.
USE: fragrance base.
BENEFITS: antioxidant; moisturizing; lovely floral scent.
CAUTION: potential irritant if sensitive to the source botanical.
USED IN: creams; lotions; moisturizers; balms.

Blending Emulsifiers

Beeswax, stearic acid and emulsifying wax can be used as the sole emulsifier in a formulation. This is not the case for carnauba, candelilla and floral waxes. It is highly recommended that these waxes make up no more than 25 percent of the total emulsifying content of a formulation. This is the best way to create a stable emulsion.

Here's an example: If a formulation calls for 20 grams of an emulsifier, you can use 5 grams of a floral wax and the remaining 15 grams should be beeswax, stearic acid or emulsifying wax.

Carrier Oils, Plant Butters and Infusions

CARRIER OILS

Carrier oils differ from essential oils in several key ways. Carrier oils are extracted (rather than distilled) from particular parts of plants such as the seeds or kernels. And, unlike essential oils, they don't evaporate when exposed to air and they're relatively odorless.

Carrier oils play a major role in creams and lotions and, when chosen wisely, will nourish and moisturize your skin. Matching carrier oils to skin type — bearing in mind the product's purpose — is one of the most important tasks you'll face when developing your own personal care products.

Protecting Your Skin with Carrier Oils

Your skin is a protective barrier that interacts with water, soaps, chemicals and weather conditions on a daily basis. This exposure can modify the skin's integrity and affect its appearance. Daily wear and tear lead to skin that looks unhealthy and is overly sensitive, dry and chapped, or subject to problematic conditions such as dermatitis, rosacea and acne.

Pure cold-pressed oils have natural protective properties that can help fight the disruptions your skin encounters from day to day. In other words, when used properly, they can help your skin maintain its proper balance, and they can also help it recover from upset equilibrium.

How do oils accomplish this? Oils are emollient, which means they are softening. They are rich in components such as essential fatty acids (EFAs), fat-soluble vitamins, plant sterols and carotenoids, all of which help skin to repair itself and protect its elasticity. They also help your skin to maintain its protective barrier. And research now shows that some components of these oils, much like similar constituents in essential oils, have antimicrobial and antifungal properties, which can help skin fight off infection.

Cold-Pressed and Organic Oils

Ideally you should be using organic or wild-crafted carrier oils, since they contain a minimal amount of chemical residue. It's also preferable to use cold-pressed oils, which retain a higher proportion of nutrients than they would if they had been exposed to heat during the extraction process.

Additional Components in Carrier Oils

Carrier oils may contain quantities of other fatty acids such as myristic, pentadecanoic, heptadecanoic or eicosenoic (arachidic) acid, as well as compounds such as vitamin E and squalane, all of which have therapeutic properties. For more on some of these ingredients, see page 55.

Carotenoids

Carrier oils contain a wide range of carotenoids, which are powerful antioxidants that help keep skin healthy and young. Some common carotenoids include beta-carotene (found primarily in orange vegetables) and lycopene (found in tomatoes.) Carotenoids provide the oil with its pigment and with some unique therapeutic properties. For example, there is growing evidence that topically applying carotenoids can help to prevent UV-induced skin aging. Oils rich in color, such as rosehip seed, argan and hempseed oils, are abundant in carotenoids.

ESSENTIAL FATTY ACIDS

All oils are composed of fatty acids. Essential fatty acids (EFAs) are specific fats that your body uses as developmental building blocks. Every cell and organ is wrapped in a fatty membrane, which means that you need EFAs to keep your body healthy. These fats also maintain a barrier on the outermost surface of your skin, which keeps it protected and hydrated.

A formulation's end product will be determined by the type of carrier oil you use, as its fatty acid content will affect your product's emollient and cleansing properties, as well as its viscosity. The three types of fatty acids are saturated fatty acids, monounsaturated fatty acids and polyunsaturated fatty acids.

EFAs Battle Bugs

Agents that kill microorganisms or limit their growth are known as antimicrobials. In the past, pharmaceutical and cosmetic companies didn't pay much attention to the antimicrobial properties of fatty acids. However, studies are now demonstrating that fatty acids have potent abilities to kill certain viruses, bacteria and fungi that can cause skin infections as well as acne breakouts. There is a lack of clarity about how exactly they do this, but new research indicates that they may be able to disrupt the cell membranes of the different microorganisms. Thus, using products that contain naturally derived fatty acids may help to protect your skin from certain bacterial, viral or fungal assaults.

What Is a Penetration Enhancer?

Certain fatty acids help to alter the stratum corneum (that's the very outer layer of the skin — the top layer of the epidermis), thereby allowing certain ingredients to reach the deeper layers of the epidermis. Adding a penetration enhancer to a formulation helps to deliver vitamins, antioxidants, humectants and other elements into the upper layers of the skin. Palmitic acid and oleic acid are examples of penetration enhancers.

SATURATED FATTY ACIDS

Oils high in saturated fatty acids (SFAs) remain solid at room temperature. Thus, carrier oils with a high level of saturated fats are heavy and have a buttery texture. SFAs are used in skin-care products as thickening agents. They also add therapeutic value: some SFAs are beneficial for inhibiting skin infections, while others promote wound healing.

SIGNIFICANT SFAS

Lauric Acid

Studies show that lauric acid is antibacterial, which means that it helps prevent skin infections, as well as acne breakouts. That makes it ideal for cleansing formulations targeted toward preventing those conditions. This saturated fatty acid is abundant in coconut and palm kernel oils.

Myristic Acid

Like lauric acid, myristic acid is antibacterial, and as a result it is beneficial for preventing skin infections. Oils high in myristic acid also act as surfactants — they help dissolve dirt and grime — making them a great addition to cleansers. This SFA is found mostly in coconut and palm kernel oils, and in trace amounts in grapeseed oil.

Palmitic Acid

Palmitic acid is found naturally on the epidermis (the top layer of the skin), where it helps to maintain the skin's moisture levels. Carrier oils with a high concentration of palmitic acid are useful in moisturizers, as this SFA is a very effective emollient. The acid helps other ingredients penetrate into the skin, and it is also a good thickening agent, which makes it useful in products where a creamy texture is desired. High concentrations of palmitic acid are found in palm kernel oil and cocoa butter; a fair amount is found in oils such as almond, sunflower and grapeseed.

Stearic Acid

This fatty acid is naturally found on the top layer of the skin. Stearic acid has been found to have anti-inflammatory properties and to promote wound healing. It is commonly used as an emulsifying agent when creating cream-based formulations. Stearic acid is found naturally in plant butters, particularly cocoa and shea butters.

MONOUNSATURATED AND POLYUNSATURATED FATTY ACIDS

Oils that contain high levels of monounsaturated and polyunsaturated fatty acids (MUFAs and PUFAs) remain liquid at room temperature, which produces lighter-textured creams, lotions and serums. Many MUFAs and PUFAs make great cleansing agents, and they have wonderful emollient properties.

SIGNIFICANT MUFAS AND PUFAS

Oleic Acid

Oleic acid is a MUFA with antiviral and antifungal properties, so it can help prevent skin infections caused by viruses or fungi. It is often used in commercial products as a penetration enhancer to facilitate the absorption of drug compounds. Therefore it's reasonable to assume that it may increase the absorption of essential oils into the body. Oils high in oleic acid, such as sweet almond, avocado, apricot kernel, marula and argan, are well suited for dry skin.

Palmitoleic Acid

This MUFA is beneficial for products targeted at aging skin. Palmitoleic acid has antibacterial capabilities, which makes it useful for formulations aimed at fighting skin infections. It is found mainly in avocado oil and in trace amounts in other oils such as grapeseed, jojoba and hazelnut.

Gamma-Linolenic Acid

A PUFA, gamma-linolenic acid is very effective at soothing the skin, making it ideal for treating atopic eczema, psoriasis and various other skin conditions. It is typically found in borage, evening primrose, hempseed and rosehip seed oils.

Linoleic Acid

Linoleic acid is a natural component of the skin's sebum. It helps to strengthen the protective barrier on the top layer of skin and guard against water loss, which makes it a very effective moisturizer. Additionally, linoleic acid is recommended for use in treatments for problematic oily skin, because it's been shown to help unblock pores. This PUFA is found in most carrier oils, usually constituting 30 to 89 percent of their total fatty acid content. It is abundant in sunflower, sesame seed and grapeseed oils.

Alpha-Linolenic Acid

This PUFA (also referred to simply as linolenic acid) has been shown to help regulate inflammation. Carrier oils that have high amounts of alpha linoleic acid are beneficial for treating inflamed skin conditions such as eczema, psoriasis, rosacea and a variety of rashes. It is found in rosehip, hemp and sesame seed oils.

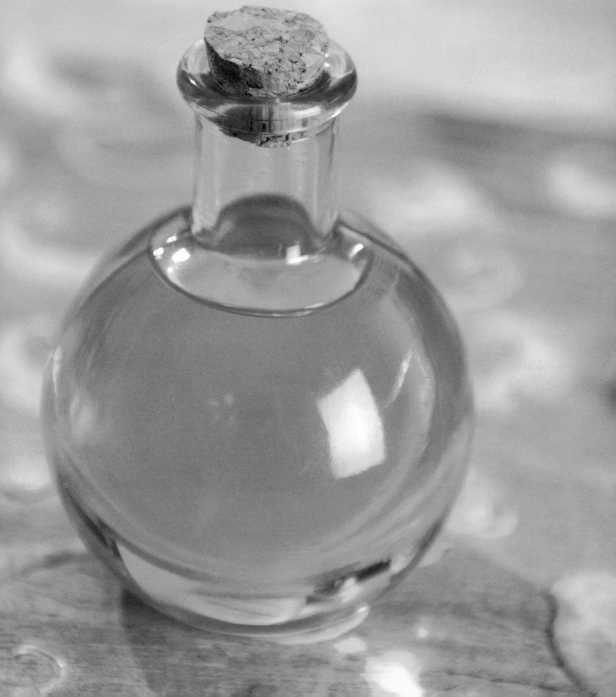

Carrier Oils
for Personal
Care Products

Sweet Almond Oil

Botanical name: *Prunus amygdalus dulcis*

Botanical family: Rosaceae

Typical Fatty Acid Composition

SATURATED FATTY ACIDS	MONOUNSATURATED FATTY ACIDS	POLYUNSATURATED FATTY ACIDS	ADDITIONAL COMPONENTS
Palmitic acid 7–10%	Oleic acid 60–65%	Linoleic acid 30–35%	Vitamin E
Stearic acid 2–4%		Alpha-linolenic acid 1–2%	Squalane
Myristic acid 0.5–1%			

Uses

Sweet almond oil is ideal for dry, chapped, scaly skin; mature skin; and conditions such as eczema, psoriasis and dermatitis.

Compounding

Sweet almond oil is a terrific base oil to use in natural care products. In formulations it can be used as 50 to 100% of the carrier oil. It can be compounded with other oils in a ratio of 80:20. Blending sweet almond oil with rosehip, avocado, hempseed or calendula or carrot-infused oils will enhance its therapeutic properties.

Sweet almond oil is obtained from the nut kernel of the sweet almond tree (the same one that produces the almonds we eat) through cold pressing and subsequent refining. It is pale yellow and scented with soft nutty notes. Sweet almond oil is produced mainly in Spain, Morocco and India. Its shelf life is 8 to 12 months.

Benefits

Sweet almond oil is rich in oleic and linoleic acids, making it a beneficial emollient and skin conditioner. It is also rich in the antioxidant vitamin E, as well as squalane, a lipid that protects the natural oils in the skin. It is good source of manganese, an essential supplement for suppressing premature aging, soothing irritation and preventing blemishes. Manganese can also shield the skin from UV damage, suggesting that the oil may have photo-protective effects. The high level of vitamin E also helps to prevent UV-related damage, including the formation of fine lines.

Apricot Kernel Oil

Botanical name: *Prunus armeniaca*

Botanical family: Rosaceae

Typical Fatty Acid Composition

SATURATED FATTY ACIDS	MONOUNSATURATED FATTY ACIDS	POLYUNSATURATED FATTY ACIDS	ADDITIONAL COMPONENT
Palmitic acid 5–6%	Oleic acid 60–65%	Linoleic acid 30–35%	Vitamin E
Stearic acid 1–2%	Palmitoleic acid 1%	Alpha-linolenic acid 1–2%	
Arachidic acid 1–2%	Eicosenoic acid 1–2%		

Uses

Apricot kernel oil is best used in formulations for oily, combination or sensitive skin.

Compounding

In formulations, apricot kernel oil is a lovely oil to use in serums, lotions and moisturizers as 100% of the carrier oil, or it can be compounded with other oils or butters at a ratio of 80:20. Blending apricot kernel oil with 20% of either rosehip, argan, avocado or hemp oil will create a phytonutrient-enriched blend that will leave you with soothed, glowing skin.

Apricot kernel oil is a pale yellow, light-textured oil obtained from the dry kernels of apricot fruit through hydraulic cold pressing. The apricot tree grows in warm climate regions, and the oil is produced mainly in Kenya and Italy. It has a shelf life of 8 to 12 months.

Benefits

Apricot kernel oil is often used in the cosmetics industry as a light moisturizer because it quickly absorbs into skin. It's a good source of oleic acid, a MUFA known for its excellent penetration capabilities (see page 56), as well as its ability to protect your skin from moisture loss. In addition to its high MUFA content, this oil is rich in vitamin E, which helps the skin to repair itself.

Numerous carrier oils, such as sweet almond, apricot kernel, argan, avocado, camellia seed, hazelnut and marula, contain a high percentage of oleic acid, which has been shown to have antifungal properties. Fungal infections on the skin, such as seborrheic dermatitis, are a problem for many people. If you are having problems with skin infections of this nature, using a carrier oil with a high percentage of oleic acid in your formulations may help with keeping such infections under control, particularly if paired with essential oils that have similar properties.

Argan Oil

Botanical name: *Argania spinosa*

Botanical family: Sapotaceae

Typical Fatty Acid Composition

SATURATED FATTY ACIDS	MONOUNSATURATED FATTY ACIDS	POLYUNSATURATED FATTY ACIDS	ADDITIONAL COMPONENTS
Palmitic acid 12–15%	Oleic acid 45–50%	Linoleic acid 30–35%	Vitamin E
Myristic acid 1–2%		Alpha-linolenic acid 1–2%	Squalane
Arachidic acid 1–2%			

Uses

Argan oil is suitable for all skin types — dry, oily, combination or sensitive. It is also a good choice for use in hair products.

Compounding

Argan oil is relatively expensive, so it should be used carefully. When making facial serums, it can be used as up to 100% of the carrier oil, but when making body products, I recommend blending it with 30% of either apricot kernel or jojoba oil.

This oil is extracted from the nut of the argan tree, which grows primarily in the southwestern part of Morocco, in an area designated as a UNESCO biosphere reserve. Recently argan trees have been planted in deserts in Israel to create additional sustainable crops.

Two types of argan oil are produced: one for personal care products, which is extracted from the raw kernels, and an edible version, where the kernel is roasted prior to oil extraction. The roasting of the kernel gives culinary argan oil a very strong, nutty scent that is not suitable for skin care, whereas the cosmetic-grade oil has a mild scent. Cosmetic argan oil has a shelf life of 12 to 18 months from the date of production.

Benefits

Argan oil is rich in vitamin E and squalane, two powerful antioxidants. This oil improves skin elasticity and is very moisturizing. It also protects and softens skin and provides anti-aging benefits, such as reducing hyperpigmentation. Also, the oil assists in wound healing and helps to prevent acne by reducing sebum production.

Avocado Oil

Botanical name: *Persea americana*

Botanical family: Lauraceae

Typical Fatty Acid Composition

SATURATED FATTY ACIDS	MONOUNSATURATED FATTY ACIDS	POLYUNSATURATED FATTY ACIDS	ADDITIONAL COMPONENTS
Palmitic acid 12–16%	Oleic acid 65–70%	Linoleic acid 10–15%	Vitamin A
	Palmitoleic acid 5–10%	Alpha-linolenic acid 1–2%	Vitamin D
			Vitamin E

Uses

Avocado oil is best used in products for very dry, chapped skin, scar tissue and stretch marks. It's also well suited to products for dry hair.

Compounding

Avocado oil should be used as 30% or less of the carrier oil in formulations for the face. In products for the hands, legs and feet, it can be used at 100%. However, this oil is very thick, so it is advisable to compound it with other oils in a ratio of 70:30. Suggested other oils include almond and grapeseed.

In contrast to most other vegetable oils, avocado oil is obtained not from the seed but from the flesh of the fruit of the avocado tree. In most cases it is obtained through mechanical cold pressing with a hydraulic press or by centrifuge extraction. Avocado oil is rich in chlorophyll, which gives it a green color. Originating in south-central Mexico, it is now produced mainly in Kenya, Israel, New Zealand and South Africa. It has a shelf life of 12 to 18 months.

Benefits

Avocado is rich in vitamin E, as well as beta carotene (a carotenoid). Its rich emollient properties make it ideal for very dry, mature skin or stretch marks and for use in hair care. It may also help with skin injuries; in one animal study, avocado oil was found to promote faster healing of topically treated wounds. And a German study, published in the journal *Dermatology*, found that a topical mixture of avocado oil and vitamin B_{12} was beneficial in treating plaque psoriasis.

Borage Oil

Botanical name: *Borago officinalis*

Botanical family: Boraginaceae

Typical Fatty Acid Composition

SATURATED FATTY ACIDS	MONOUNSATURATED FATTY ACIDS	POLYUNSATURATED FATTY ACIDS
Palmitic acid 15–20%	Oleic acid 15–20%	Linoleic acid 35–40%
Stearic acid 10–15%	Erucic acid 2–3%	Gamma-linolenic acid 25–30%
Arachidic acid 3–4%		

Uses

Borage oil is best used in formulations that address dry, sensitive or inflamed skin.

Compounding

In formulations, borage oil can be used as 10 to 30% of the carrier oil.

IRRITATION ALERT

Borage oil penetrates into damaged skin at a higher rate than into normal skin, which can cause irritation. Avoid using on injured skin.

Borage oil is derived from the seeds of borage, a large plant with bright blue star-shaped flowers that is found throughout Europe and North Africa and naturalized to North America. Today the golden yellow or pale green oil is produced mainly in Canada, England, New Zealand and China. It is extracted by cold-pressing the seeds, which produces a relatively low yield. It has a short shelf life of only 6 to 8 months.

Benefits

Borage oil is very rich in gamma-linolenic acid (GLA), an important fat that helps keep skin healthy and helps to reduce inflammation (borage seed oil has the highest amount of GLA of all the seed oils). This oil is often used in topical applications for eczema, topical dermatitis and psoriasis, to reduce dryness and inflammation. There's also evidence that applying borage oil to skin reduces itching. In addition, its skin-repairing activity makes it a good oil to use in after-sun formulations.

Borage oil and evening primrose oil both contain GLA and in most cases can be used interchangeably. The exception is when treating sensitive skin, in which case evening primrose oil should be used.

Camellia Seed Oil

Botanical name: *Camellia sinensis*

Botanical family: Theaceae

Typical Fatty Acid Composition

SATURATED FATTY ACIDS	MONOUNSATURATED FATTY ACIDS	POLYUNSATURATED FATTY ACIDS
Palmitic acid 6–9%	Oleic acid 72–80%	Linoleic acid 6–14%
Stearic acid 2–3%	Nervonic acid 1–2%	Alpha-linolenic acid 1–2%
	Eicosenoic acid 1–2%	

Uses

Camellia seed oil is ideal for all types of skin and hair-care products.

Compounding

Camellia seed oil is a thick oil with a lovely texture that can be compounded with most other carrier oils. In formulations I recommend compounding camellia seed oil with apricot kernel, grapeseed or jojoba oil in a ratio between 30:70 and 50:50. It can be used as 100% of the carrier oil in formulations for facial serums.

Camellia seed oil is also known as tea oil, since it comes from the tea plant, *Camellia sinensis*. The oil is produced by pulverizing and cold-pressing the seeds into a viscous light green oil. Camellia seed oil is produced in China and Japan. It has a short shelf life of 6 to 8 months.

Benefits

Camellia seed oil is high in oleic acid — an excellent emollient and skin healer — which makes it a very good choice for dry, chapped skin and for treating conditions such as psoriasis, eczema and burns. This oil's moisturizing properties also make it ideal for mature skin, so it's well suited for anti-aging formulations. It can be used in moisturizers, serums, creams, lotions, balms and body oils.

Numerous carrier oils, such as sweet almond, apricot kernel, argan, avocado, camellia seed, hazelnut and marula, contain a high percentage of oleic acid, which has been shown to have antifungal properties. Fungal infections on the skin, such as seborrheic dermatitis, are a problem for many people. If you are having problems with skin infections of this nature, using a carrier oil with a high percentage of oleic acid in your formulations may help with keeping such infections under control, particularly if paired with essential oils that have similar properties.

Coconut Oil

Botanical name: *Cocos nucifera*

Botanical family: Arecaceae

Typical Fatty Acid Composition

SATURATED FATTY ACIDS		MONOUNSATURATED FATTY ACIDS	POLYUNSATURATED FATTY ACIDS
Lauric acid 45–52%	Capric acid 5–10%	Oleic acid 5–10%	Linoleic acid 1–2%
Myristic acid 13–19%	Caprylic acid 5–10%		
Palmitic acid 10–15%	Stearic acid 1–3%		

Uses

This lightweight oil is suitable for all skin types and can be used in formulations for the face, body, hair and scalp.

Compounding

In formulations, extra virgin coconut oil can be used as 100% of the carrier oil.

Allergy Alert

Although coconuts are technically a fruit, coconut oil could potentially pose a problem for people with tree-nut allergies. If you have such an allergy, avoid using coconut oil in your personal care products.

Extra virgin coconut oil is extracted either by pressing the fresh white meat of the coconut or by drying the meat first and then cold-pressing it. It has a sweet scent and is very stable, giving it a shelf life of 2 years.

Benefits

Coconut oil is an excellent moisturizer, making it a popular carrier oil to use in personal care products. It's naturally antibacterial, thanks in part to lauric and myristic acids. Lauric acid is abundant in coconut oil; this fatty acid is commonly used as a base for cleansers and is also known for its skin-soothing properties. Myristic acid is a good cleansing agent as well.

The caprylic acid in coconut oil is a potent antifungal, meaning that it can help prevent and treat fungal infections. There's also evidence that coconut oil has UV-protective qualities, making it ideal for sunscreen formulations; estimates of the oil's SPF vary but are usually within the range of 4 to 8%.

Fractionated Coconut Oil

This clear, light oil is produced by removing the long-chain fatty acids from coconut oil through a hot extraction method. It is rich in medium-chain fatty acids, which help repair damaged skin and protect against moisture loss. It is most often used in conjunction with other carrier oils to reduce the oily feel of a product. Since it does not stain sheets, it is a convenient massage oil.

Evening Primrose Oil

Botanical name: *Oenothera biennis*

Botanical family: Onagraceae

Typical Fatty Acid Composition

SATURATED FATTY ACIDS	MONOUNSATURATED FATTY ACIDS	POLYUNSATURATED FATTY ACIDS
Palmitic acid 6–10%	Oleic acid 5–10%	Linoleic acid 70–75%
Stearic acid 2–10%		Gamma-linolenic acid 5–10%

Uses

Evening primrose oil is suitable for all skin types. It is particularly beneficial for aging, inflamed or sensitive skin.

Compounding

In formulations, evening primrose oil can be used as 10 to 30% of the carrier oil.

Evening primrose is a light yellow oil with a subtle marine scent. It's extracted by cold-pressing and filtering the seeds of the evening primrose plant. Evening primrose originated throughout eastern and central North America and eventually spread to subtropical climates around the world. Today the oil is produced mainly in China. It has a short shelf life of 6 to 8 months.

Benefits

Evening primrose oil is a rich source of gamma-linolenic acid, an important fat that is known for its ability to help prevent and treat inflammatory skin conditions. Research shows that evening primrose oil can calm symptoms of inflamed skin; one study found improvement in scaling, dryness, redness and itching after participants applied the oil.

Topical application of the oil can help ease symptoms of psoriasis and eczema and is excellent for caring for wounds. The powerful skin-repairing activity of this oil also makes it well suited for after-sun formulations.

Borage oil and evening primrose oil both contain GLA and in most cases can be used interchangeably. The exception is when treating sensitive skin, in which case evening primrose oil should be used.

Grapeseed Oil

Botanical name: *Vitis vinifera*

Botanical family: Vitaceae

Typical Fatty Acid Composition

SATURATED FATTY ACIDS	MONOUNSATURATED FATTY ACIDS	POLYUNSATURATED FATTY ACIDS	ADDITIONAL COMPONENT
Myristic acid 5–10%	Oleic acid 15–20%	Linoleic acid 65–70%	Vitamin E
Palmitic acid 5–10%	Palmitoleic acid 1%	Alpha-linolenic acid 1–2%	
Stearic acid 5–10%			

Uses

Grapeseed oil is suitable for oily and combination skins. It can be used in formulations for face, body, hair and scalp.

Compounding

In formulations, grapeseed oil can be used as 100% of the carrier oil. It is ideal for compounding with other oils to increase the volume of a formulation.

Grapeseed oil is obtained from the seeds of grapes. The green, scentless oil is a by-product of the wine industry and is extracted by expeller pressing of the grape seeds, followed by further refinement. Grapeseed oil is produced mainly in Italy, France, Portugal, Chile and Argentina. It has a shelf life of 12 to 18 months.

Benefits

Grapeseed oil is rich in linoleic acid, which is known for its moisturizing properties, as well as for its ability to heal wounds. It is generally a safe choice for all skin types, since it has a very low risk of allergy. The oil is commonly used by massage therapists because of its light texture, lack of scent and easy absorption into the skin.

Hazelnut Oil

Botanical Name: *Corylus avellana*

Botanical family: Betulaceae

Typical Fatty Acid Composition

SATURATED FATTY ACIDS	MONOUNSATURATED FATTY ACIDS	POLYUNSATURATED FATTY ACIDS
Palmitic acid 5-10%	Oleic acid 75-80%	Linoleic acid 10-15%
Stearic acid 3-6%	Palmitoleic acid 1-2%	Alpha-linolenic acid 1-2%
Arachidic acid 1-2%		

Uses

Hazelnut oil is best suited for oily or combination skin.

Compounding

In formulations, hazelnut oil can be used as 50 to 100% of the carrier oil. It's a good choice for adding volume to products, and it is particularly well suited for facial products, especially masks. Keep in mind that it has a heavier scent, which can dominate the final product.

ALLERGY ALERT

If you suffer from a nut allergy, do not use hazelnut oil in your personal care products.

This oil is obtained from the fresh nuts of the hazelnut tree. The oil is extracted by cold pressing, followed by filtration, refining and deodorization. Hazelnut oil is deep yellow in color, with a strong, nutty scent. The oil is produced mainly in Turkey. It has a short shelf life of 6 to 8 months.

Benefits

The texture of hazelnut oil is thick and smooth. It's known for its astringent properties, which make it ideal for unclogging pores in oily or combination skin. It's also a good source of linoleic acid, which helps to moisturize skin and to heal wounds. This oil can penetrate the top layer of the skin because of its very high oleic acid content, so it's a good carrier oil to use if you want to boost the properties of a particular essential oil.

Numerous carrier oils, such as sweet almond, apricot kernel, argan, avocado, camellia seed, hazelnut and marula, contain a high percentage of oleic acid, which has been shown to have antifungal properties. Fungal infections on the skin, such as seborrheic dermatitis, are a problem for many people. If you are having problems with skin infections of this nature, using a carrier oil with a high percentage of oleic acid in your formulations may help with keeping such infections under control, particularly if paired with essential oils that have similar properties.

Hempseed Oil

Botanical name: *Cannabis sativa*

Botanical family: Cannabaceae

Typical Fatty Acid Composition

SATURATED FATTY ACIDS	MONOUNSATURATED FATTY ACIDS	POLYUNSATURATED FATTY ACIDS	ADDITIONAL COMPONENTS
Palmitic acid 5–10%	Oleic acid 10–20%	Linoleic acid 45–65%	Vitamin E
Stearic acid 2–4%		Alpha-linolenic acid 14–28%	Cannabidiol (CBD)
		Gamma-linolenic acid 5–10%	Trace amounts of tetrahydro-cannabinol (THC)

Uses

Hempseed oil is best used in formulations for dry skin, eczema- and psoriasis-inflamed skin and sensitive or aging skin.

Compounding

In formulations, hempseed oil can be used as 10% of the carrier oil. Blend hempseed oil with grapeseed or apricot kernel oil.

Hempseed oil is derived from the hemp plant, which is cultivated around the world. It's often confused with the marijuana plant but is quite different.

Hempseed oil is dark green in color (because of its high chlorophyll content) and has a sweet, herbaceous scent. It has a short shelf life of 6 to 8 months. In the past 20 years, it has been recognized for its use in natural cosmetics; it has a unique composition of fatty acids that provide outstanding emollient properties, which help keep moisture in the skin.

Benefits

This oil is a rich source of linoleic acid and provides a good amount of gamma-linolenic acid; research shows that topical applications of these fatty acids can help reduce fine lines and other signs of aging, making this a wonderful oil for mature skin. Hempseed is also packed with skin-protecting antioxidants, making it a good choice for after-sun products.

CBD and THC

Cannabidiol (CBD) is a component found in cannabis plants; it is non-psychoactive, meaning that it does not alter brain function. Evidence shows that this compound has many benefits when it comes to skin care, especially when treating inflammation. It makes up between 18 and 20% of hempseed oil.

Tetrahydrocannabinol (THC) is found in trace amounts in hempseed oil (0.3%, on average). However, the use of the oil in skin-care products is limited in most countries because THC is considered to be a psychoactive compound. Its use in a product is restricted to less than 10% of the total formulation.

Jojoba Oil

Botanical name: *Simmondsia chinensis*

Botanical family: Simmondsiaceae

Typical Fatty Acid Composition

SATURATED FATTY ACIDS	MONOUNSATURATED FATTY ACIDS	POLYUNSATURATED FATTY ACIDS
Stearic acid 5–10%	Erucic acid 12–15%	Linoleic acid 1%
Palmitic acid 3–6%	Oleic acid 5–15%	
Behenic acid 1–2%	Palmitoleic acid 1–2%	
	Nervonic acid 1–2%	
	Eicosenoic Acid 65–80%	

Uses

Jojoba oil is suitable for all skin types.

Compounding

In formulations, jojoba can be used as 50 to 100% of the carrier oil. Blend it with argan, marula or rosehip seed oil.

Jojoba is a heavy-textured liquid wax that is usually identified as jojoba oil. The golden yellow, lightly scented oil is extracted from the seeds of jojoba, a desert shrub. This oil is produced mainly in Israel, the United States (specifically Arizona) and Argentina. It has a shelf life of 2 years.

Benefits

Jojoba is a balancing, emollient oil suitable for all types of skin. It's commonly used as a carrier oil because of its long shelf life. Jojoba has anti-inflammatory effects and can be used in formulations for a variety of skin conditions, including infections and skin aging, as well as wound healing. This ability to reduce inflammation also makes it suitable for use in sunscreens and after-sun care products.

Jojoba and Rosacea

A study published in the *British Journal of Dermatology* found that patients with rosacea had lower levels of eicosenoic acid in their skin. This may explain why using jojoba oil on rosacea-infected skin offers relief from symptoms of inflammation.

Marula Oil

Botanical name: *Sclerocarya birrea*

Botanical family: Anacardiaceae

Typical Fatty Acid Composition

SATURATED FATTY ACIDS	MONOUNSATURATED FATTY ACIDS	POLYUNSATURATED FATTY ACIDS
Palmitic acid 10–15%	Oleic acid 70–80%	Linoleic acid 5–10%
Stearic acid 5–10%	Eicosenoic acid 1–2%	Alpha-linolenic acid 1–2%
Myristic acid 1–5%		
Arachidic acid 1–3%		

Uses

Marula oil is best used in formulations for sensitive skin. It's also well suited for dry, oily or combination skin formulations, as well as hair products.

Compounding

Because of the high price of this oil, it's advisable to compound it in a ratio of 70:30 with oils such as apricot kernel or jojoba when creating body or hair products. Use marula oil as 100% of the carrier oil when creating facial serums.

Marula oil comes from the kernel of a tree that is indigenous to Namibia, Botswana, Zambia and Zimbabwe. Kernels of the marula tree have been found in prehistoric caves, alongside tools that are similar to those still used today to extract the oil. The oil has been used for ages to prevent skin from breaking out and to keep it hydrated. Today marula oil is produced in South Africa. It has a shelf life of 12 to 18 months.

Benefits

Evidence-based studies have concluded that topically applied marula oil has protective properties and can help skin retain moisture. This is attributed to its high levels of oleic and palmitic acids, which are both excellent emollients.

Numerous carrier oils, such as sweet almond, apricot kernel, argan, avocado, camellia seed, hazelnut and marula, contain a high percentage of oleic acid, which has been shown to have antifungal properties. Fungal infections on the skin, such as seborrheic dermatitis, are a problem for many people. If you are having problems with skin infections of this nature, using a carrier oil with a high percentage of oleic acid in your formulations may help with keeping such infections under control, particularly if paired with essential oils that have similar properties.

Rosehip Seed Oil

Botanical name: *Rosa rubiginosa*

Botanical family: Rosaceae

Typical Fatty Acid Composition

SATURATED FATTY ACIDS	MONOUNSATURATED FATTY ACIDS	POLYUNSATURATED FATTY ACIDS
Palmitic acid 4–5%	Oleic acid 10–15%	Linoleic acid 40–50%
Stearic acid 3–6%	Eicosenoic acid 1–2%	Alpha-linolenic acid 30–35%
Myristic acid 1–2%		

Uses

Rosehip seed oil is best used in formulations targeted to aging skin and for treating inflammatory skin conditions.

Compounding

In formulations, rosehip seed oil can be used as 30% of the carrier oil. Blending rosehip seed oil with 70% jojoba oil is especially helpful for treating skin inflammation, rashes and acne.

This bright red oil is extracted from the seeds of the fruit ("hip") of the wild rose bush. Known in Spanish as *rosa mosqueta*, it is native to the southern Andes Mountains; the oil is now produced mainly in Chile. It has a short shelf life of 6 to 8 months.

Benefits

This oil is high in alpha-linolenic acid, which is well-known for helping to reduce skin inflammation. Research indicates that rosehip seed oil is suitable for treating aging skin, fine lines and hyperpigmentation caused by sun damage. There's also evidence that it has a significant therapeutic effect on ulcerative wounds.

Sesame Seed Oil

Botanical name: *Sesamum indicum*

Botanical family: Pedaliaceae

Typical Fatty Acid Composition

SATURATED FATTY ACIDS	MONOUNSATURATED FATTY ACIDS	POLYUNSATURATED FATTY ACIDS	ADDITIONAL COMPONENT
Stearic acid 11%	Oleic acid 5-10%	Linoleic acid 40-45%	Vitamin E
Palmitic acid 5-20%		Alpha-linolenic acid 40-45%	

Uses

Sesame oil is suitable for all skin types.

Compounding

In formulations, sesame oil can be used as 100% of the carrier oil.

Sesame seed oil is obtained from the seeds of the sesame plant, an annual herb native to the tropics. The oil is extracted from either the raw seeds, which produce a light-colored oil, or from roasted seeds, which produce a darker oil. Sesame oil has been used for thousands of years in cooking and in cosmetics. It is produced in India and China and has a shelf life of 12 months.

Benefits

Sesame seed oil has many therapeutic properties and can be used in a variety of products. Its antibacterial and anti-parasitic properties make it a good addition to hair and scalp-care formulations to treat dandruff and head lice. It's best used in formulations for hair and scalp, and it's also a great choice for baby skin-care products, as a massage oil or in formulations to protect against diaper rash.

Sesame oil's astringent properties help improve the look of large pores, as well as dull, aging skin. It has been shown to shield skin from the damaging effects of chlorine and windburn and is also mildly sun-protective.

Sunflower Seed Oil

Botanical name: *Helianthus annuus*

Botanical family: Asteraceae

Typical Fatty Acid Composition

SATURATED FATTY ACIDS	MONOUNSATURATED FATTY ACIDS	POLYUNSATURATED FATTY ACIDS	ADDITIONAL COMPONENTS
Palmitic acid 5–10%	Oleic acid 15–20%	Linoleic acid 70–75%	Vitamin E
Stearic acid 4%	Palmitoleic acid 1–2%	Alpha-linolenic acid 1–2%	Squalane

Uses

Sunflower oil is suitable for all skin types.

Compounding

In formulations, sunflower oil can be used as 100% of the carrier oil, or it can be compounded with other, richer oils such as rosehip seed, borage, hempseed or evening primrose. It is also ideal for compounding with infused oils such as carrot and calendula.

Sunflower seed oil is obtained by cold-pressing the seeds of the sunflower, which is then followed by conventional refining. The oil is light yellow in color, with a subtle scent. Sunflower seed oil is produced in Italy, Argentina, China and the Netherlands. It has a short shelf life of 6 to 8 months.

Benefits

Sunflower seed oil is a non-greasy emollient suitable for all skin types, but especially for sensitive skin. Its high levels of linoleic acid give this oil strong skin-protective properties; studies conducted on infants (who don't yet have a fully developed skin barrier) showed that sunflower seed oil was able to prevent different types of infection. In addition, one study of adults with dermatitis found that topical application of the oil resulted in a decrease in skin's water loss and cleared up the scaly dermatitis-related lesions. The fact that this oil is not greasy makes it well suited for use as a natural massage oil, and in moisturizers, lotions, ointments and bath products.

Plant Butters

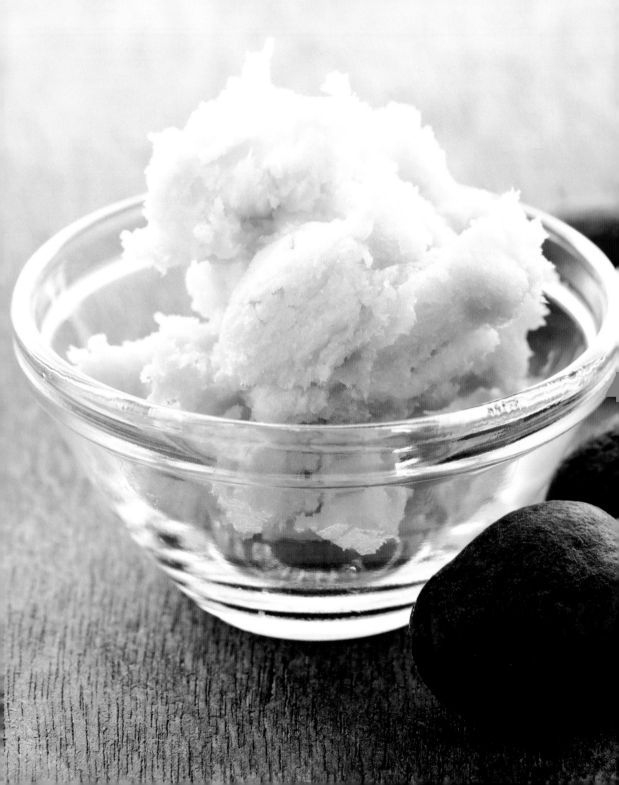

Cocoa Butter

Botanical name: *Theobroma nucifera*

Botanical family: Malvaceae

Typical Fatty Acid Composition

SATURATED FATTY ACIDS	MONOUNSATURATED FATTY ACIDS	POLYUNSATURATED FATTY ACIDS
Stearic acid 35–40%	Oleic acid 35–40%	Linoleic acid 2–5%
Palmitic acid 25–30%		
Lauric acid 5–10%		

Uses

Cocoa butter is suitable for all skin types.

Compounding

In formulations, cocoa butter can be used as 10 to 90% of the carrier base.

IRRITATION ALERT

Cocoa butter may cause irritation to sensitive skin. Also, avoid using it if you have an allergy to cocoa.

Cocoa butter comes from the beans of the cocoa tree. Cocoa is grown mainly in West Africa (Ghana, Ivory Coast, Nigeria), Malaysia, Brazil, Central America, India and Sri Lanka. The butter is pale yellow, with a distinctive chocolate scent. (It is also available in a deodorized form, which has a neutral smell.) It has a shelf life of 12 months.

Benefits

Cocoa butter is wonderful for soothing and softening skin. It protects the skin from dehydration and can also be used to improve elasticity. In formulations, cocoa butter can act as a mild emulsifier; it has rich emollient properties and adds a creamy texture to a product. Cocoa butter is a terrific addition to formulations that require a thicker base, such as body butters, scrubs and lip balms. It may also be added to lotions and moisturizers to create a thicker texture than an oil.

Shea Butter

Botanical name: *Vitellaria paradoxa*

Botanical family: Sapotaceae

Typical Fatty Acid Composition

SATURATED FATTY ACIDS	MONOUNSATURATED FATTY ACIDS	POLYUNSATURATED FATTY ACIDS
Stearic acid 35–50%	Oleic acid 35–70%	Linoleic acid 5–10%
Palmitic acid 5–10%		

Uses

Shea butter is suitable for all skin types.

Compounding

In formulations, shea butter can be used as 10 to 90% of the carrier base. (Note that this butter can cause a formulation to become granular in texture as it ages.)

Shea butter comes from the nuts of the shea tree. In its raw form it has a slightly greenish yellow tint and a very strong scent. Shea butter is often refined (deodorized and bleached) to use in commercial cosmetic products. The butter is produced in West Africa and has a shelf life of 12 months.

Shea butter is a terrific addition to formulations that require a thicker base, such as body butters, scrubs and lip balms. It may also be added to lotions and moisturizers to create a thicker texture than an oil.

Benefits

This butter is recognized for its wound-healing and skin-repairing properties, which are likely a result of its high levels of stearic acid — studies have shown that stearic acid assists in recovery from burns and wounds. Shea butter is also soothing and moisturizing, and it's been shown to have a wrinkle-reducing effect, making it a great addition to anti-aging formulations.

SENSITIVITY ALERT

Shea butter is unlikely to trigger an allergic reaction in people with nut allergies. However, such people may be sensitive to products containing shea butter, so use it with caution.

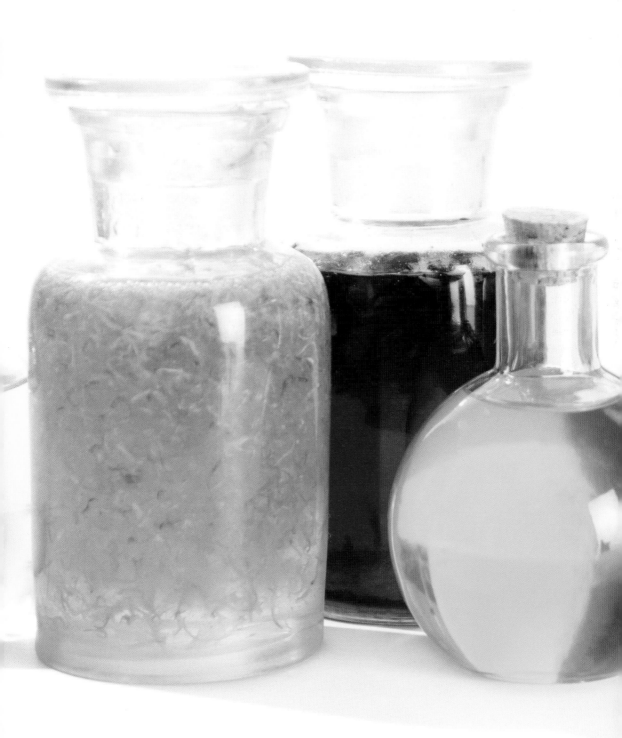

Infusions

Infusing carrier oils, vinegars, glycerin or alcohol with ingredients such as herbs, spices, flowers or tea will enrich your formulations with beneficial nutrients that essential oils simply can't provide. Creating an herbal infusion extracts bioactive components, such as carotenoids and phenols, from the particular plant used. In addition to adding extra healing properties to your products, these herbal infusions can add wonderful scents.

Below you'll find some of my favorite ingredients that I use to create infusions. You can find most of them at health food stores or online (for recommended online retailers, see the list of suppliers on page 371). You can buy fresh or dried herbals, but I recommend growing fresh herbs yourself, if possible (for instance, I grow my own marigolds).

ARNICA

Botanical name: *Arnica montana*

Botanical family: Asteraceae

Arnica is a perennial herbaceous plant that grows in Europe and North America. It has a long-stemmed bright yellow daisy-like flower. The herb is found to be anti-inflammatory, which is why it is used in classical homeopathic remedies to topically treat bruises, wounds, rashes and sunburns. It's also used as a pain reliever; randomized controlled studies have found that arnica helps reduce swelling in post-operative patients. Arnica can be used in foot and hand balms, creams for bruising, and body oils for muscular aches and pains.

CALENDULA

Botanical name: *Calendula officinalis*

Botanical family: Asteraceae

Calendula, also known as marigold, is a short-lived herbaceous plant that grows in warm European climates throughout the year, and in the northern hemisphere, including North America, from early summer to late fall. The plant has vivid bright orange daisy-like flowers on tall, weed-like stems. Calendula flower petals are found to be helpful in treating inflammation and wounds. Marigolds are also packed with carotenoids, which act as antioxidants in the body and defend against aging free radicals; this is why calendula is widely used in formulas for sun protection and repair.

ST. JOHN'S WORT

Botanical name: *Hypericum perforatum*

Botanical family: Hypericaceae

St. John's wort is an herbaceous perennial plant, often considered to be an invasive weed, that grows throughout Europe and North America. It has short stems with yellow star-like flowers. Interestingly, when it is infused in alcohol, it instantly turns red, while with oils it takes some time for it to turn a dark auburn. The characteristic red color of St. John's wort is the result of one of its chemical components, hypericin, which is currently being researched for its potential to fight viruses. In traditional aromatherapy, St. John's wort is used for nerve- and virus-related conditions such as shingles, herpes and other inflamed-skin disorders. Use it in ointments, balms, oils and creams.

CARROT ROOT

Botanical name: *Daucus carota*

Botanical family: Apiaceae

The carrot is a bright orange root vegetable native to Europe and cultivated all over the world. Carrot-root infusions are rich in carotenoids, which have significant skin-healing properties and benefit inflamed and aging skin. This is why carrot root is widely used in formulas for sun protection and repair. (Do not confuse carrot root–infused oil with carrot seed essential oil, which is derived from distillation of the plant's seed, not the root.) Use it in preparations such as moisturizers, body creams, lotions, balms and massage oils.

CHAMOMILE

Botanical Names: *Matricaria recutita (M. chamomilla)* and *Chamaemelum nobile*

Botanical Family: Asteraceae

This small white flower grows in many parts of the world. The two species of chamomile, *Matricaria recutita* (German chamomile) and *Chamaemelum nobile* (Roman chamomile), produce essential oils that are very different from one another in terms of their therapeutic properties. However, when it comes to the herb, the two species are very similar in action.

Chamomile tea is a common beverage that is recognized for its calming effect on the nervous system and digestive tract. Topically applied through an herbal infusion, chamomile demonstrates these same comforting anti-inflammatory and skin-soothing properties. Chamomile herbal infusions can be used in toners, moisturizers, bath products and balms.

HIBISCUS

Botanical name: *Hibiscus* species

Botanical family: Malvaceae

Hibiscus flowers are large and trumpet-shaped and can vary in color. Hibiscus is rich in phenols, which are plant-based molecules with powerful antioxidant properties. One of hibiscus's major antioxidants is quercetin, which, when used in an oil-delivery system, can penetrate the top layers of skin without producing irritation. Quercetin also helps sun-damaged skin, reduces degradation of elastin, and improves the appearance of skin and scars. Use in formulations targeted to aging skin and in skin-repairing moisturizers.

SAFFRON

Botanical name: *Crocus sativus*

Botanical family: Iridaceae

This precious spice is a perennial bulb with purple flowers. Cultivated throughout the Middle East and Asia, saffron has been used in food and cosmetics since ancient times. Saffron has been shown to enhance the moisturizing effects of skin-care products. It also exhibits powerful anti-aging properties. Use it in facial masks, cleansers, toners and moisturizers.

Expert Tip

Saffron is a very expensive spice and many vendors sell fake versions. To check for genuine saffron, place the dried threads in water. If the color infuses slowly into the water, you can be sure it's the real deal; if a yellow pigment diffuses quickly, it is likely colored corn silk.

TURMERIC ROOT

Botanical name: *Curcuma longa*

Botanical family: Zingiberaceae

Turmeric root is native to Asia. One of its major active compounds is curcumin, a yellow-pigmented polyphenol that is a powerful antioxidant; it has also been shown to help with inflammation and fight infection.

Turmeric root helps relieve bruises and sores and inflammatory skin conditions. It is also found to be a tightening and firming agent. Use it in facial masks, cleansers, toners and moisturizers.

WHITE TEA

Botanical name: *Camellia sinensis*

Botanical family: Theaceae

White tea is made from the buds and young leaves of the *Camellia sinensis* plant. Unlike other teas, it is minimally processed, so it is a soft gray in color. White tea is high in a type of flavonoid called catechins, known for their disease-fighting antioxidant properties. In cosmetics, white tea is used as an anti-aging ingredient and is reported to be beneficial as a germ-fighting antiseptic. Use it in facial masks, cleansers, toners and moisturizers.

GREEN TEA

Botanical name: *Camellia sinensis*

Botanical family: Theaceae

Green tea is made from the leaves of the *Camellia sinensis* plant. It is quickly heated and dried to prevent too much oxidation from occurring. As the name suggests, it is green in color. The slight oxidation means that it contains fewer antioxidants than white tea. However, green tea remains known for its antioxidant properties, which are particularly beneficial in after-sun products. This tea is also used in treatments for dry skin and inflammation. Use it in facial masks, cleansers, toners and moisturizers.

Warm Oil-Based Herbal Infusion

When making an oil-based infusion, always use fresh, cold-pressed oils with a long shelf life in order to avoid rancidity. Use the infused oil as an additive to oil-based formulations such as creams, lotions, serums and balms.

Makes about 13 oz (375 mL)

Tip

This makes a fairly large quantity. If you prefer, reduce the yield to produce half or even one quarter of the amount.

- Bowl-style double boiler
- Glass jar (14 oz/400 mL) sprayed with 70% ethyl alcohol

1½ cups (375 mL)	sesame seed, coconut or jojoba oil
5 tbsp (90 mL)	dried or fresh herb of choice
20 drops (1 mL)	vitamin E
20 drops (1 mL)	antimicrobial synergy of choice (see pages 36 to 38)

1. Set a heatproof glass bowl over a saucepan of simmering (212°F/100°C) water. Add oil and herbs and stir to combine. Let simmer over very low heat for 3 to 4 hours (the water in the saucepan may evaporate, so check regularly and refill as needed).
2. Remove bowl from heat. Using a fine-mesh sieve set over prepared jar, strain infused oil. Use the back of a spoon to press against the herbs to extract as much of their essence as possible. Discard solids.
3. Add vitamin E and synergy. Seal tightly and shake well. Properly stored (see page 219), the infusion will keep for up to 6 months. Shake before using.

Making Herbal Infusions

Numerous carriers can be infused with herbs and other plant-based ingredients. Oils are commonly used — I recommend sesame, coconut and jojoba oils for their long shelf life. In addition to oils, you can use glycerin, apple cider vinegar or alcohol. These last two are natural preservatives, so in addition to adding therapeutic benefit to your formulations, they will extend their shelf life as well.

Classic Oil-Based Herbal Infusion

When making an oil-based infusion, always use fresh, cold-pressed oils in order to avoid rancidity. Use these infusions as an additive to oil-based formulations such as creams, lotions, serums and balms.

Makes about
13 oz (375 mL)

Tip

This makes a fairly large quantity. If you prefer, reduce the yield to produce half or even one quarter of the amount.

• 2 glass jars (14 oz/400 mL) sprayed with 70% ethyl alcohol

5 tbsp (90 g)	dried herb of choice
1½ cups (375 mL)	sweet almond, sunflower, sesame seed, jojoba or extra virgin olive oil
20 drops (1 mL)	vitamin E
20 drops (1 mL)	antimicrobial synergy of choice (see pages 36 to 38)

1. Place herbs in one prepared jar and cover with oil, leaving about 2 inches (5 cm) headspace and ensuring that they are completely submerged in oil. Seal jar tightly and shake well. Store in a cool, dark place for 3 to 4 weeks.
2. Using a fine-mesh sieve set over second prepared jar, strain infused oil. Use the back of a spoon to press against the herbs to extract as much of their essence as possible. Discard solids.
3. Add vitamin E and synergy and stir well. Seal jar tightly. Properly stored (see page 219), the infusion will keep for up to 6 months. Shake before using.

Oils and Herbals

There are two basic methods for infusing oil with herbs: warming the oil to speed up the process or allowing a longer time for the benefits to slowly infuse in room-temperature oil. You will need to strain your infusions and since much of the oil is absorbed by the herbs, you need to press them in the strainer to extract as much of their valuable ingredients as possible.

Herbal Infusion in Glycerin

Use this as an additive to oil-based formulations such as creams, lotions, serums, balms, toners and body washes.

Tip
This makes a fairly large quantity. If you prefer, reduce the yield to produce half or even one quarter of the amount.

- 2 glass jars (14 oz/400 mL) sprayed with 70% ethyl alcohol

5 tbsp (90 g)	fresh herb of choice (see Tip, below), chopped finely
1½ cups (375 mL)	glycerin
20 drops (1 mL)	vitamin E
20 drops (1 mL)	antimicrobial synergy of choice (see pages 36 to 38)

1. Place herbs in one prepared jar and add glycerin, leaving about 2 inches (5 cm) headspace. Seal jar tightly and shake well. Store in a cool, dry place for 1 to 2 weeks.
2. Using a fine-mesh sieve set over second prepared jar, strain infused oil. Use the back of a spoon to press against the herbs to extract as much of their essence as possible. Discard solids.
3. Add vitamin E and synergy. Seal jar tightly. Properly stored (see page 219), the infusion will keep for up to 6 months. Shake before using.

Expert Tip

You can also use dried herbs to make glycerin-based infusions. However, fresh herbs are ideal, since they have their own natural moisture that enables the active compounds and pigments to dissolve in the glycerin base. If you are using dried herbs, add 2 tbsp (30 mL) filtered water for every ⅓ cup (75 mL) of herb.

Apple Cider Vinegar Herbal Infusion

Use in toners and body and hair-wash formulations.

Makes 2 cups (500 mL)

Tip

This makes a fairly large quantity. If you prefer, reduce the yield to produce half or even one quarter of the amount.

Makes 2 cups (500 mL)

- 2 glass jars (18 oz/500 mL) sprayed with 70% ethyl alcohol

6 tbsp (120 g)	fresh herb of choice, chopped finely
2 cups (500 mL)	apple cider vinegar

1. Place herbs in one prepared jar. Add apple cider vinegar, pressing down on the herbs to make sure they are completely covered with liquid (shake slightly to make sure). Seal jar tightly and set aside in a cool, dark place for 1 to 2 weeks.
2. Using a fine-mesh sieve set over second prepared jar, strain infused vinegar. Use the back of a spoon to press against the herbs to extract as much of their essence as possible. Discard solids. Seal jar tightly. Properly stored (see page 219), the infusion will keep for up to 6 months.

Alcohol-Based Herbal Infusion

Alcohol is a natural preservative. Use an alcohol-based herbal infusion as an additive to oil-based formulations such as creams, lotions, serums and balms, toners and body washes to add preservative capabilities. Hypersensitive individuals may have reactions to alcohol, in which case they should use a different method for making herbal infusions.

Makes 2 cups (500 mL)

Tip
This makes a fairly large quantity. If you prefer, reduce the yield to produce half or even one quarter of the amount.

- 2 glass jars (18 oz/500 mL) sprayed with 70% ethyl alcohol

6 tbsp (120 g)	fresh herb of choice, chopped finely
2 cups (500 mL)	grain alcohol

1. Place herbs in one prepared jar. Add alcohol, pressing down on the herbs to make sure they are completely covered with liquid. Seal tightly and set aside in a cool, dark place for 1 to 2 weeks.
2. Using a fine-mesh sieve set over second prepared jar, strain infused alcohol. Use the back of a spoon to press against the herbs to extract as much of their essence as possible. Discard solids. Seal jar tightly. Properly stored (see page 219), the infusion will keep for up to 6 months.

CAUTION

Herbal infusions are very potent and get stronger with age. These preparations are meant for use only on the skin.

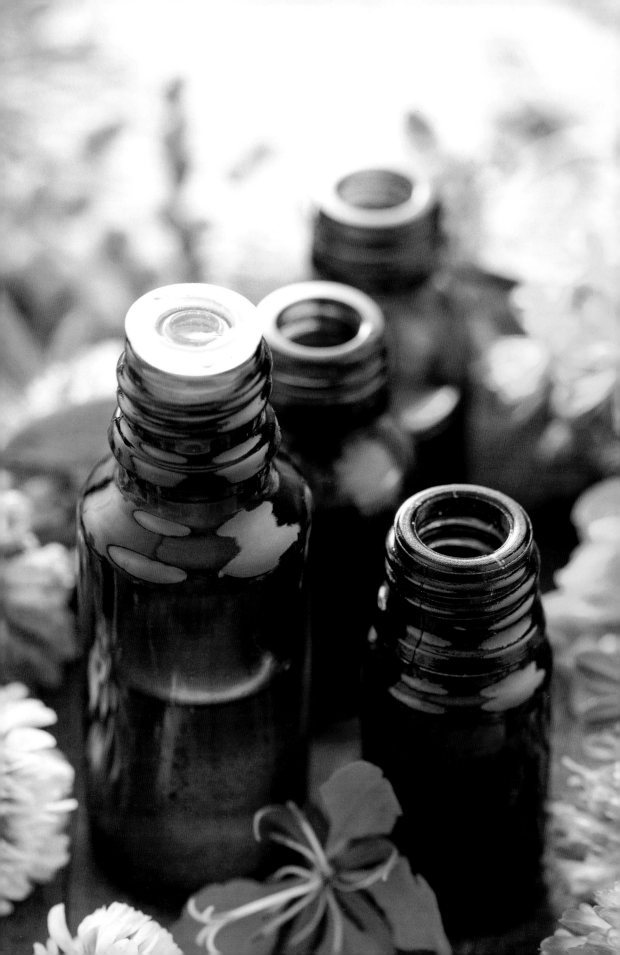

PART 3

Essential Oils

All About Essential Oils

WHAT ARE ESSENTIAL OILS?

Essential oils play a significant role in natural personal care products. Not only do they add the enhancement of scent, they are also rich in a wide variety of therapeutic properties. I'm not overstating it when I say that every drop of an essential oil contains a unique natural pharmacy.

Essential oils may be defined as aromatic essences that are extracted from plants by various means. These oils are minute chemical structures that are metabolized within aromatic plants, which create these structures in the process of adapting to their environment. The aromatic compounds help to ensure the plant's survival by protecting it from pathogens and by deterring insects and animals from eating it. When people use essential oils, these constituents perform similar functions, such as stopping infections, healing wounds and boosting immunity.

Essential oils are volatile, meaning that they evaporate into the air, even at room temperature and oxidize when exposed to air. Each oil contains between 30 and 100 bioactive chemicals, and each is unique by virtue of its distinctive chemical composition.

PRODUCING ESSENTIAL OILS

Essential oils can be produced in various ways. Here are some common methods.

Steam Distillation

In steam distillation, botanical material is placed in a still and hot steam is used to break up the delicate membranes that contain the aromatic oils. The essential oil is isolated and then collected. Steam distillation is a very common method of extraction, and also the most economical way of producing essential oils. The disadvantage of this method is that heat may degrade the original plant constituents. High-quality oils are monitored very carefully to avoid over-processing.

Cold Expression

In cold expression, the essential oil is forced from the plant material by using strong mechanical pressure, without applying any kind of heat. This method is usually used with citrus fruit to produce essential oils and with seeds and nuts to produce carrier oils. One of the benefits of this method is that the aroma of the essential oil remains close to the scent of the original fruit. This method also preserves more of the natural therapeutic constituents in carrier oils.

Carbon Dioxide Extraction

In this method of extraction, carbon dioxide (CO_2) gas is pressurized to the point where it becomes a liquid. This extremely cold liquid then dissolves the botanical material. When the pressure of the CO_2 is allowed to fall, it returns to a gaseous state and the essential oil can be collected.

Chemical Solvent Extraction

Chemical extraction involves removing the aromatic compounds from botanical material by using solvents such as hexane, as well as evaporation. During this process, nonvolatile materials such as waxes and pigments are also extracted. This method is commonly used when the plant has a very low yield of essential oil or for oils that yield resinous components. It delivers fine fragrances, but the solvents that are used may remain in the oils, which could lead to sensitization.

What Is an Absolute?

Absolutes are similar to essential oils in that both are extracted from plants. However, absolutes are created using a different method of solvent extraction that produces a distinctive result: an absolute contains both the aromatic compounds of the plant and some semi-solid material such as waxes and pigments. A plant's absolute may be more fragrant than its essential oil precisely because it contains this additional material. Rose absolute and jasmine absolute are good examples; they are commonly used in perfumes for their strong fragrance.

Enfleurage

This method involves placing freshly picked flowers between two glass plates, each of which is covered with a layer of pure, odorless animal or vegetable fat. The botanicals are left in contact with the fat until the fat is infused with their extracts. This process is repeated with new flower petals until the fat is saturated, at which point it is washed with alcohol to separate the floral extract (the fat is then used to make soap). Once the alcohol evaporates, the essential oil remains. Because this method is costly and time-consuming and produces small batches, it is used only for flowers that yield very low amounts of oil.

Sustainability and Essential Oils

Plants do not produce large quantities of essential oil. That makes them a valuable resource that should not be taken for granted. As someone who relies on plant-sourced medicine, I know that it is crucial that we protect the sources. It is so important that you use essential oils with consciousness and with sustainability in mind. I can't stress enough the need for taking care of our plants — and our planet. Be prudent with essential oils in order to sustain the plant kingdom.

USING ESSENTIAL OILS IN NATURAL PRODUCTS

When using essential oils, it's important to understand the properties of their individual constituents to ensure their safe and effective use. In the next section you will find detailed profiles of individual oils and guidelines for their use in natural products. Each profile also provides the botanical name and family of the plant. This is vital information, because many plants have similar common names. You need to know the botanical name of a plant to be certain that you are purchasing and using the correct essential oil.

Before moving on to the next section, we'll review the basic classification of plants so that you can understand why some essential oils have similar names — Roman and German chamomile, for example — but different therapeutic effects. You'll also find an outline of important safety considerations for using essential oils in your personal care products. Finally we'll take a look at how topical application of essential oils can help calm the mind and relieve stress.

Know Your Plants

Oils from the same type of plant can vary in their chemical composition. It can be especially confusing when two plants have similar names but different properties. Take Roman chamomile and German chamomile, for example. Both are produced from plants in the Asteraceae family, but they belong to different genera and species. They also differ in their therapeutic properties: Roman chamomile has a more relaxing, sedating effect, while German chamomile is known for reducing inflammation.

Plants are classified (in descending order) according to family, genus, species and variety. Let's review what these terms mean.

Family

The plant kingdom is divided into orders and then into families, which represent the next highest order of classification. Plants are assigned to a family based on common botanical features and similar characteristics. Family names usually end in -ae; Lamiaceae (formerly Labiatae), for example, is known as the mint family.

Genus

The genus refers to closely related plants and often includes more than one species. Often the name will describe some aspect of the plant — the color of the flowers or the size or shape of the leaves — or it may be named after the place where it was found. For example, *Lavandula* is a genus in the Lamiaceae family that is commonly known as lavender.

Species

Although they have the same ancestry and nearly identical structure and behavior, there are differences between species in the same genus. Together, the genus and species name can refer to only one particular plant; this combined name is thus the most effective way to identify an individual plant. For example, *Lavandula angustifolium* (formerly known as *L. officinalis*) and *Lavandula latifolia* are two species in the *Lavandula* genus. The former is the most common species and what we often refer to as "true lavender."

Variety

In some cases, a species is further divided into subspecies that contain very similar plants. These plants are known as varieties. Numerous varieties can be created from a species through plant cultivation; these are often hybrids called cultivars (that is, cultivated varieties). The variety name follows the genus and species name, with the abbreviation "var." or "subsp." before it. Cultivar names are preceded by an "x" instead.

What Is a Chemotype?

Chemotypes are plants of the same genus and species that have different chemical constituents in their essential oils. A plant's chemotype can vary because of many different factors, including the soil of the region in which it was cultivated and the climate of that region. Basil is an example of a plant that has chemotypes; its essential oils are usually identified by chemotype, such as linalool, eugenol or camphor, among others. Knowing an essential oil's chemotype is important, as it can affect not only its therapeutic properties but also safety considerations. With basil, for example, only the linalool chemotype is safe for use in personal care products (see page 96 for more information).

The Power of Essential Oils

As the very essence of plants, essential oils are incredibly potent. When applied topically, a wide range of the constituents in essential oils are able to penetrate the stratum corneum (the top layer of skin) and through the rest of the layers of the epidermis to reach the middle layer of skin, the dermis. Once there, these molecules can make their way into the capillaries and eventually into the bloodstream.

It's important to make sure that you don't exceed the recommended maximum amount of an essential oil that can be added to a formulation. You don't want to overexpose yourself to an essential oil, because this could lead to irritation or even sensitization.

Too Much of a Good Thing

After years of formulating personal care products, I've concluded that excessive use of essential oils is counterproductive. Most people use numerous products throughout the day, from cleansers and moisturizers to deodorants and bath products. If each of these products contains a significant amount of one particular essential oil, they'll likely be overexposed to that oil by the end of the day. That is why most of my formulations do not exceed a dilution of 3 percent, meaning that the essential oil does not make up more than 3 percent of the formulation.

General Precautions for Using Essential Oils

Contrary to popular belief, a skin reaction to an essential oil does not mean that your body is "detoxing." If your skin becomes irritated in response to topical application, you should stop using that oil immediately.

Serious allergic reactions to essential oils are extremely rare. However, if you experience a severe reaction, seek appropriate medical attention.

Safety Guidelines

- Do not ingest essential oils.
- Do not apply essential oils directly to the skin. Avoid contact with eyes and mucous membranes.
- Do not add an essential oil directly to bathwater. It will accumulate on top of the water and have the potential to irritate the skin.
- Before using an essential oil for the first time, conduct a skin patch test (see page 27).
- Avoid strong sunlight or sun beds after topically applying phototoxic essential oils, such as citrus oils.
- Avoid applying essential oils immediately after perspiring or after using a sauna.
- Store essential oils away from extreme cold or heat, light and moisture.
- Essential oils are flammable. Do not use near an open flame.
- Keep essential oils out of reach of children.

Quality in Essential Oils

With the increased popularity of aromatherapy, more and more companies are creating low-grade products for sale. This is unfortunate, because the quality of an oil is paramount to its safety as well as to its healing properties. ("Perfume-grade" oils, for example, are laboratory synthetics that have an aroma but lack any therapeutic value.) Using good-quality oils in your personal care products will allow you to achieve maximum results. It's preferable that you select just a few of high quality rather than use a wide range of low-quality essential oils.

The quality of an essential oil depends on many factors, including the plant's environment and geographical location, weather conditions, soil type, age of the plant and month — even the time of day — that it was harvested. Production methods and manufacturing equipment also have a big impact.

Another factor is contamination by pesticides and adulterants, which may include other essential oils and chemicals, both natural and synthetic. This can increase an oil's toxicity. Unfortunately, adulteration is very common. The quantity of essential oils available within the botanical world is limited, which makes them very expensive. Producers are tempted to stretch yields by adding synthetics or other similar materials. This leads to a cheaper oils of inferior quality. Detecting adulteration is difficult, even with the help of gas chromatography testing. Therefore, purchase your oils from a reputable supplier. For recommendations, see my list on page 371.

ESSENTIAL OILS AND THE MIND-SKIN CONNECTION

Have you ever experienced goose bumps when you're afraid or a flushed face when you feel angry? That is your skin communicating an emotional response.

The nerves in your skin are continuously responding to a wide variety of stimuli. These nerves carry messages to your central nervous system, and vice versa. It's not surprising, then, that many skin diseases are classified as psychosomatic — emotional stressors can trigger conditions such as psoriasis, eczema, acne and even premature aging. Unfortunately, most of these conditions have an aesthetic impact that increases stress, further aggravating symptoms.

In short, stress affects not only your emotional state but also your skin's appearance and behavior. Enter essential oils. Many studies have shown that essential oils can help to calm the body and relieve symptoms of stress. That's one reason why they're such a valuable addition to personal care products.

When you inhale the scent of an essential oil, that aroma is transported to your brain. From there it travels to your limbic system, the network in the brain that controls emotional response. Essential oils are able to travel across these biological pathways when they are inhaled or when they are applied directly to the skin.

Lavender and clary sage oils in particular have been shown to calm the nervous system. Neroli essential oil has been found to decrease cortisol levels and to lower blood pressure. These are just a few of the essential oils that have been identified as particularly soothing. Adding such essential oils to your personal care products has the added benefit of supporting a calm mind and a more relaxed body.

Psycho-dermatology

The mind–skin connection is now being taken seriously by the medical profession. These days, more and more dermatologists are recognizing that chronic skin conditions may have a strong psychological connection. In the burgeoning field of psychodermatology, dermatologists and psychologists are working together to come up with treatment plans for patients. The understanding is that stress and anxiety can exacerbate existing skin problems, and vice versa — severe skin problems often trigger psychological distress.

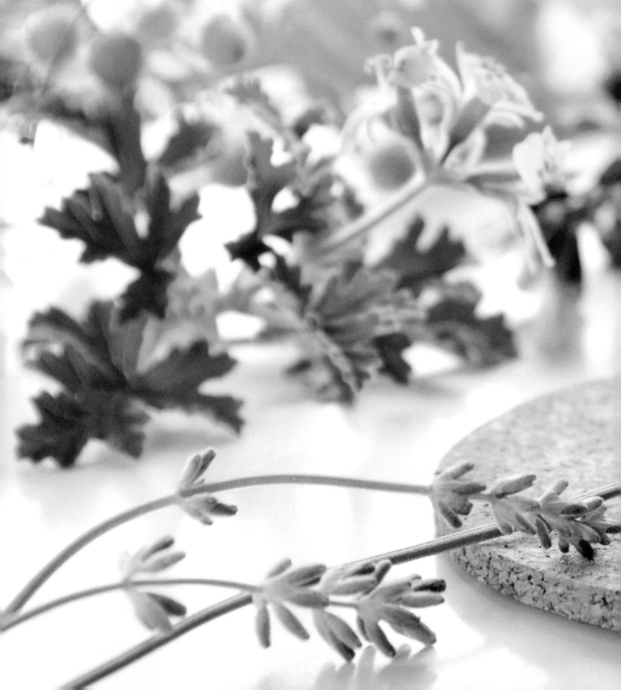

Essential Oils
for Personal
Care Products

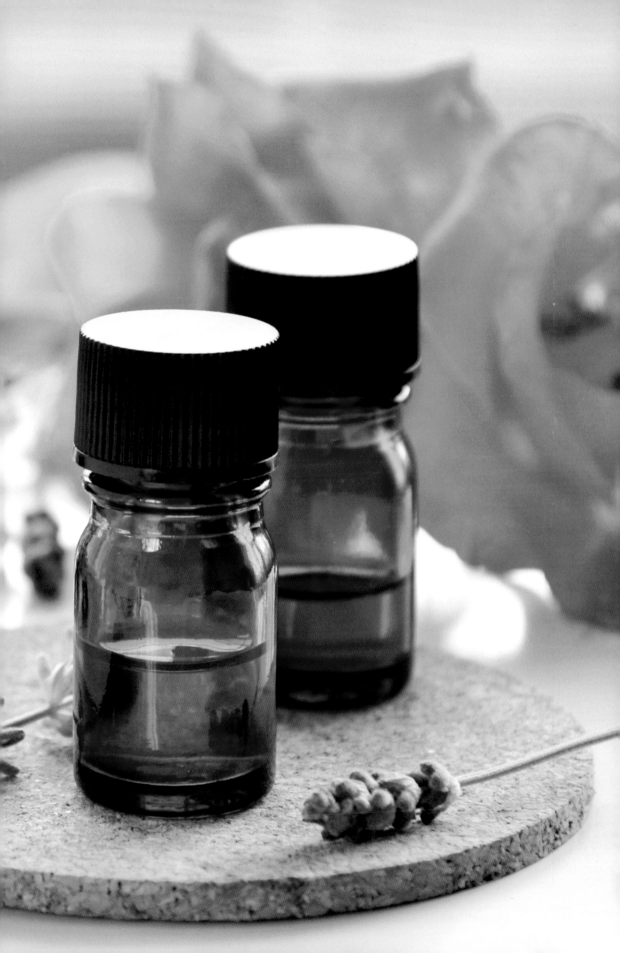

Sweet Basil (Linalool Type)

Botanical Name: *Ocimum basilicum*

Botanical Family: Lamiaceae

Habitat: native to Africa and Asia; cultivated worldwide

Aroma: soft, warm, spicy base notes

KNOW THE VARIETY

There are several major chemotypes of basil (see page 91 for more on chemotypes), each of which varies in its major chemical components. When making your own personal care products, you should always choose the linalool-type sweet basil; look for "*Ocimum basilicum* ct. linalool" on labels. Avoid other types, such as exotic basil (*Ocimum basilicum* ct. methyl chavicol), for example.

Another way to identify the type of basil is by scent. Sweet basil linalool type has a soft, sweet, herbaceous scent, with only a hint of clove, whereas clove dominates the scent of the other basil chemotypes.

Description of the Plant

Basil is a sweet-smelling perennial plant that grows in many regions of the world. The leaves are dark emerald-green pointed ovals. The flowering tops of the plant are greenish to pink-white in color. The herb itself is popular for culinary use.

EXTRACTION: steam distillation of the leaves and flowers

Using Sweet Basil Oil in Natural Products

Sweet basil essential oil has a tonic-like effect on the skin: it is stimulating and helps increase blood circulation. It has also been found to contain strong antioxidants. Additionally, its eugenol and methyl chavicol content make it a potent antimicrobial, meaning that it can help kill or slow the spread of microorganisms. It is particularly well suited for use in disinfecting ointments, lotions and creams for the hands and feet.

CAUTION: There are several chemotypes of basil. When making personal care products, it is important to use the linalool type.

PRECAUTIONS: This oil is non-irritating when applied at or below the maximum recommended dilutions, unless you have a pre-existing sensitivity to any of its components (such as linalool, which makes up a large percentage). Do not use during pregnancy or while breastfeeding. Properly stored, sweet basil oil has a shelf life of up to 2 years.

Main Chemical Constituents of Sweet Basil Essential Oil

LINALOOL (55-70%) This constituent absorbs through the skin and helps relieve swelling and inflammation. It is a pain-reliever as well as an antimicrobial. Linalool has many beneficial properties — for instance, it is calming and sedating — but at high concentrations it can cause an allergic reaction (see page 31 and Oxidation Alert, page 108).

METHYL CHAVICOL (25-30%) Studies show that this constituent is an antimicrobial that can help inhibit skin infections.

EUCALYPTOL (3-5%) This constituent acts as a penetration enhancer (see page 54). It has also been shown to have antimicrobial and antifungal properties. When inhaled, it acts as a decongestant that helps to release phlegm.

EUGENOL (1-2%) This compound is responsible for the oil's distinctive clove scent. It's good at killing bacteria, which makes this oil very useful as an antiseptic treatment. Eugenol has many beneficial properties, but it is a known sensitizer (see page 27.)

SENSITIVITY ALERT

Sweet basil essential oil contains eugenol, and overexposure to eugenol can lead to sensitization. Do not use this oil in products for prolonged periods of time, and always stick to the recommended dilutions.

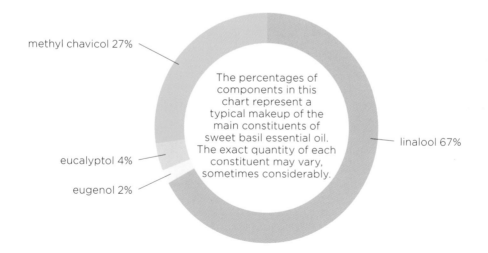

methyl chavicol 27%

eucalyptol 4%

eugenol 2%

linalool 67%

The percentages of components in this chart represent a typical makeup of the main constituents of sweet basil essential oil. The exact quantity of each constituent may vary, sometimes considerably.

GUIDELINES FOR USING

Sweet Basil Essential Oil in Personal Care Products

SKIN CARE: A dilution of up to 1% can be used in products that are left on the skin, while hand and foot products can contain up to a 2% dilution. Sweet basil is suitable for most skin types, with the exception of sensitive skin, which may react to the high levels of eugenol and methyl chavicol.

BENEFITS

- warming
- stimulating
- antibacterial
- antifungal

CONDITIONS

- oily skin
- acne
- bacterial infections
- fungal infections
- insect bites
- dull, tired skin

PRODUCT	SKIN TYPE / CONDITION	QUANTITY
FACE		
Moisture creams	all skin types, excluding sensitive skin	1% (6 drops in 30 mL)
Facial masks	all skin types, excluding sensitive skin	1% (6 drops in 30 mL)
Toners	all skin types, excluding sensitive skin	1% (6 drops in 30 mL)
Cleansers	oily skin and acne	1% (6 drops in 30 mL)
Exfoliants	oily skin and acne	1% (6 drops in 30 mL)
BODY		
Massage oils		1% (6 drops in 30 mL)
Body oils and lotions		1% (6 drops in 30 mL)
Exfoliants		1–2% (6–12 drops in 30 mL)
HANDS AND FEET		
Ointments		1–2% (6–12 drops in 30 mL)
Lotions/butters		1–2% (6–12 drops in 30 mL)
HAIR AND SCALP		
Shampoos and conditioners*		1% (6 drops in 30 mL)
Hair serums		1% (6 drops in 30 mL)

* Exposing oils to heat and water will cause them to oxidize at a faster rate. Consider packaging shampoos and conditioners in flip-top or pump bottles to help reduce oxidation.

Benzoin

Botanical Name: *Styrax benzoin*

Botanical family: Styracaceae

Habitat: native to the rainforests of Vietnam, Laos and Indonesia

Aroma: warm vanilla base notes

Description of the Plant

The benzoin tree is an aromatic evergreen that grows up to 115 feet (34 m) tall. The tree is found in the tropical rainforest and woodland swamps in and around Malaysia and Indonesia. It produces a thick resin that can be accessed only by making deep incisions in the bark of the tree.

EXTRACTION: solvent extraction from the resin, usually using alcohol or benzene

Using Benzoin in Natural Products

Benzoin is commonly used as an alternative to vanilla in perfumes and deodorants. Because of its excellent wound-healing capabilities, it's also used to treat dry, chapped, itchy skin. This oil's benzoic acid content has preservative properties, so it can be used to extend the shelf life of your personal care products. It hardens easily, creating a granular texture. To counteract this tendency, when using it in a formulation, mix the essential oil in $1/2$ tsp (2 mL) carrier oil before adding to the mixture. Use it in moisture gels for problem skin, or for ointments, lotions and butters for extremely dry skin.

PRECAUTIONS: This oil is non-irritating when applied at or below the maximum recommended dilutions. Benzoin is classified as a skin sensitizer and should be used with caution on hypersensitive skin. Avoid use during pregnancy. Properly stored, benzoin essential oil has a shelf life of up to 2 years.

KNOW THE VARIETY

Benzoin (*Styrax benzoin*) is commonly used in aromatherapy. Benzoin Sumatra (*Styrax tonkinensis*) is used by the perfume industry for its vanilla-like scent.

Main Chemical Constituents of Benzoin Essential Oil

BENZYL BENZOATE (60–65%) This constituent is known for its disinfecting properties, which is useful in formulations meant for fighting germs and viruses. It's also been shown to stop the spread of scabies, a contagious skin disease that causes itching and raised red spots. Benzyl benzoate has many beneficial properties, but it is sensitizing (see page 27).

BENZOIC ACID (15–20%) This constituent also has disinfecting properties. It is known as an effective preservative.

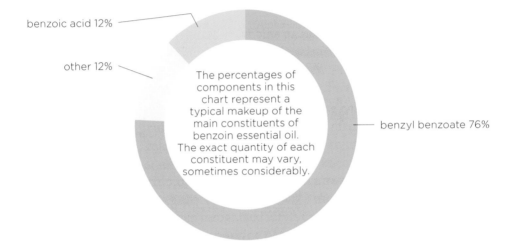

benzoic acid 12%

other 12%

benzyl benzoate 76%

The percentages of components in this chart represent a typical makeup of the main constituents of benzoin essential oil. The exact quantity of each constituent may vary, sometimes considerably.

GUIDELINES FOR USING

Benzoin Essential Oil in Personal Care Products

SKIN CARE: A dilution of up to 2% can be used in products that are left on the skin.

BENEFITS

- calming
- relaxing
- antibacterial

CONDITIONS

- dry, chapped skin
- acne
- inflamed skin
- itchy skin

PRODUCT	SKIN TYPE / CONDITION	QUANTITY
FACE		
Moisture gels	acne, wounds and inflamed skin	1% (6–8 drops in 30 mL)
Eye creams	all skin types	0.5% (3 drops in 30 mL)
Facial masks	all skin types	1% (6 drops in 30 mL)
Toners	all skin types	1% (6 drops in 30 mL)
Cleansers	all skin types	1% (6 drops in 30 mL)
Exfoliants	all skin types	1% (6 drops in 30 mL)
Lip balms		1–2% (30 mL per batch)
BODY		
Massage oils		1–2% (6–12 drops in 30 mL)
Body lotions		1–2% (6–12 drops in 30 mL)
Ointments		1–2% (6–12 drops in 30 mL)
HANDS AND FEET		
Ointments		2% (12 drops in 30 mL)
Lotions/butters		2% (12 drops in 30 mL)
HAIR AND SCALP		
Shampoos and conditioners*		1–3% (6–18 drops in 30 mL)
Hair serums	dandruff	1% (6 drops in 30 mL)

* Exposing oils to heat and water will cause them to oxidize at a faster rate. Consider packaging shampoos and conditioners in flip-top or pump bottles to help reduce oxidation.

Bergamot

Botanical name: *Citrus bergamia*

Botanical family: Rutaceae

Habitat: native to tropical Asia; now cultivated in Italy

Aroma: deep herbaceous and citrus top notes

OXIDATION ALERT

Bergamot essential oil contains a significant amount of d-limonene. This is one of the most commonly found constituents in fruit and it gives the bergamot orange and other citrus fruits their distinctive scent. However, it oxidizes quite quickly. This can lead to skin irritation (see page 27). When using in formulations, be particularly conscious of keeping any products containing this essential oil away from heat, water and light.

Description of the Plant

The bergamot orange tree grows to a height of 16 feet (5 m). This citrus tree has dark green leaves and fragrant star-shaped flowers. The essential oil is derived from the rind of the small, bitter fruit. Today it is extensively cultivated in Calabria, Italy.

EXTRACTION: cold expression of the peel of the nearly ripe fruit

Using Bergamot Oil in Natural Products

Inhaling bergamot essential oil will calm and relax the nervous system. Thus, using the oil in your personal care products will reduce stress and promote relaxation. Bergamot has also demonstrated strong antifungal activity when applied topically, meaning that it can help prevent and treat fungal infections on the skin. Use it in formulations targeted at oily, acne-prone skin.

CAUTION: Bergamot essential oil contains furocoumarins, which are organic chemical compounds known to promote phototoxicity on the skin. If you will be exposing your skin to the sun or other UV radiation, use furocoumarin-free bergamot essential oil in your personal care products — look for "FCF" on the label.

PRECAUTIONS: This oil is non-irritating when applied at or below the maximum recommended dilutions. Properly stored, bergamot essential oil has a shelf life of 6 to 8 months.

Main Chemical Constituents of Bergamot Essential Oil

LINALYL ACETATE (35–40%) This constituent gives bergamot essential oil its scent. It absorbs through the skin and helps prevent and treat skin inflammation. It also has antispasmodic effects, so it can help relax muscles and relieve cramps.

D-LIMONENE (20–30%) This is one of the most commonly found constituents in fruit, and it gives the bergamot orange and other citrus fruits their distinctive citrus scent. D-limonene is absorbed into the skin but it oxidizes quickly which will lead to skin irritation.

LINALOOL (20–26%) This constituent absorbs through the skin and helps relieve swelling and inflammation. It is a pain-reliever as well as an antimicrobial. Linalool has many beneficial properties, but at high concentrations it can cause an allergic reaction (see page 31). Also, when oxidized, it can lead to irritation.

BETA-PINENE (6–19%) This constituent has strong antimicrobial properties and is also very good at preventing skin infections. B-pinene carries a low risk of allergy, but when oxidized can lead to irritation.

GAMMA-TERPINENE (6–9%) This constituent has strong antibacterial properties, which can help prevent skin infections. It also slows down oxidization of linoleic acid, so it can act as a preservative when added to carrier oils.

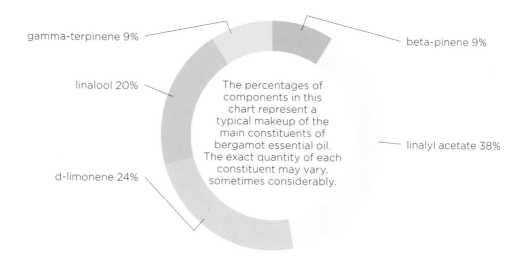

gamma-terpinene 9%

beta-pinene 9%

linalool 20%

d-limonene 24%

linalyl acetate 38%

The percentages of components in this chart represent a typical makeup of the main constituents of bergamot essential oil. The exact quantity of each constituent may vary, sometimes considerably.

GUIDELINES FOR USING

Bergamot Essential Oil in Personal Care Products

SKIN CARE: A dilution of up to 3% can be used in products that are left on the skin.

BENEFITS

- stimulating
- uplifting
- deodorizing
- tonic
- antifungal

CONDITIONS

- acne
- cold sores
- oily skin
- tired skin
- athlete's foot

PRODUCT	SKIN TYPE / CONDITION	QUANTITY
FACE		
Moisture gels	acne	1–2% (6–12 drops in 30 mL)
Facial masks	oily skin and acne	1–2% (6–12 drops in 30 mL)
Toners	oily skin and acne	2% (12 drops in 30 mL)
Cleansers	oily skin and acne	2–3% (12–18 drops in 30 mL)
Exfoliants	oily skin and acne	2–3% (12–18 drops in 30 mL)
Lip balms		2–3 % (12–18 drops in 30 mL)
BODY		
Massage oils		1–3% (6–18 drops in 30 mL)
Body lotions		1–3% (6–18 drops in 30 mL)
Deodorants		1–3% (6–18 drops in 30 mL)
Exfoliants		1–2% (6–12 drops in 30 mL)
Body butters		2–3% (12–18 drops in 30 mL)
HANDS AND FEET		
Foot balms		2–3% (12–18 drops in 30 mL)
HAIR AND SCALP		
Shampoos and conditioners*		1–3% (6–18 drops in 30 mL)
Leave-in conditioning balms for scalp treatment*		1–2% (6–12 drops in 30 mL)

* Exposing oils to heat and water will cause them to oxidize at a faster rate. Consider packaging shampoos and conditioners in flip-top or pump bottles to help reduce oxidation.

Cajuput

Botanical name: *Melaleuca cajuputi*

Botanical family: Myrtaceae

Habitat: cultivated in Malaysia, Australia and other tropical regions

Aroma: fresh and light, with camphor base notes

Description of the Plant

The cajuput tree is a tall evergreen that can grow up to 90 feet (27 m). The tree has a flexible, spongy white bark that flakes off easily. It is native to Australia.

EXTRACTION: steam distillation of fresh leaves and twigs

Using Cajuput in Natural Products

Cajuput is used for its ability to decongest skin, as well as for its antimicrobial properties. These properties make this oil a terrific addition to skin-care products that address oily and acne-prone skin. The scent of cajuput is very refreshing, making it a good essential oil to use in morning cleansers. Also, its warming properties make it a wonderful addition to massage oils. Note that cajuput essential oil has a camphor scent, caused by its eucalyptol content.

CAUTION: Cajuput essential oil has a tendency to oxidize quickly, which can lead to skin irritation.

PRECAUTIONS: This oil is non-irritating when applied at or below the maximum recommended dilutions. Do not use while pregnant or breastfeeding. Properly stored, the shelf life of cajuput essential oil is 2 years.

OXIDATION ALERT

Cajuput essential oil contains a significant amount of alpha-pinene, which oxidizes quite quickly. This can lead to skin irritation. Be particularly conscious of keeping any products containing high ranges of this essential oil away from heat, water and light.

Main Chemical Constituents of Cajuput Essential Oil

ALPHA-PINENE (45–55%) This constituent is known for its ability to relieve pain and inflammation and for being a potent antimicrobial, which can help prevent and treat skin infections. When oxidized, it can lead to skin irritation.

EUCALYPTOL (30–35%) This constituent acts as a penetration enhancer (see page 54). It has also been shown to have antimicrobial and antifungal properties. When inhaled, it acts as a decongestant that helps to release phlegm.

ALPHA-TERPINENE (7–10%) This constituent has strong antifungal and antibacterial activity, meaning that it can prevent or slow the growth of fungi and bacteria.

TERPINEN-4-OL (3–4%) This constituent is a potent antibacterial agent. It is also an anti-inflammatory and absorbs easily into the skin. Studies show that terpinen-4-ol is effective at clearing skin infections and relieving acne. It's also effective against skin mites and yeast infections on the skin.

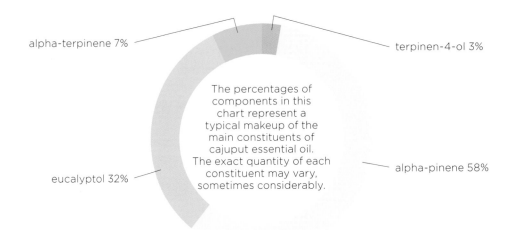

alpha-terpinene 7%

terpinen-4-ol 3%

The percentages of components in this chart represent a typical makeup of the main constituents of cajuput essential oil. The exact quantity of each constituent may vary, sometimes considerably.

eucalyptol 32%

alpha-pinene 58%

GUIDELINES FOR USING

Cajuput Essential Oil in Personal Care Products

SKIN CARE: A dilution of up to 3% can be used in products that are left on the skin.

BENEFITS

- refreshing
- antibacterial
- antifungal

CONDITIONS

- acne
- oily skin
- fungal infections
- insect bites
- blotchy skin

PRODUCT	SKIN TYPE / CONDITION	QUANTITY
FACE		
Moisture creams	oily skin and acne	1% (6 drops in 30 mL)
Facial masks	oily skin and acne	1% (6 drops in 30 mL)
Toners	oily skin and acne	1–2% (6–12 drops in 30 mL)
Cleansers	oily skin and acne	1–3% (6–18 drops in 30 mL)
Exfoliants	oily skin and acne	1–2% (6–12 drops in 30 mL)
Lip balms		1–2% (6–12 drops in 30 mL)
BODY		
Massage oils		2–3% (12–18 drops in 30 mL)
Body lotions		2–3% (12–18 drops in 30 mL)
Exfoliants		1–2% (6–12 drops in 30 mL)
HANDS AND FEET		
Ointments		2–3% (12–18 drops in 30 mL)
Lotions/butters		2–3% (12–18 drops in 30 mL)
HAIR AND SCALP		
Shampoos and conditioners*		3% (18 drops in 30 mL)
Scalp serums		1% (6 drops in 30 mL)

* Exposing oils to heat and water will cause them to oxidize at a faster rate. Consider packaging shampoos and conditioners in flip-top or pump bottles to help reduce oxidation.

Cardamom

Botanical name: *Elettaria cardamomum*

Botanical family: Zingiberaceae

Habitat: native to India, Pakistan, Bangladesh, Indonesia and Nepal; cultivated in India, Cambodia, Guatemala and El Salvador

Aroma: deep green, spicy camphor base note

OXIDATION ALERT

Cardamom essential oil contains a significant amount of linalool, a constituent that absorbs through the skin and helps relieve swelling and inflammation. It is a pain-reliever as well as an antimicrobial. Linalool has a calming floral scent that has many beneficial properties, but at high concentrations it can cause an allergic reaction. Also, when oxidized it can lead to irritation (see page 27). Be particularly conscious of keeping any products containing this essential oil away from heat, water and light.

Description of the Plant

Cardamom is a shrub that grows up to 13 feet (4 m) in height. It has very long leaves and yellow flowers with purple tips. The fruit of the shrub contains many green seeds, which are a popular culinary ingredient.

EXTRACTION: steam distillation of the seeds, gathered just before the fruit is ripe

Using Cardamom Oil in Natural Products

Cardamom essential oil has a warm, spicy aroma and unique therapeutic properties. The oil has a lovely effect on the skin, toning and cleansing it at the same time and helping give it a youthful appearance. This makes it ideal for using on mature skin, as well as on oily and acne-prone skin. Note that cardamom has a very powerful scent — due to its high levels of eucalyptol — so it's advisable to use it sparingly.

CAUTION: Cardamom essential oil has a tendency to oxidize quickly, which can lead to skin irritation.

PRECAUTIONS: This oil is non-irritating when applied at or below the maximum recommended dilutions. Do not use while pregnant or breastfeeding. Properly stored, the shelf life of cardamom essential oil is 2 years.

Main Chemical Constituents of Cardamom Essential Oil

ALPHA-TERPINYL ACETATE (40–45%) This constituent has a strong antifungal effect, meaning that it can prevent or slow the growth of fungus infections.

EUCALYPTOL (30–35%) This constituent acts as a penetration enhancer (see page 54). It has also been shown to have antimicrobial and antifungal properties. When inhaled, it acts as a decongestant that helps to release phlegm.

LINALOOL (10–15%) This constituent absorbs through the skin and helps relieve swelling and inflammation. It is a pain-reliever as well as an antimicrobial. Linalool has many beneficial properties — for instance, it is calming — but at high concentrations it can cause an allergic reaction (see page 31) and when oxidized can lead to irritation (see page 108).

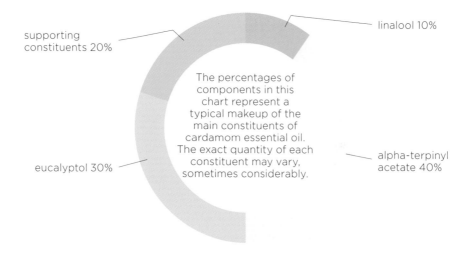

supporting constituents 20%

linalool 10%

The percentages of components in this chart represent a typical makeup of the main constituents of cardamom essential oil. The exact quantity of each constituent may vary, sometimes considerably.

eucalyptol 30%

alpha-terpinyl acetate 40%

GUIDELINES FOR USING

Cardamom Essential Oil in Personal Care Products

SKIN CARE: A dilution of up to 3% can be used in products that are left on the skin.

BENEFITS

- stimulating
- antibacterial
- antifungal

CONDITIONS

- oily skin
- dull-looking skin
- athlete's foot
- aging skin
- insect bites

PRODUCT	SKIN TYPE / CONDITION	QUANTITY
FACE		
Moisture creams	oily skin and acne	1% (6 drops in 30 mL)
Facial masks	oily skin and acne	1% (6 drops in 30 mL)
Toners	oily skin and acne	1–2% (6–12 drops in 30 mL)
Cleansers	oily skin and acne	1–2% (6–12 drops in 30 mL)
Exfoliants	oily skin and acne	1–2% (6–12 drops in 30 mL)
Lip balms		1–2% (6–12 drops in 30 mL)
BODY		
Massage oils		1–2% (6–12 drops in 30 mL)
Body lotions		1–2% (6–12 drops in 30 mL)
Deodorants		1–2% (6–12 drops in 30 mL)
Exfoliants		1–2% (6–12 drops in 30 mL)
HANDS AND FEET		
Ointments		1–2% (6–12 drops in 30 mL)
Lotions/butters		1–2% (6–12 drops in 30 mL)
HAIR AND SCALP		
Shampoos and conditioners*		3% (18 drops in 30 mL)
Scalp serums		1% (6 drops in 30 mL)

* Exposing oils to heat and water will cause them to oxidize at a faster rate. Consider packaging shampoos and conditioners in flip-top or pump bottles to help reduce oxidation.

Carrot Seed

Botanical name: *Daucus carota*

Botanical family: Apiaceae

Habitat: cultivated worldwide; the essential oil produced mainly in the Netherlands, Hungary and France

Aroma: spicy and herbaceous middle notes

Description of the Plant

Carrots are grown as annuals. The plant consists of a crown of feathery leaves that rise directly from the top of the orange-red taproot, which grows below ground. Carrot seeds come from the flowers of the carrot.

EXTRACTION: steam distillation of the dried seed

Using Carrot Seed Oil in Natural Products

Carrot seed essential oil is beneficial for a wide variety of skin conditions and can be used on all skin types. Its major chemical constituent, carotol, is a potent antifungal that can prevent or slow the growth of fungus infections. This makes it quite suitable for anti-dandruff shampoos and conditioners. It also has mild anti-inflammatory properties, which makes it a wonderful addition to formulations that treat eczema and psoriasis. The beta-caryophyllene in carrot seed essential oil has skin-lightening properties, which helps improve dull-looking skin. And alpha-pinene has strong antibacterial effects that boost the germ-killing properties of this wonderful essential oil.

CAUTION: Carrot seed essential oil contains trace amounts of furocoumarins, which are organic chemical compounds known to promote phototoxicity on the skin. If you will be exposing your skin to the sun or other UV radiation, do not use a skin-care product containing carrot seed essential oil.

PRECAUTIONS: Do not confuse carrot seed essential oil with carrot-infused oil or cold-expressed carrot seed oil (see above right). Carrot seed essential oil is non-irritating when applied at or below the maximum recommended dilutions. Avoid use during pregnancy and breastfeeding. Properly stored, carrot seed essential oil has a shelf life of 2 years.

KNOW YOUR CARROT

Three carrot derivatives are used in aromatherapy. The dried root is infused into an oil (see page 79), which creates an orange herbal infusion that is rich in skin-repairing beta-carotene. The carrot seeds can be cold-pressed to extract an oil that is rich in monounsaturated fatty acids, or they can be steam distilled to yield an essential oil. This section refers to carrot seed essential oil.

OXIDATION ALERT

The alpha-pinene in carrot seed essential oil will cause it to oxidize particularly quickly. This can lead to skin irritation. Keep any products containing high ranges of this oil away from heat, water and light.

Main Chemical Constituents of Carrot Seed Essential Oil

CAROTOL (75–85%) This constituent is unique to carrot seed essential oil. Laboratory studies have shown that it has a strong antifungal effect, meaning that it can prevent or slow the growth of fungus.

BETA-CARYOPHYLLENE (8–10%) This constituent has been found to have an ability to relieve pain and inflammation. It also has potential as a skin-lightening agent.

ALPHA-PINENE (6–8%) This constituent is known for its ability to relieve pain and inflammation, and for being a potent antimicrobial that can help prevent and treat skin infections. When oxidized, it can lead to skin irritation.

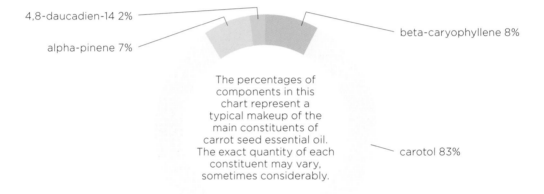

4,8-daucadien-14 2%

alpha-pinene 7%

beta-caryophyllene 8%

The percentages of components in this chart represent a typical makeup of the main constituents of carrot seed essential oil. The exact quantity of each constituent may vary, sometimes considerably.

carotol 83%

Carrot Seed Essential Oil in Personal Care Products

SKIN CARE: A dilution of up to 2% can be used in products that are left on the skin.

BENEFITS

- stimulating
- antibacterial
- antifungal

CONDITIONS

- acne
- psoriasis
- dull skin
- eczema
- aging skin
- dandruff

PRODUCT	SKIN TYPE / CONDITION	QUANTITY
FACE		
Moisture creams	all skin types	1–2% (6–12 drops in 30 mL)
Facial masks	all skin types	1–2% (6–12 drops in 30 mL)
Toners	all skin types	1–2% (6–12 drops in 30 mL)
Cleansers	all skin types	1–2% (6–12 drops in 30 mL)
Exfoliants		1–2% (6–12 drops in 30 mL)
Lip balms		2% (12 drops in 30 mL)
BODY		
Massage oils		1–2% (6–12 drops in 30 mL)
Body lotions		1–2% (6–12 drops in 30 mL)
Exfoliants		1–2% (6–12 drops in 30 mL)
HANDS AND FEET		
Ointments		2% (12 drops in 30 mL)
Lotions/butters		2% (12 drops in 30 mL)
HAIR AND SCALP		
Shampoos and conditioners*		2% (12 drops in 30 mL)

* Exposing oils to heat and water will cause them to oxidize at a faster rate. Consider packaging shampoos and conditioners in flip-top or pump bottles to help reduce oxidation.

German Chamomile

Botanical name: *Matricaria recutita* (also known as *M. chamomilla*)

Botanical family: Asteraceae

Habitat: cultivated in Eastern Europe and Egypt

Aroma: deep, flat herbal base notes

KNOW THE VARIETY

There are two main varieties of chamomile essential oil, each with its own therapeutic properties. German chamomile (*Matricaria recutita*), also called blue chamomile, has a distinctive blue color, attributed to the component chamazulene. Roman chamomile (*Anthemis nobilis*) yields only a very small amount of chamazulene (see page 117 for more on this oil).

A less common variety is Moroccan chamomile. Buyer beware: Moroccan chamomile mixed with chamazulene is often sold as German or blue chamomile at a much lower price than real thing. Always request a gas chromatography report when purchasing German chamomile.

Description of the Plant

German chamomile is an annual herb with long, erect, feathery stems that grow 2 to 3 feet (0.6 to 0.9 m) tall. The daisy-like flowers have rounded heads that distinguish them from Roman chamomile flowers, which have flat heads. The herb is popular in culinary applications and is best known as a tea.

EXTRACTION: steam distillation of the flowers (chamazulene, which causes the deep blue color of the oil, is not a constituent of the flower but develops during the process of extraction)

Using German Chamomile Oil in Natural Products

Both the herb and the essential oil are used often in skin care. The essential oil has wonderful anti-inflammatory properties. It is used to help repair inflamed skin, which makes it ideal for after-sun treatments as well as products that treat rashes, burns and other wounds. Its high alpha-bisabolol content makes it effective as a natural skin lightener. German chamomile is an expensive essential oil, and therefore recommended for use in leave-on products such as moisturizers, creams, lotions and ointments.

CAUTION: German chamomile essential oil has a tendency to oxidize quickly, which can lead to skin irritation.

PRECAUTIONS: Individuals with a ragweed allergy may be sensitive to this oil, and to other oils in the Asteraceae family. Use cautiously when pregnant or breastfeeding. Properly stored, German chamomile essential oil has a shelf life of up to 2 years.

Main Chemical Constituents of German Chamomile Essential Oil

ALPHA-BISABOLOL (50-60%) This constituent is known for its ability to treat skin inflammation. It also has a strong antifungal effect, meaning that it can prevent or slow the growth of fungus infections. Furthermore, there's evidence that alpha-bisabolol can help reduce skin hyperpigmentation and reduce the healing time for burns.

CHAMAZULENE (15-20%) This constituent has strong anti-inflammatory properties. It's also a potent antimicrobial that can help prevent and treat skin infections.

FARNESENE (15-20%) Studies show that this constituent is an antimicrobial that can help inhibit skin infections.

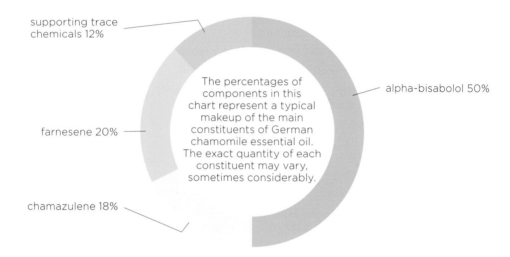

supporting trace chemicals 12%

alpha-bisabolol 50%

farnesene 20%

chamazulene 18%

The percentages of components in this chart represent a typical makeup of the main constituents of German chamomile essential oil. The exact quantity of each constituent may vary, sometimes considerably.

German Chamomile Essential Oil in Personal Care Products

SKIN CARE: A dilution of up to 2% can be used in products that are left on the skin.

BENEFITS

- anti-inflammatory
- antibacterial
- antifungal

CONDITIONS

- inflamed skin
- wounds
- burns
- dry, itchy skin
- scars
- acne

PRODUCT	SKIN TYPE / CONDITION	QUANTITY
FACE		
Moisture gels	acne, wounds and inflamed skin	1% (6 drops in 30 mL)
Eye creams	all skin types	0.5% (3 drops in 30 mL)
Facial masks	acne, wounds and inflamed skin	1% (6 drops in 30 mL)
Toners	acne, wounds and inflamed skin	1–2% (9 drops in 30 mL)
Cleansers	acne, wounds and inflamed skin	1–2% (12 drops in 30 mL)
Lip balms		1–2% (6–12 drops in 30 mL)
BODY		
Massage oils		1–2% (6–12 drops in 30 mL)
Body lotions		1–2% (6–12 drops in 30 mL)
Ointments		1–2% (6–12 drops in 30 mL)
HANDS AND FEET		
Ointments		2–3% (12–18 drops in 30 mL)
Lotions/butters		2–3% (12–18 drops in 30 mL)
HAIR AND SCALP		
Hair serums		1% (6 drops in 30 mL)

Roman Chamomile

Botanical name: *Chamaemelum nobile*

Botanical family: Asteraceae

Habitat: native to southern and western Europe; cultivated in Great Britain, Belgium, Hungary, Italy and France

Aroma: deep, sweet, full-bodied base notes

Description of the Plant

Roman chamomile is a perennial herb with small daisy-like flowers that can grow up to 10 inches (25 cm) tall. The flowers have feathery stems and flat heads that distinguish them from German chamomile flowers, which have rounded heads (for more differences between Roman and German chamomile, see "Know the Variety," page 114). The herb is popular for culinary uses; it is best known as a tea.

EXTRACTION: steam distillation of the flowers

Using Roman Chamomile Oil in Natural Products

Roman chamomile is renowned for its calming, sedative-like effects, which may be attributed to the angelates that are its principal components. Research confirms that this oil soothes the nervous system, but we do not understand why this happens. Since angelates are major constituents of this oil, we can probably assume that they contribute to this effect. It's a terrific addition to a wide variety of skin-care products and is particularly well suited to relaxing massage oils. Roman chamomile is also well-known for its anti-inflammatory properties, which can help ease inflamed skin and muscle aches. Use it in creams, lotions and moisture gels for irritated skin and rashes, and in soothing balms and butters for tired feet.

PRECAUTIONS: Individuals with a ragweed allergy may be sensitive to this oil, and to other oils in the Asteraceae family. Use cautiously when pregnant or breastfeeding. Properly stored, Roman chamomile essential oil has a shelf life of up to 2 years.

OXIDATION ALERT

Roman chamomile essential oil contains a significant amount of alpha-pinene, which oxidizes quite quickly. This can lead to skin irritation. Be particularly conscious of keeping any products containing high ranges of this essential oil away from heat, water and light.

Main Chemical Constituents of Roman Chamomile Essential Oil

ISOBUTYL ANGELATE (40-45%) Not much is known about this constituent, but it may be a factor that gives Roman chamomile its sedative and calming properties.

ALPHA-PINENE (20-25%) This constituent is known for its ability to relieve pain and inflammation, and for being a potent antimicrobial that can help prevent and treat skin infections. When oxidized, it can lead to skin irritation.

METHYLBUTYL ANGELATE (19-25%) Not much is known about this constituent, but it may be the factor that gives Roman chamomile its sedative and calming properties.

ISOAMYL ANGELATE (5-8%) We don't know much about this constituent but believe that it may help to calm the nervous system.

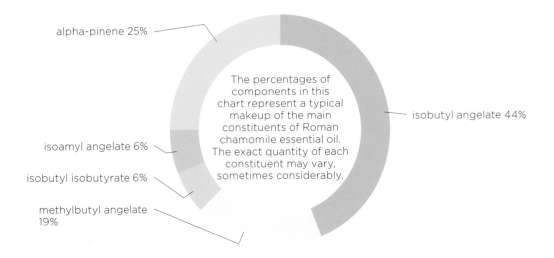

The percentages of components in this chart represent a typical makeup of the main constituents of Roman chamomile essential oil. The exact quantity of each constituent may vary, sometimes considerably.

alpha-pinene 25%

isobutyl angelate 44%

isoamyl angelate 6%

isobutyl isobutyrate 6%

methylbutyl angelate 19%

Roman Chamomile Essential Oil in Personal Care Products

SKIN CARE: A dilution of up to 3% can be used in products that are left on the skin.

BENEFITS

- calming and soothing
- suitable for all skin types

CONDITIONS

- rashes
- irritated skin
- acne

PRODUCT	SKIN TYPE / CONDITION	QUANTITY
FACE		
Moisture gels	all skin types	1–2% (6–12 drops in 30 mL)
Facial masks	all skin types	1–2% (6–12 drops in 30 mL)
Toners	all skin types	2% (12 drops in 30 mL)
Cleansers	all skin types	2–3% (12–18 drops in 30 mL)
Exfoliants	all skin types	2–3% (12–18 drops in 30 mL)
Lip balms		2–3% (12–18 drops in 30 mL)
BODY		
Massage oils		1–2% (6–12 drops in 30 mL)
Body lotions		1–2% (6–12 drops in 30 mL)
Deodorants		1–2% (6–12 drops in 30 mL)
Exfoliants		1–2% (6–12 drops in 30 mL)
HANDS AND FEET		
Balms and butters		2–3% (12–18 drops in 30 mL)
HAIR AND SCALP		
Anti-dandruff shampoos*		1–3% (6–18 drops in 30 mL)
Leave-in conditioning balms for scalp treatment*		1–2% (6–12 drops in 30 mL)

* Exposing oils to heat and water will cause them to oxidize at a faster rate. Consider packaging shampoos and conditioners in flip-top or pump bottles to help reduce oxidation.

Citronella

Botanical name: *Cymbopogon nardus*

Botanical family: Poaceae

Habitat: native to Asia; now cultivated in Sri Lanka, India and Indonesia

Aroma: bold citrus, curbed by flat base notes

Description of the Plant

Citronella essential oil comes from a species of *Cymbopogon*, better known as lemongrass. This fragrant perennial tropical grass has smooth, drooping leaves that are about 3 feet (1 m) in length.

EXTRACTION: steam distillation of the leaves

Using Citronella Oil in Natural Products

Citronella is known for its insect-repellent properties. This essential oil contains citronellol and geraniol, both of which help ward off bacterial and fungal infections. Citronella acts as an effective deodorant in personal care products; it's also used in skin care for oily, acne-prone and combination skin types.

CAUTIONS: Citronella contains a fair amount of borneol, which, when used in amounts higher than the recommended dilutions, can cause nausea. It also contains a high level of citronellal, which is a known allergen and may cause skin irritation in some individuals.

PRECAUTIONS: This oil is non-irritating when applied at or below the maximum recommended dilutions. However, do not use when pregnant or breastfeeding. Properly stored, citronella essential oil has a shelf life of 2 years.

Main Chemical Constituents of Citronella Essential Oil

CITRONELLAL (23–25%) This constituent has proven antimicrobial abilities. However, it is classified as a skin allergen and may cause irritation.

CITRONELLOL (19–25%) This constituent has proven antibacterial abilities. It's also what contributes to the oil's rose-like scent.

GERANIOL (19–25%) This constituent also contributes to the oil's rose-like scent. Geraniol has strong antifungal and antibacterial activity, meaning that it can prevent or slow the growth of fungi and bacteria. It has many beneficial properties, but at high concentrations it can be a skin irritant and sensitizer, or even lead to an allergic reaction (see page 27).

BORNEOL (13–15%) This constituent is a natural insect repellent, which can help prevent diseases carried by mosquitoes and other pests.

BETA-CARYOPHYLLENE (8–10%) This constituent is known for its ability to relieve pain and inflammation. It also has potential as a skin-lightening agent.

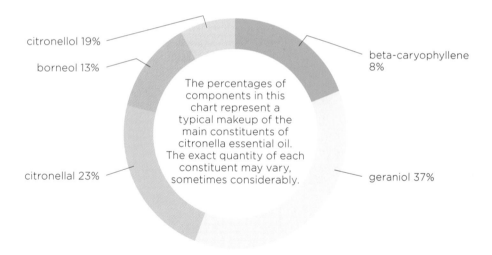

citronellol 19%

borneol 13%

beta-caryophyllene 8%

The percentages of components in this chart represent a typical makeup of the main constituents of citronella essential oil. The exact quantity of each constituent may vary, sometimes considerably.

citronellal 23%

geraniol 37%

Citronella Essential Oil in Personal Care Products

SKIN CARE: A dilution of up to 3% can be used in products that are left on the skin.

BENEFITS

- deodorizing
- antibacterial
- antifungal

CONDITIONS

- acne
- oily skin
- dull skin
- cold sores
- insect bites
- athlete's foot

PRODUCT	SKIN TYPE / CONDITION	QUANTITY
FACE		
Moisture gels	acne	1% (6 drops in 30 mL)
Facial masks	oily skin and acne	1–2% (6–12 drops in 30 mL)
Toners	oily skin and acne	1–2% (6–12 drops in 30 mL)
Cleansers	oily skin and acne	1–3% (6–18 drops in 30 mL)
Exfoliants	oily skin and acne	1–2% (6–12 drops in 30 mL)
Lip balms		2–3% (12–18 drops in 30 mL)
BODY		
Massage oils		1–2% (6–12 drops in 30 mL)
Body lotions		1–2% (6–12 drops in 30 mL)
Deodorant		1–2% (6–12 drops in 30 mL)
Insect repellent		1–3% (6–18 drops in 30 mL)
HANDS AND FEET		
Antifungal foot balm		2–3% (12–18 drops in 30 mL)
HAIR AND SCALP		
Anti-dandruff shampoos*		1–3% (6–18 drops in 30 mL)
Leave-in hair conditioning balms for scalp treatment*		1–2% (6–12 drops in 30 mL)

* Exposing oils to heat and water will cause them to oxidize at a faster rate. Consider packaging shampoos and conditioners in flip-top or pump bottles to help reduce oxidation.

Clary Sage

Botanical name: *Salvia sclarea*

Botanical family: Lamiaceae

Habitat: native to the Mediterranean; now cultivated worldwide

Aroma: herbaceous, sweet and floral middle and base notes

Description of the Plant

Clary sage is a strongly aromatic herb that grows up to 3 feet (1 m) in height. It has hairy leaves and small purple or blue flowers. The herb is cultivated for its essential oil in France, Britain and Morocco.

EXTRACTION: steam distillation of the flowers

Using Clary Sage Oil in Natural Products

The essence of clary sage calms the nervous system while gently repairing the skin. The linalyl acetate in this essential oil contributes to a toning effect on the skin and helps to relax muscles. Clary sage is a wonderful addition to a wide range of personal care products. It is especially well suited for night creams, moisturizers and serums because of its ability to help relax the body.

CAUTIONS: Clary sage essential oil has sedative properties that can enhance the intoxicating effects of alcohol.

PRECAUTIONS: This oil is non-irritating when applied at or below the maximum recommended dilutions. Do not use when pregnant or while breastfeeding. Properly stored, clary sage essential oil has a shelf life of 2 years.

Main Chemical Constituents of Clary Sage Essential Oil

LINALYL ACETATE (65–70%) This constituent absorbs through the skin and helps prevent and treat skin inflammation. It also has antispasmodic effects, so it can help relax muscles and relieve cramps.

LINALOOL (15–20%) This constituent absorbs through the skin and helps relieve swelling and inflammation. It is a pain-reliever as well as an antimicrobial. Linalool has many beneficial properties — for instance, it is calming — but at high concentrations it can cause an allergic reaction (see page 31) and when oxidized can lead to irritation.

ALPHA-TERPINEOL (3–5%) This constituent has strong antibacterial properties, which can help prevent skin infections.

GERANIOL (4–5%) This constituent has strong antifungal and antibacterial activity, meaning that it can prevent or slow the growth of fungi and bacteria. Geraniol has many beneficial properties, but at high concentrations it can be a skin irritant and sensitizer, or even lead to an allergic reaction (see page 27).

BETA-CARYOPHYLLENE (4–6%) This constituent is known for its ability to relieve pain and inflammation. It also has potential as a skin-lightening agent.

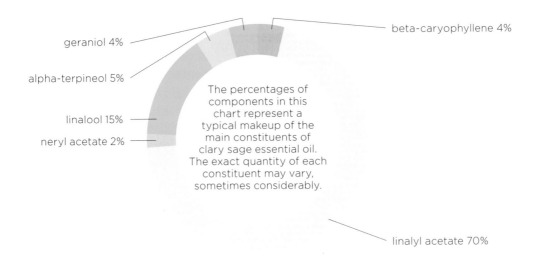

geraniol 4%

alpha-terpineol 5%

beta-caryophyllene 4%

linalool 15%

neryl acetate 2%

The percentages of components in this chart represent a typical makeup of the main constituents of clary sage essential oil. The exact quantity of each constituent may vary, sometimes considerably.

linalyl acetate 70%

GUIDELINES FOR USING

Clary Sage Essential Oil in Personal Care Products

SKIN CARE: A dilution of up to 3% can be used in products that are left on the skin.

BENEFITS

- calming and relaxing
- suitable for all skin types
- deodorizing

CONDITIONS

- acne
- aging skin
- dandruff
- oily skin

PRODUCT	SKIN TYPE / CONDITION	QUANTITY
FACE		
Moisture gels	all skin types	1–2% (6–12 drops in 30 mL)
Facial masks	all skin types	1–2% (6–12 drops in 30 mL)
Toners	all skin types	2% (12 drops in 30 mL)
Cleansers	all skin types	2–3% (12–18 drops in 30 mL)
Exfoliants	all skin types	2–3% (12–18 drops in 30 mL)
Lip balms		2–3% (12–18 drops in 30 mL)
BODY		
Massage oils		1–2% (6–12 drops in 30 mL)
Body lotions		1–2% (6–12 drops in 30 mL)
Deodorants		1–2% (6–12 drops in 30 mL)
Exfoliants		1–3% (6–18 drops in 30 mL)
HANDS AND FEET		
Balms and butters		2–3% (12–18 drops in 30 mL)
HAIR AND SCALP		
Shampoos and conditioners*	1–3% (6–18 drops in 30 mL)	
Leave-in conditioning balms for scalp treatment*		1–2% (6–12 drops in 30 mL)

* Exposing oils to heat and water will cause them to oxidize at a faster rate. Consider packaging shampoos and conditioners in flip-top or pump bottles to help reduce oxidation.

Frankincense

Botanical name: *Boswellia carterii*

Botanical family: Burseraceae

Habitat: native to the Red Sea region; now grows wild throughout northeast Africa

Aroma: oriental, herbaceous and balsamic base and middle notes

OXIDATION ALERT

Frankincense essential oil contains a significant amount of both alpha-pinene and l-limonene, which oxidize quite quickly. This can lead to skin irritation (see page 27). When using it in formulations, be particularly conscious of keeping any products containing this essential oil away from heat and water.

Description of the Plant

The ancient *Boswellia carterii* is a small tree that grows in rocky areas. To harvest frankincense, a deep incision is made in the trunk of the tree and a 5-inch (13 cm) piece of bark is peeled off. Small milky droplets of resin are exuded from the stripped wood; when dried, the resin has traditionally been used as incense. The oil is pale yellow in color.

EXTRACTION: steam distillation of the resin

Using Frankincense Oil in Natural Products

Frankincense is one of the leading essential oils in skin care and cosmetics. It has a wonderful ability to treat wounds and is frequently recommended for toning and rejuvenating mature skin, which makes it a great addition to anti-aging products. The beta-caryophyllene in this oil makes it effective as a natural skin lightener in creams, cleansers, toners, masks and exfoliants. In addition, this essential oil is a potent antimicrobial, which makes it a good choice for acne formulations, as well as for balms aimed at treating fungal foot infections.

CAUTIONS: The alpha-pinene and the l-limonene in frankincense essential oil will cause it to oxidize particularly quickly, which may lead to skin irritation. Additionally, this oil has been shown to interact with certain psychotropic drugs and may increase grogginess.

PRECAUTIONS: Frankincense is non-irritating when applied at or below the maximum recommended dilutions. Avoid during pregnancy and breastfeeding. Properly stored, the shelf life of frankincense essential oil ranges between 1 and 2 years.

Main Chemical Constituents of Frankincense Essential Oil

ALPHA-PINENE (58-60%) Known for its ability to relieve pain and inflammation, it is a potent antimicrobial that can help prevent and treat skin infections.

L-LIMONENE (18-20%) L-limonene is found in many conifer essential oils and when oxidized can lead to irritation.

SABINENE (10-15%) This constituent has antimicrobial properties.

BETA-CARYOPHYLLENE (7-10%) This constituent is known for its ability to relieve pain and inflammation. It also has potential as a skin-lightening agent.

BETA-PINENE (3-5%) This constituent, which carries a low risk of allergy, has strong antimicrobial properties and is very good at preventing skin infections. When oxidized it can lead to skin irritations.

GERANYL ACETATE (1-5%) This constituent has antispasmodic effects, so it can help relax muscles and relieve cramps.

MYRCENE (1-3%) This antioxidant is non-irritating and non-allergenic. It has sedative properties that help calm the nervous system.

TERPINEN-4-OL (1-3%) This is a potent antibacterial agent that is also anti-inflammatory. It can help clear skin infections and relieve acne and is effective against skin mites and yeast infections on the skin.

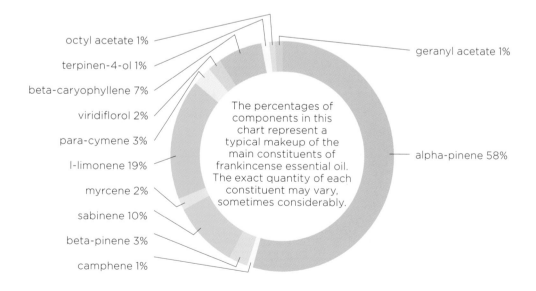

octyl acetate 1%
terpinen-4-ol 1%
beta-caryophyllene 7%
viridiflorol 2%
para-cymene 3%
l-limonene 19%
myrcene 2%
sabinene 10%
beta-pinene 3%
camphene 1%

geranyl acetate 1%

The percentages of components in this chart represent a typical makeup of the main constituents of frankincense essential oil. The exact quantity of each constituent may vary, sometimes considerably.

alpha-pinene 58%

GUIDELINES FOR USING

Frankincense Essential Oil in Personal Care Products

SKIN CARE: A dilution of up to 3% can be used in products that are left on the skin.

BENEFITS

- antibacterial
- toning
- suitable for all skin types

CONDITIONS

- bacterial and fungal infections
- acne
- scar tissue
- fine lines

PRODUCT	SKIN TYPE / CONDITION	QUANTITY
FACE		
Moisture creams	all skin types and mature skin	1–2% (6–12 drops in 30 mL)
Facial masks	all skin types and mature skin	1–2% (6–12 drops in 30 mL)
Toners	all skin types and mature skin	2% (12 drops in 30 mL)
Cleansers	all skin types and mature skin	2–3% (12–18 drops in 30 mL)
Exfoliants	all skin types and mature skin	2–3% (12–18 drops in 30 mL)
BODY		
Massage oils		1–2% (6–12 drops in 30 mL)
Body lotions		1–2% (6–12 drops in 30 mL)
Exfoliants		1–3% (6–18 drops in 30 mL)
HANDS AND FEET		
Foot balms and butters		2–3% (12–18 drops in 30 mL)
HAIR AND SCALP		
Leave-in conditioning balms for scalp treatment*		1–2% (6–12 drops in 30 mL)

* Exposing oils to heat and water will cause them to oxidize at a faster rate. Consider packaging shampoos and conditioners in flip-top or pump bottles to help reduce oxidation.

Geranium

Botanical name: *Pelargonium* species

Botanical family: Geraniaceae

Habitat: native to South Africa; cultivated worldwide

Aroma: full-bodied herbaceous and rose middle notes

Description of the Plant

There are more than 250 species of geranium (*Pelargonium*); the ones used for essential oils are cultivated in Egypt, France, China, Algeria, South Africa, Morocco and Spain. Geraniums are woody perennial plants that reach a height of about 3 feet (1 m). The plants have fragrant, deeply ridged green leaves and small pink flowers.

EXTRACTION: steam distillation of the leaves, stalks and flowers

Using Geranium Oil in Natural Products

When used subtly, geranium essential oil adds a fresh rose scent to personal care products. It tones and relieves blotchy and bloated skin, which makes it well suited for skin aggravated by hormonal imbalances. It's also frequently used in formulations to reduce the appearance of cellulite.

Geranium essential oil has strong antibacterial and antifungal properties, meaning that it can prevent or slow the growth of bacteria and fungi. It also has a cooling and relaxing effect on muscle tissue, so it can help the smooth muscles of the face and body. This makes the oil effective in anti-aging formulations; use it in lotions, toners and face creams.

> **SENSITIVITY ALERT**
>
> Overexposure to geranium essential oil may cause an allergic reaction. This reaction is due to one of its major chemical constituents, geraniol (see page 30).

CAUTION: When inhaled, the geraniol in geranium has been found to elevate enzymes in the liver; this may be the reason why overexposure to this essential oil can cause headaches and nausea. Furthermore, geranium essential oil may enhance the penetration of topical drugs, so do not use it on skin treated with topical drugs.

PRECAUTIONS: Overexposure to geranium essential oil may irritate sensitive skin. Avoid using while pregnant or breastfeeding. Properly stored, this essential oil has a shelf life of 2 years.

Main Chemical Constituents of Geranium Essential Oil

CITRONELLOL (38-40%) This constituent has proven antibacterial abilities. It is what contributes to the oil's rose-like scent.

GERANIOL (20-30%) This constituent also contributes to the oil's rose-like scent. Geraniol has strong antifungal and antibacterial activity, meaning that it can prevent or slow the growth of fungi and bacteria. Geraniol has many beneficial properties, but at high concentrations it can be a skin irritant and sensitizer, or even lead to an allergic reaction (see page 27).

ISOMENTHONE (9-10%) This constituent contributes to the cooling effect on the skin; it also relaxes smooth muscles.

CITRONELLYL FORMATE (8-10%) This constituent has a relaxing effect and contributes to the sweet floral fragrance.

GERANYL FORMATE (5-6%) This constituent has a relaxing effect and contributes to the sweet floral fragrance.

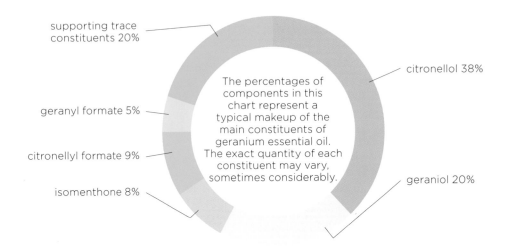

supporting trace constituents 20%

citronellol 38%

The percentages of components in this chart represent a typical makeup of the main constituents of geranium essential oil. The exact quantity of each constituent may vary, sometimes considerably.

geranyl formate 5%

citronellyl formate 9%

isomenthone 8%

geraniol 20%

GUIDELINES FOR USING

Geranium Essential Oil in Personal Care Products

SKIN CARE: A dilution of up to 3% can be used in products that are left on the skin.

BENEFITS

- toning
- deodorizing
- antibacterial
- antifungal

CONDITIONS

- oily skin
- skin infections
- dull skin
- aging skin
- cellulite
- body odor

PRODUCT	SKIN TYPE / CONDITION	QUANTITY
FACE		
Moisture creams and gels	all skin types	1% (6 drops in 30 mL)
Facial masks	all skin types	1% (6 drops in 30 mL)
Toners	all skin types	1–2% (6–12 drops in 30 mL)
Cleansers	all skin types	1–2% (6–12 drops in 30 mL)
Exfoliants	all skin types	1–2% (6–12 drops in 30 mL)
BODY		
Massage oils		1–2% (6–12 drops in 30 mL)
Body lotions		1–2% (6–12 drops in 30 mL)
Exfoliants		1–2% (6–12 drops in 30 mL)
HANDS AND FEET		
Creams		1–2% (6–12 drops in 30 mL)
HAIR AND SCALP		
Shampoos and conditioners*		3% (18 drops in 30 mL)
Leave-in hair serums		1% (6 drops in 30 mL)

* Exposing oils to heat and water will cause them to oxidize at a faster rate. Consider packaging shampoos and conditioners in flip-top or pump bottles to help reduce oxidation.

Ginger

Botanical name: *Zingiber officinale*

Botanical family: Zingiberaceae

Habitat: native to Asia; cultivated in tropical regions

Aroma: dry, bold base notes

Description of the Plant

Ginger is a perennial plant that grows to a height of about 2 feet (60 cm). It has long, narrow, reed-like green leaves and yellow flowers that stem from the aromatic rhizomes (roots). Gingerroot is popular for culinary applications.

EXTRACTION: steam distillation of the dried rhizome

Using Ginger Oil in Natural Products

Ginger essential oil is used mainly for inflammation-related conditions, such as muscle aches and pains. It has a warming effect on skin and promotes blood circulation; a combination of ginger essential oil and massage will stimulate blood flow, making this a perfect addition to sports massage oils. Added to skin-care products, it has a rejuvenating effect, which makes this oil well suited to mature skin. Use in morning cleansers, moisturizers and masks.

PRECAUTIONS: Ginger essential oil may irritate sensitive skin; use in low concentrations. This oil may be mildly phototoxic if applied in high concentrations. Do not use while pregnant or breastfeeding. Properly stored, ginger essential oil has a shelf life of 2 years.

Main Chemical Constituents of Ginger Essential Oil

ZINGIBERENE (46–48%) This constituent contributes to ginger's aroma and has strong anti-inflammatory properties. Zingiberene has been shown to be moderately irritating to the skin.

AR-CURCUMENE (16–21%) This compound has potent anti-inflammatory properties. It's also antibacterial, which can help prevent and treat bacterial infections.

CAMPHENE (6–10%) The odor of this compound is similar to that of camphor. Camphene acts as an antifungal, meaning that it can prevent or slow the growth of fungi. It also has antioxidant properties.

BETA-BISABOLENE (6–8%) This compound has a balsamic fragrance. One study found that beta-bisabolene had a toxic effect on human cancer cells. It can be slightly irritating to skin.

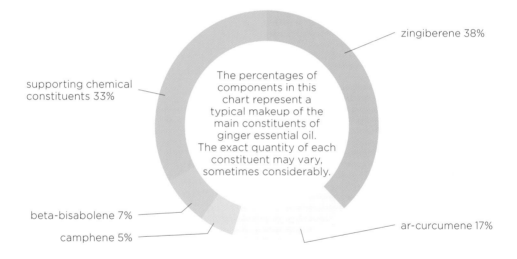

zingiberene 38%

supporting chemical constituents 33%

The percentages of components in this chart represent a typical makeup of the main constituents of ginger essential oil. The exact quantity of each constituent may vary, sometimes considerably.

beta-bisabolene 7%

camphene 5%

ar-curcumene 17%

GUIDELINES FOR USING

Ginger Essential Oil in Personal Care Products

SKIN CARE: A dilution of up to 3% can be used in products that are left on the skin.

BENEFITS

- warming
- stimulating
- antibacterial

CONDITIONS

- pale and tired-looking skin
- oily skin
- aging skin
- acne

PRODUCT	SKIN TYPE / CONDITION	QUANTITY
FACE		
Moisture creams	mature skin	1–2% (6–12 drops in 30 mL)
Facial masks	mature skin	1–2% (6–12 drops in 30 mL)
Toners	mature skin	1–2% (6–12 drops in 30 mL)
Cleansers	all skin types	1–2% (6–12 drops in 30 mL)
Exfoliants		1–2% (6–12 drops in 30 mL)
BODY		
Massage oils		1–2% (6–12 drops in 30 mL)
Body lotions		1–2% (6–12 drops in 30 mL)
Exfoliants		1–2% (6–12 drops in 30 mL)
HANDS AND FEET		
Creams	tired and aching	2–3% (12–18 drops in 30 mL)
HAIR AND SCALP		
Shampoos and conditioners*		1–3% (6–18 drops in 30 mL)
Serums	inflamed scalp	1–2% (6–12 drops in 30 mL)

* Exposing oils to heat and water will cause them to oxidize at a faster rate. Consider packaging shampoos and conditioners in flip-top or pump bottles to help reduce oxidation.

Grapefruit

Botanical name: *Citrus x paradisi*

Botanical family: Rutaceae

Habitat: native to tropical Asia and the West Indies; cultivated in California, Florida, Brazil and Israel

Aroma: evanescent bittersweet citrus top notes

Description of the Plant

The grapefruit tree grows to a height of 16 feet (5 m) and has dark green leaves and fragrant star-shaped flowers. The tree yields a large, round bittersweet fruit with a thick yellow peel.

EXTRACTION: cold expression of the fruit's peel

Using Grapefruit Oil in Natural Products

Grapefruit essential oil is wonderfully stimulating and uplifting. In aromatherapy it's usually used for treating depression and anxiety. This essential oil also has an invigorating effect on the body. As a result, it is recommended for hair and body products that are used in the morning. These same stimulating properties help make the face look supple and toned, which is why grapefruit oil is ideal for anti-aging products. In addition, grapefruit essential oil has strong antimicrobial properties, which makes it ideal for cleansers, toners, creams and masks for oily and acne-prone skin.

CAUTIONS: Grapefruit essential oil contains trace amounts of furocoumarins, which are organic chemical compounds known to promote phototoxicity on the skin. If you will be exposing your skin to the sun or other UV radiation, do not use a skin-care product containing grapefruit essential oil.

PRECAUTIONS: Grapefruit essential oil is non-irritating when applied at or below the maximum recommended dilutions. However, the high level of d-limonene in this oil makes it prone to oxidization, which may cause sensitization. Use cautiously when pregnant or breastfeeding. Properly stored, grapefruit essential oil has a shelf life of 6 to 8 months.

OXIDATION ALERT

Grapefruit essential oil contains a significant amount of D-limonene. This is one of the most commonly found constituents in fruit and it gives citrus fruits their distinctive citrus scent. However, it oxidizes quite quickly, which can lead to skin irritation. Be particularly conscious of keeping any products containing this essential oil away from heat, water and light.

Main Chemical Constituents of Grapefruit Essential Oil

D-LIMONENE (80–85%) This is one of the most commonly found constituents in fruit, and it gives grapefruit and other citrus fruits their distinctive scent. D-limonene oxidizes quite quickly, which can lead to skin irritation (see page 27).

ALPHA-PINENE (2%) This constituent is known for its ability to relieve pain and inflammation, and for being a potent antimicrobia that can help prevent and treat skin infections. When oxidized, it can lead to skin irritation.

MYRCENE (2%) This non-irritating, non-allergenic constituent is an antioxidant. It has sedative properties, which help calm and soothe the nervous system.

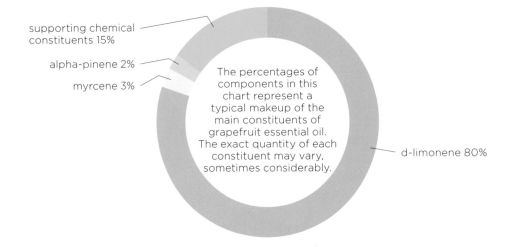

supporting chemical constituents 15%

alpha-pinene 2%

myrcene 3%

The percentages of components in this chart represent a typical makeup of the main constituents of grapefruit essential oil. The exact quantity of each constituent may vary, sometimes considerably.

d-limonene 80%

Grapefruit Essential Oil in Personal Care Products

SKIN CARE: A dilution of up to 2% can be used in products that are left on the skin. A dilution of up to 3% can be used in rinse-off products.

BENEFITS

- toning
- stimulating and invigorating
- antibacterial

CONDITIONS

- bacterial infections
- oily skin
- acne
- congested skin
- cellulite

PRODUCT	SKIN TYPE / CONDITION	QUANTITY
FACE		
Moisture creams and gels	oily skin and acne	1% (6 drops in 30 mL)
Facial masks	oily skin and acne	1% (6 drops in 30 mL)
Toners	oily skin and acne	1% (6 drops in 30 mL)
Cleansers	oily skin and acne	1% (6 drops in 30 mL)
Exfoliants		1% (6 drops in 30 mL)
BODY		
Massage oils		1–2% (6–12 drops in 30 mL)
Body lotions		1–2% (6–12 drops in 30 mL)
Exfoliants		1–2% (6–12 drops in 30 mL)
Deodorants		1–2% (6–12 drops in 30 mL)
HANDS AND FEET		
Nail-whitening and cuticle repair oils		1–2% (6–12 drops in 30 mL)
HAIR AND SCALP		
Shampoos and conditioners*		3% (18 drops in 30 mL)

* Exposing oils to heat and water will cause them to oxidize at a faster rate. (The d-limonene in grapefruit essential oil will cause it to oxidize particularly quickly.) Consider packaging shampoos and conditioners in flip-top or pump bottles to help reduce oxidation.

Helichrysum

Botanical name: *Helichrysum italicum*

Botanical family: Asteraceae

Habitat: native to the Mediterranean region; now cultivated in Italy, the Balkans, Spain and France

Aroma: honey and curry base notes

AN EXPENSIVE OIL

Helichrysum is an expensive oil and, as such, is not recommended for wash-off hair products. If you do use it in shampoos and conditioners, be sure to pack those products in flip-top or pump bottles to help reduce oxidation from exposure to water and heat.

Description of the Plant

Helichrysum is a strongly aromatic herb that grows up to 2 feet (60 cm) high. It has flat, oblong leaves and bright yellow daisy-like flowers. There are hundreds of species of *Helichrysum*, which is why it's commonly referred to by other names such as everlasting and immortelle. It's also known as curry plant because of the strong scent of its leaves.

EXTRACTION: steam distillation of the flowering plant

Using Helichrysum in Natural Products

In traditional aromatherapy, helichrysum is known for its diverse skin-healing abilities. That's why it's often used to treat conditions such as burns, chapped skin and rosacea. It's also noted for repairing scar tissue. Use this essential oil in nighttime moisture creams, serums, lotions and toners to help repair skin after sun exposure or to reduce the look of scars.

PRECAUTIONS: Helichrysum essential oil is non-irritating when applied at or below the maximum recommended dilutions. Overexposure can lead to mild skin irritation. Do not use while pregnant or breastfeeding. Properly stored, helichrysum essential oil has a shelf life of up to 2 years.

Main Chemical Constituents of Helichrysum Essential Oil

NERYL ACETATE (20-25%) This constituent is non-irritating and has a calming, relaxing effect.

ALPHA- AND GAMMA-CURCUMENE (15-20% EACH) These curcuminoid compounds have strong anti-inflammatory capabilities that promote wound healing and skin repair. They also have potent antioxidant properties.

ITALIDONE (3-5%) Helichrysum's ability to help heal wounds and bruising is attributed to this constituent. However, more evidence is required to substantiate this claim.

BETA-CARYOPHYLLENE (2-4%) This constituent is known for its ability to relieve pain and inflammation. It also has potential as a skin-lightening agent.

CHAMAZULENE (2-3%) This constituent has strong anti-inflammatory properties. It's also a potent antimicrobial that can help prevent skin infections.

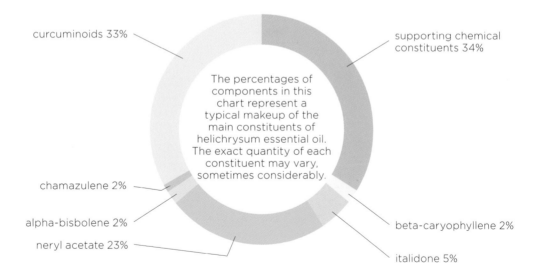

curcuminoids 33%

supporting chemical constituents 34%

The percentages of components in this chart represent a typical makeup of the main constituents of helichrysum essential oil. The exact quantity of each constituent may vary, sometimes considerably.

chamazulene 2%

alpha-bisbolene 2%

neryl acetate 23%

beta-caryophyllene 2%

italidone 5%

Helichrysum Essential Oil in Personal Care Products

SKIN CARE: A dilution of up to 3% can be used in products that are left on the skin. There is no need to rinse them off.

BENEFITS

- skin repair
- suitable for all skin types
- antibacterial

CONDITIONS

- sensitive skin
- acne
- burns
- rosacea

PRODUCT	SKIN TYPE / CONDITION	QUANTITY
FACE		
Moisture creams	all skin types	1–2% (6–12 drops in 30 mL)
Facial masks	all skin types	1–2% (6–12 drops in 30 mL)
Toners	all skin types	1–2% (6–12 drops in 30 mL)
Cleansers	all skin types	1–2% (6–12 drops in 30 mL)
BODY		
Massage oils		1–2% (6–12 drops in 30 mL)
Body lotions		1–2% (6–12 drops in 30 mL)
HANDS AND FEET		
Ointments		2–3% (12–18 drops in 30 mL)
Lotions/butters		2–3% (12–18 drops in 30 mL)
HAIR AND SCALP		
Shampoos*		1–3% (6–18 drops in 30 mL)
Serums	inflamed scalp	1–2% (6–12 drops in 30 mL)

* Exposing oils to heat and water will cause them to oxidize at a faster rate. Consider packaging shampoos and conditioners in flip-top or pump bottles to help reduce oxidation.

Jasmine

Botanical names: *Jasminum grandiflorum, J. sambac*

Botanical family: Oleaceae

Habitat: many species grown around the world; common jasmines used in aromatherapy cultivated in Egypt and India

Aroma: deep, sweet, amber middle base notes (*J. grandiflorum*); light, sweet, amber middle base notes (*J. sambac*)

Jasmine Absolute

It is virtually impossible to find pure jasmine essential oil, as the yield from the plant is so minute. Therefore, this section refers to jasmine absolute (see page 89 for more on absolutes).

Description of the Plant

Jasmine grows as an evergreen shrub or vine that can climb up to 30 feet (9 m) high. It has fragrant waxy white flowers. The peak growing season is from March to July.

EXTRACTION: solvent extraction of the flowers

Using Jasmine Absolute in Natural Products

The lovely scent of the jasmine flower is what makes this absolute a wonderful addition to your skin-care products. The sweet fragrance helps reduce stress and anxiety. In addition, the benzyl benzoate in jasmine is effective against scabies, a skin disorder marked by raised, itchy red spots. Use it in cleansers, lotions, balms, body washes, shampoos and conditioners.

CAUTION: Jasmine absolute is expensive, which is why some companies cut it with benzyl acetate and benzyl benzoate. This creates a thick, viscous oil with a cloying, overpowering fragrance.

PRECAUTIONS: Jasmine absolute is obtained by solvent extraction, so overexposure may lead to skin irritation. Avoid use during pregnancy and when breastfeeding. Properly stored, jasmine absolute has a shelf life of up to 2 years.

KNOW THE VARIETY

Two principal species of jasmine are used to create an absolute: *Jasminum grandiflorum* (royal or Spanish jasmine) and *Jasminum sambac* (tea jasmine). The two vary in their fragrance as well as in their chemical makeup. For example, *J. sambac* has higher levels of linalool and lower levels of benzyl acetate.

SENSITIVITY ALERT

Jasminum sambac absolute contains a high level of linalool. If you have been overexposed to linalool, you may react to its presence in jasmine.

Main Chemical Constituents of Jasmine Absolute (*Jasminum sambac*)

LINALOOL (13-20%) This constituent absorbs through the skin and helps relieve swelling and inflammation. It is a pain-reliever as well as an antimicrobial. Linalool has many beneficial properties, but at high concentrations it can cause an allergic reaction (see page 31) and when oxidized it can lead to irritation (see Oxidation Alert, page 108).

BENZYL ACETATE (10-20%) This constituent contributes to jasmine's sweet, exotic floral fragrance. (A synthetic version is found in many commercial products to give them that distinctive jasmine scent.) Some laboratory studies found that high levels of benzyl acetate were linked to pancreatic cancer; it is advisable to use oils high in benzyl acetate at low concentrations (1% of a formulation). Note that *Jasminum grandiflorum* has higher levels of benzyl acetate than *J. sambac*.

FARNESENE (10-13%) This antimicrobial helps prevent and treat skin infections. It's also known to reduce skin inflammation.

METHYL JASMONATE (1-3%) This compound, along with jasmone, contributes to the fragrance of this absolute.

BENZYL BENZOATE (1-2%) This constituent has disinfecting properties, so it is useful in formulations targeted at fighting germs and viruses. It's also been shown to stop the spread of scabies, a contagious skin disease. Benzyl benzoate has many beneficial properties, but it is sensitizing (see page 27).

JASMONE (1-2%) This compound, along with methyl jasmonate, contributes to the fragrance of the absolute.

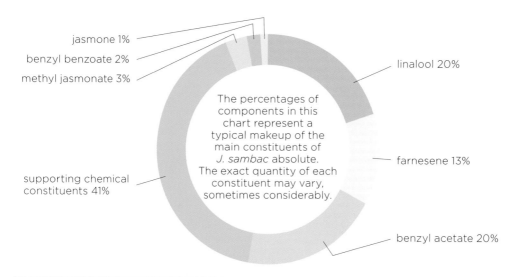

jasmone 1%
benzyl benzoate 2%
methyl jasmonate 3%
linalool 20%
The percentages of components in this chart represent a typical makeup of the main constituents of *J. sambac* absolute. The exact quantity of each constituent may vary, sometimes considerably.
farnesene 13%
supporting chemical constituents 41%
benzyl acetate 20%

GUIDELINES FOR USING

Jasmine Absolute
in Personal Care Products

SKIN CARE: A dilution of up to 3% can be used in products that are left on the skin. However, it's advisable to use lower dilutions of this absolute, as its extraction method may leave residues that can irritate skin.

BENEFITS

- calming and soothing
- suitable for most skin types, excluding sensitive skin
- deodorizing
- antibacterial

CONDITIONS

- dry skin
- fine lines
- tense muscles

PRODUCT	SKIN TYPE / CONDITION	QUANTITY
FACE		
Moisture gels	all skin types	1% (6 drops in 30 mL)
Facial masks	all skin types	1% (6 drops in 30 mL)
Toners	all skin types	1% (6 drops in 30 mL)
Cleansers	all skin types	1% (6 drops in 30 mL)
Exfoliants	all skin types	1% (6 drops in 30 mL)
Lip balms		1% (6 drops in 30 mL)
BODY		
Massage oils		1% (6 drops in 30 mL)
Body lotions		1% (6 drops in 30 mL)
Deodorants		1% (6 drops in 30 mL)
HANDS AND FEET		
Foot balms and butters		1% (6 drops in 30 mL)
HAIR AND SCALP		
Shampoos and conditioners*		1–3% (6–18 drops in 30 mL)
Leave-in conditioning balms for scalp treatment*		1–2% (6–12 drops in 30 mL)

* Exposing oils to heat and water will cause them to oxidize at a faster rate. Consider packaging shampoos and conditioners in flip-top or pump bottles to help reduce oxidation.

Juniper Berry

Botanical name: *Juniperus communis*

Botanical family: Cupressaceae

Habitat: native to the northern hemisphere, including Scandinavia, Siberia, Canada, northern Europe and northern Asia; essential oil produced mainly in Italy, France, Austria, Spain and Germany.

Aroma: evanescent fluid-like pine middle and top notes

OXIDATION ALERT

Juniper berry essential oil contains a significant amount of alpha-pinene, which oxidizes quite quickly. This can lead to skin irritation. Be particularly conscious of keeping any products containing high ranges of this essential oil away from heat, water and light.

Description of the Plant

Juniper is a prickly evergreen shrub or small tree that grows to a height of 40 feet (12 m). It has blue-green needle-like leaves, green-yellow flowers and small berries.

EXTRACTION: steam distillation of the crushed dried berries

Using Juniper Berry Oil in Natural Products

Juniper berry essential oil contains a fair amount of myrcene. Found in trace quantities in many essential oils, it is known for its ability to calm and soothe the nervous system. The alpha-pinene in this oil acts as an antimicrobial that can help stave off skin infections.

Juniper berry is ideal for treating oily skin conditions such as congested pores, as well as varicose veins. Use in personal care products such as cleansers, exfoliants, facial masks, body washes, shampoos and conditioners.

CAUTION: Some companies produce juniper essential oil from the needles and twigs of the tree, which results in a low-grade, heavily scented essential oil that can irritate skin.

PRECAUTIONS: Juniper berry essential oil is non-irritating when applied at or below the maximum recommended dilutions. Do not use during pregnancy or when breastfeeding. Properly stored, juniper berry essential oil has a shelf life of up to 2 years.

Main Chemical Constituents of Juniper Berry Essential Oil

ALPHA-PINENE (44-48%) This constituent is known for its ability to relieve pain and inflammation, and for being a potent antimicrobial that can help prevent and treat skin infections. When oxidized, it can lead to skin irritation.

MYRCENE (10-12%) This non-irritating, non-allergenic constituent is an antioxidant. It has sedative properties that help calm and soothe the nervous system.

SABINENE (10-12%) This constituent has antimicrobial properties, and it's responsible for the oil's spicy, woody scent.

BETA-PINENE (3-5%) This constituent has strong antimicrobial properties and is also very good at preventing skin infections. Beta-pinene carries a low risk of allergy.

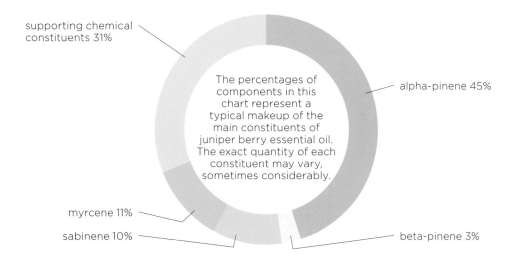

supporting chemical constituents 31%

alpha-pinene 45%

The percentages of components in this chart represent a typical makeup of the main constituents of juniper berry essential oil. The exact quantity of each constituent may vary, sometimes considerably.

myrcene 11%

sabinene 10%

beta-pinene 3%

GUIDELINES FOR USING

Juniper Berry Essential Oil in Personal Care Products

SKIN CARE: A dilution of up to 2% can be used in products that are left on the skin.

BENEFITS

- calming and relaxing
- antibacterial

CONDITIONS

- dandruff
- oily skin
- combination skin
- acne

PRODUCT	SKIN TYPE / CONDITION	QUANTITY
FACE		
Moisture gels	oily skin and acne	1% (6 drops in 30 mL)
Facial masks	oily skin and acne	1% (6 drops in 30 mL)
Toners	oily skin and acne	1.5% (9 drops in 30 mL)
Cleansers	oily skin and acne	2% (12 drops in 30 mL)
Exfoliants	all skin types	1% (6 drops in 30 mL)
BODY		
Massage oils		1–2% (6–12 drops in 30 mL)
Body lotions		1–2% (6–12 drops in 30 mL)
Body scrubs		1–2% (6–12 drops in 30 mL)
HANDS AND FEET		
Creams		1–3% (6–18 drops in 30 mL)
HAIR AND SCALP		
Shampoos and conditioners*	dandruff	3% (18 drops in 30 mL)
Scalp serums		1% (6 drops in 30 mL)

* Exposing oils to heat and water will cause them to oxidize at a faster rate. Consider packaging shampoos and conditioners in flip-top or pump bottles to help reduce oxidation.

Lavender

Botanical name: *Lavandula angustifolia*

Botanical family: Lamiaceae

Habitat: indigenous to the Mediterranean region; now cultivated worldwide

Aroma: fresh, soft herbaceous violet floral middle notes

Description of the Plant

This medium-tall (about $1^1/_2$ feet/0.6 m) plant has gray-green downy leaves and similarly colored stems. The essential oil is extracted from the flowers. Lavender essential oil was originally produced only in Provence, France. However, many small farmers in North America now grow the plant for essential oil production. This means there are many sources and varieties of lavender, each with a unique chemical composition.

EXTRACTION: steam distillation of the flowers

Using Lavender Oil in Natural Products

Lavender is one of the most popular essential oils in aromatherapy. It has a lovely scent and a calming and relaxing effect on the nervous system. It also has antibacterial and antifungal properties and soothes physical trauma.

CAUTIONS: Some types of lavender are not suitable for use on skin because they contain higher levels of camphor and eucalyptol, which severely dries the skin. Before using lavender in skin-care products — especially if they are intended for sensitive and damaged skin — ensure that the oil's camphor and eucalyptol levels are below 2% (see page 148).

PRECAUTIONS: Lavender essential oil is non-irritating when applied at or below the maximum recommended dilutions, unless you have a pre-existing sensitivity to any of its components. It is known to dissolve in sweat, and under the influence of sunlight it becomes an irritant; this may lead to allergic reactions, even in non-sensitive individuals. Use cautiously when pregnant or breastfeeding.

Properly stored, lavender essential oil has a shelf life of up to 2 years.

KNOW THE VARIETY

There are numerous types of lavender, and some are not suitable for skin-care products. When making skin-care products, use an essential oil derived from lavender grown at high altitudes. Pure high-altitude lavender, which is rich in esters and alcohols, does not contain high levels of camphor and eucalyptol, which can be irritants (see Cautions, left).

SENSITIVITY ALERT

Synthetic linalool is a fragrance that is very commonly used in mainstream products such as detergents, fabric softeners, air fresheners and cosmetics. If you have been overexposed to linalool, you may react to its presence in essential oils such as lavender.

Main Chemical Constituents of Lavender Essential Oil

LINALYL ACETATE (38-44%) This constituent absorbs through the skin and helps prevent and treat skin inflammation. It also has antispasmodic effects, so it can help relax muscles and relieve cramps.

LINALOOL (37-40%) This constituent absorbs through the skin and helps relieve swelling and inflammation. It is a pain-reliever as well as an antimicrobial. Linalool has many beneficial properties, but at high concentrations it can cause an allergic reaction (see page 31). It may also lead to irritation when oxidized (see Oxidation Alert, page 108).

BORNEOL (5-6%) This is a natural insect repellent that can help prevent disease carried by mosquitoes and other pests.

BETA-CARYOPHYLLENE (4-6%) This constituent has the ability to relieve pain and inflammation. It also has potential as a skin-lightening agent.

TERPINEN-4-OL (4-6%) This is a potent antibacterial agent; studies show that it's effective at clearing skin infections and relieving acne. Also, it's effective against skin mites and yeast infections on the skin. It is an anti-inflammatory and is easily absorbed into the skin.

EUCALYPTOL (2%) This pungent compound acts as a penetration enhancer (see page 54). It has also been shown to have antimicrobial and antifungal properties. When inhaled, eucalyptol acts as a decongestant that helps to release phlegm. However, applying skin-care products that contain high amounts of eucalyptol to the face can not only dry the skin but also affect the respiratory tract. Keep this in mind when formulating products for children and people with sensitivities.

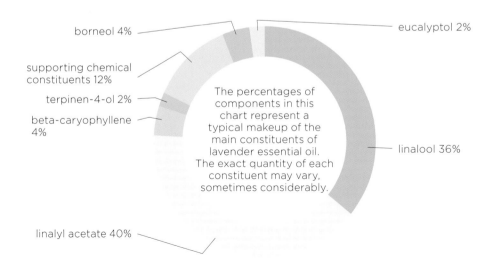

borneol 4%

supporting chemical constituents 12%

terpinen-4-ol 2%

beta-caryophyllene 4%

eucalyptol 2%

The percentages of components in this chart represent a typical makeup of the main constituents of lavender essential oil. The exact quantity of each constituent may vary, sometimes considerably.

linalool 36%

linalyl acetate 40%

GUIDELINES FOR USING

Lavender Essential Oil in Personal Care Products

SKIN CARE: A dilution of up to 3% can be used in products that are left on the skin.

BENEFITS

- calming and relaxing
- suitable for all skin types
- antibacterial
- antifungal
- anti-inflammatory

CONDITIONS

- acne
- inflamed skin
- sunburn
- eczema
- psoriasis

PRODUCT	SKIN TYPE / CONDITION	QUANTITY
FACE		
Moisture gels	all skin types	1–2% (6–12 drops in 30 mL)
Facial masks	all skin types	1–2% (6–12 drops in 30 mL)
Toners	all skin types	2% (12 drops in 30 mL)
Cleansers	all skin types	2–3% (12–18 drops in 30 mL)
Exfoliants	all skin types	2–3% (12–18 drops in 30 mL)
Lip balms		2–3% (12–18 drops in 30 mL)
BODY		
Massage oils		1–2% (6–12 drops in 30 mL)
Body lotions		1–2% (6–12 drops in 30 mL)
Body butters		2–3% (12–18 drops in 30 mL)
Deodorants		1–2% (6–12 drops in 30 mL)
HANDS AND FEET		
Foot balms and butters		2–3% (12–18 drops in 30 mL)
HAIR AND SCALP		
Shampoos and conditioners*		1–3% (6–18 drops in 30 mL)
Leave-in hair conditioning balms*		1–3% (6–18 drops in 30 mL)

* Exposing oils to heat and water will cause them to oxidize at a faster rate. Consider packaging shampoos and conditioners in flip-top or pump bottles to help reduce oxidation.

Lemon

Botanical name: *Citrus x limon*

Botanical family: Rutaceae

Habitat: native to Asia; now grows wild in the Mediterranean region, especially in Italy, Spain and Portugal; cultivated extensively in Italy, Israel and North and South America

Aroma: vigorous, bright citrus top notes

OXIDATION ALERT

Lemon essential oil contains a significant amount of D-limonene. This is one of the most commonly found constituents in fruit and it gives citrus fruits their distinctive citrus scent. However, it oxidizes quite quickly, which can lead to skin irritation. Be particularly conscious of keeping any products containing this essential oil away from heat, water and light.

Description of the Plant

The lemon tree grows to a height of 16 feet (5 m); it has dark green leaves and fragrant star-shaped flowers. The tree yields a sour fruit 3 to 5 inches (7.5 to 12.5 cm) long that has a thick yellow peel.

EXTRACTION: cold expression of the peel of the nearly ripe fruit

Using Lemon Essential Oil in Natural Products

The oil is recognized for its invigorating effect, which helps to promotes alertness. This makes it a lovely addition to morning cleansing routines; use the oil to create revitalizing shampoos, body washes and lotions. Lemon essential oil is slightly antibacterial and antifungal, which is beneficial for treating oily and acne-prone skin; use it in cleansers, toners and moisture gels for oily skin.

CAUTIONS: Lemon essential oil contains trace amounts of furocoumarins, which are organic chemical compounds known to promote phototoxicity on the skin. Use products containing this oil sparingly if you will be exposing skin to the sun or other UV radiation, or avoid sun exposure for 12 hours after regular application.

PRECAUTIONS: Lemon essential oil is non-irritating when applied at or below the maximum recommended dilutions. However, the oil should not be applied to damaged or sunburned skin. Use cautiously when pregnant or breastfeeding. This essential oil is prone to oxidization, which may cause sensitization. Properly stored, lemon essential oil has a shelf life of 6 to 8 months.

Main Chemical Constituents of Lemon Essential Oil

D-LIMONENE (65–70%) This is one of the most commonly found constituents in fruit, and what gives lemons and other citrus fruits their distinctive scent. D-limonene oxidizes quite quickly, which can lead to skin irritation.

GAMMA-TERPINENE (10–12%) This constituent has strong antibacterial properties that can help prevent skin infections. It also slows the oxidation of linoleic acid, so it can act as a preservative when added to carrier oils.

BETA-PINENE (10%) This constituent has strong antimicrobial properties and is also very good at preventing skin infections. Beta-pinene carries a low risk of allergy.

MYRCENE (2%) This non-irritating, non-allergenic constituent is an antioxidant. It has sedative properties that help calm and soothe the nervous system.

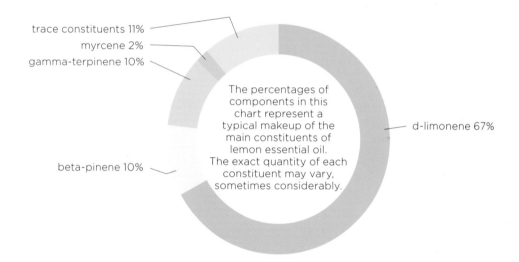

trace constituents 11%

myrcene 2%

gamma-terpinene 10%

beta-pinene 10%

d-limonene 67%

The percentages of components in this chart represent a typical makeup of the main constituents of lemon essential oil. The exact quantity of each constituent may vary, sometimes considerably.

GUIDELINES FOR USING

Lemon Essential Oil
in Personal Care Products

SKIN CARE: A dilution of up to 2% can be used in products that are left on the skin.

BENEFITS

- uplifting
- refreshing and invigorating
- antibacterial

CONDITIONS

- acne
- oily skin
- warts
- boils
- fungal infections
- cuts

PRODUCT	SKIN TYPE / CONDITION	QUANTITY
FACE		
Moisture gels	acne	1% (6 drops in 30 mL)
Facial masks	oily skin and acne	1% (6 drops in 30 mL)
Toners	oily skin and acne	1.5% (9 drops in 30 mL)
Cleansers	oily skin and acne	2% (12 drops in 30 mL)
BODY		
Massage oils		1–2% (6–12 drops in 30 mL)
Body lotions		1–2% (6–12 drops in 30 mL)
Deodorants		1–2% (6–12 drops in 30 mL)
Exfoliants		1–2% (6–12 drops in 30 mL)
HANDS AND FEET		
Nail whitening and cuticle repair oils		1–2% (6–12 drops in 30 mL)
HAIR AND SCALP		
Shampoos and conditioners*		1–3% (6–18 drops in 30 mL)

* Exposing oils to heat and water will cause them to oxidize at a faster rate. (The d-limonene in lemon essential oil will cause it to oxidize particularly quickly.) Consider packaging shampoos and conditioners in flip-top or pump bottles to help reduce oxidation.

Lemongrass

Botanical names: *Cymbopogon citratus* (West Indian lemongrass); *C. flexuosus* (East Indian lemongrass)

Botanical family: Poaceae

Habitat: native to Asia; now cultivated in the West Indies, Africa and other tropical regions

Aroma: deep citrus middle and base notes

Description of the Plant

Lemongrass is a tall, aromatic perennial grass. The fast-growing leaves can reach up to 5 feet (1.5 m) in height. The scent of this tropical grass is strong, lemony and herbaceous.

EXTRACTION: steam distillation of the partially dried leaves

Using Lemongrass Oil in Natural Products

This essential oil is highly effective at stopping excessive perspiration and is well suited to skin-care products that address bacterial and fungal infections. The high levels of citral in this oil are responsible for its sedative properties, and citral can also aid with insomnia. Thus this essential oil is ideal for use in nighttime cleansers, toners and facial masks. Note that lemongrass essential oil will dominate the scent of a skin-care product.

CAUTION: In large amounts, the citral in lemongrass essential oil may be overpowering in its sedative effect. Do not exceed the maximum recommended dilution.

PRECAUTIONS: Do not use when pregnant or breasfeeding. Properly stored, lemongrass essential oil has a shelf life of 1 year.

OXIDATION ALERT

The citral in lemongrass essential oil is a skin irritant and will also cause it to oxidize very quickly. Be particularly conscious of keeping any products containing high ranges of this oil away from heat, water and light.

Main Chemical Constituents of Lemongrass Essential Oil

CITRAL (80-85%) Neral and geranial are forms of citral. These constituents have strong antifungal and antibacterial activity, meaning that they can prevent or slow the growth of fungi and bacteria. Citral is also known for its sedative properties that help calm and soothe the nervous system. Although this component has many beneficial properties, it is a skin irritant and has a high oxidation rate (see page 29).

FARNESOL (5-8%) Farnesol is an antimicrobial that helps prevent and treat skin infections. It's also known for its ability to reduce skin inflammation. As a bonus, farnesol helps smooth fine lines and increases the skin's elasticity.

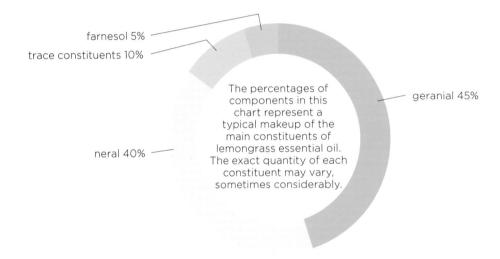

farnesol 5%

trace constituents 10%

geranial 45%

neral 40%

The percentages of components in this chart represent a typical makeup of the main constituents of lemongrass essential oil. The exact quantity of each constituent may vary, sometimes considerably.

Lemongrass Essential Oil in Personal Care Products

SKIN CARE: A dilution of up to 1% can be used in products that are left on the skin.

BENEFITS

- toning
- deodorizing
- antibacterial

CONDITIONS

- acne
- oily skin
- mature skin
- dull skin
- insect bites
- cold sores
- athlete's foot
- candida skin infections
- excessive perspiration

PRODUCT	SKIN TYPE / CONDITION	QUANTITY
FACE		
Moisture gels	acne	0.5% (3 drops in 30 mL)
Facial masks	oily skin and acne	0.5% (3 drops in 30 mL)
Toners	oily skin and acne	0.5% (3 drops in 30 mL)
Cleansers	oily skin and acne	0.5% (3 drops in 30 mL)
Exfoliants	oily skin and acne	0.5% (3 drops in 30 mL)
Lip balms		0.5% (3 drops in 30 mL)
BODY		
Massage oils		0.5% (3 drops in 30 mL)
Body lotions		1% (6 drops in 30 mL)
Deodorants		0.5% (3 drops in 30 mL)
Exfoliants		0.5% (3 drops in 30 mL)
HANDS AND FEET		
Foot balms and butters		1% (6 drops in 30 mL)
HAIR AND SCALP		
Shampoos*	dandruff	1% (6 drops in 30 mL)
Leave-in conditioning balms for scalp treatment*		0.5% (3 drops in 30 mL)

* Exposing oils to heat and water will cause them to oxidize at a faster rate. Consider packaging shampoos and conditioners in flip-top or pump bottles to help reduce oxidation.

Lime

Botanical name: *Citrus aurantifolia*

Botanical family: Rutaceae

Habitat: native to southern Asia; cultivated in many tropical and subtropical regions of the world

Aroma: bold green citrus with fleeting top notes

OXIDATION ALERT

Lime essential oil contains a significant amount of D-limonene. This is one of the most commonly found constituents in fruit and it gives citrus fruits their distinctive citrus scent. However, it oxidizes quite quickly, which can lead to skin irritation. Be particularly conscious of keeping any products containing this essential oil away from heat, water and light.

Description of the Plant

The *Citrus aurantifolia* tree grows to a height of 16 feet (5 m); it has dark green leaves and fragrant star-shaped flowers. The tree yields a round, tart fruit that has a thick green peel. Today the tree is cultivated mainly in southern Florida, Cuba, Mexico and Italy. The fruits are known as Key limes in culinary applications.

EXTRACTION: cold expression or steam distillation of the rind of the fruit (see "Cautions," below)

Using Lime Oil in Natural Products

Lime essential oil is a very good choice for treating oily skin and acne. When used in moderation, it has a calming and relaxing effect on the nervous system. It's also a great addition to massage oils, as its stimulating effects can help detox the body. Lime can be used in morning cleansers, moisturizers, toners, shampoos, conditioners, body washes and exfoliants.

CAUTIONS: Cold-expressed lime essential oil is highly phototoxic and potentially carcinogenic. The distilled version is not phototoxic and is safe to use in cosmetics. Always verify that the label on a bottle of lime essential oil says "distilled." Check the gas chromatography report as well, to make sure that the essential oil is free of coumarins.

PRECAUTIONS: The high level of d-limonene in this essential oil makes it prone to oxidization, which may cause irritation. Use cautiously when pregnant or breastfeeding. Properly stored, lime essential oil has a shelf life of 6 to 8 months.

Main Chemical Constituents of Lime Essential Oil

D-LIMONENE (65–75%) This is one of the most commonly found constituents in fruit and gives limes and other citrus fruits their distinctive citrus scent. D-limonene oxidizes quite quickly, which can lead to skin irritation.

GAMMA-TERPINENE (12–15%) This constituent has strong antibacterial properties that can help prevent skin infections. It slows down oxidization of linoleic acid and it can act as a preservative when added to carrier oils.

ALPHA-TERPINOLENE (10–12%) There's evidence that this constituent has antioxidant and antiviral properties.

MYRCENE (4–6%) This non-irritating, non-allergenic constituent is an antioxidant. It has sedative properties that help calm and soothe the nervous system.

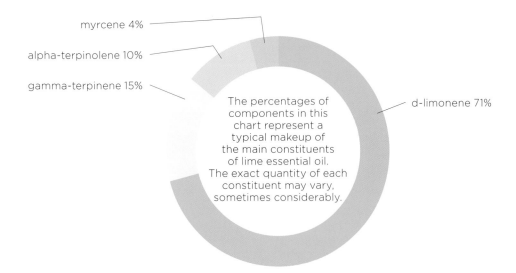

myrcene 4%

alpha-terpinolene 10%

gamma-terpinene 15%

d-limonene 71%

The percentages of components in this chart represent a typical makeup of the main constituents of lime essential oil. The exact quantity of each constituent may vary, sometimes considerably.

GUIDELINES FOR USING

Lime Essential Oil in Personal Care Products

SKIN CARE: A dilution of up to 3% can be used in products that are left on the skin.

BENEFITS

- uplifting and invigorating
- antibacterial
- toning

CONDITIONS

- acne
- bacterial infections
- viral infections
- tired-looking skin

PRODUCT	SKIN TYPE / CONDITION	QUANTITY
FACE		
Moisture creams and gels	all skin types	1% (6 drops in 30 mL)
Facial masks	all skin types	1% (6 drops in 30 mL)
Toners	all skin types	1–2% (6–12 drops in 30 mL)
Cleansers	all skin types	1–3% (6–18 drops in 30 mL)
Exfoliants	all skin types	2% (12 drops in 30 mL)
Lip balms		1–3% (6–18 drops in 30 mL)
BODY		
Massage oils		1–3% (6–18 drops in 30 mL)
Body lotions		1–3% (6–18 drops in 30 mL)
Exfoliants		1–3% (6–18 drops in 30 mL)
HANDS AND FEET		
Toning creams or ointments		1–3% (6–18 drops in 30 mL)
HAIR AND SCALP		
Shampoos and conditioners*		3% (18 drops in 30 mL)

* Exposing oils to heat and water will cause them to oxidize at a faster rate. (The d-limonene in lime essential oil will cause it to oxidize particularly quickly.) Consider packaging shampoos and conditioners in flip-top or pump bottles to help reduce oxidation.

Mandarin

Botanical name: *Citrus reticulata*

Botanical family: Rutaceae

Habitat: native to southern China

Aroma: full-bodied citrus and honey top notes

Description of the Plant

The *Citrus reticulata* tree grows up to 15 feet (4.5 m) in height. It has glossy leaves and fragrant white flowers. The tree produces mandarins — small, spherical fruits that resemble oranges but are sweeter in flavor. These citrus fruits were brought to Europe in 1805 and then to the United States in 1845, where they became known as tangerines. Today mandarins are grown mainly in Italy, Spain, Algeria, Cyprus, Greece, the Middle East and Brazil.

EXTRACTION: cold expression of the peel of the nearly ripe fruit

Using Mandarin Oil in Natural Products

Part of what differentiates mandarin from other citrus essential oils is its slightly elevated level of dimethyl anthranilate, a constituent that gives this oil its sweet scent and uplifting effect. Use it to create invigorating body lotions and massage oils. Mandarin essential oil also contains significant levels of gamma-terpinene, a constituent recognized for its ability to act as a preservative in most carrier oils. Adding mandarin essential oil to your personal care products may extend their shelf life.

CAUTIONS: Mandarin essential oil contains trace amounts of furocoumarins, which are organic chemical compounds known to promote phototoxicity on the skin. Use products containing this oil sparingly if you will be exposing your skin to the sun or other UV radiation, or avoid sun exposure for 12 hours after regular application.

PRECAUTIONS: The high level of d-limonene in this essential oil makes it prone to oxidization, which may cause sensitization. Use cautiously when pregnant or breastfeeding. Properly stored, mandarin essential oil has a shelf life of 6 to 8 months.

OXIDATION ALERT

Mandarin essential oil contains a significant amount of D-limonene. This is one of the most commonly found constituents in fruit and it gives citrus fruits their distinctive citrus scent. However, it oxidizes quite quickly, which can lead to skin irritation. Be particularly conscious of keeping any products containing this essential oil away from heat, water and light.

Main Chemical Constituents of Mandarin Essential Oil

D-LIMONENE (65–75%) This is one of the most commonly found constituents in fruit, and it gives limes and other citrus fruits their distinctive citrus scent. D-limonene is absorbed into the skin. This constituent oxidizes quite quickly, which can lead to skin irritation.

GAMMA-TERPINENE (18–20%) This constituent has strong antibacterial properties, which can help prevent skin infections. It also slows the oxidation of linoleic acid, so it can act as a preservative when added to most carrier oils.

BETA-PINENE (2–4%) This constituent has strong antimicrobial properties and is also very good at preventing skin infections. Beta-pinene carries a low risk of allergy, but when oxidized can lead to skin irritation.

MYRCENE (2–4%) This non-irritating, non-allergenic constituent is an antioxidant. It has sedative properties that help calm and soothe the nervous system.

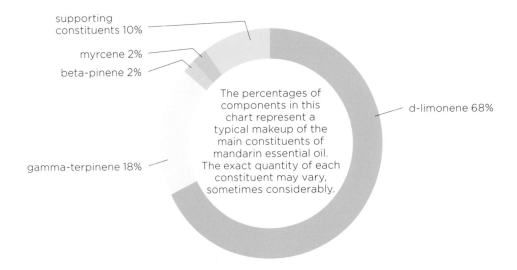

supporting constituents 10%

myrcene 2%

beta-pinene 2%

gamma-terpinene 18%

The percentages of components in this chart represent a typical makeup of the main constituents of mandarin essential oil. The exact quantity of each constituent may vary, sometimes considerably.

d-limonene 68%

GUIDELINES FOR USING

Mandarin Essential Oil in Personal Care Products

SKIN CARE: A dilution of up to 3% can be used in products that are left on the skin.

BENEFITS

- uplifting
- suitable for all skin types
- antibacterial

CONDITIONS

- acne
- fungal infections
- viral infections

PRODUCT	SKIN TYPE / CONDITION	QUANTITY
FACE		
Moisture creams and gels	all skin types	1–2% (6–12 drops in 30 mL)
Facial masks	all skin types	1–2% (6–12 drops in 30 mL)
Toners	all skin types	1–2% (6–12 drops in 30 mL)
Cleansers	all skin types	1–2% (6–12 drops in 30 mL)
Exfoliants	all skin types	1–2% (6–12 drops in 30 mL)
BODY		
Massage oils		1–3% (6–18 drops in 30 mL)
Body lotions		1–3% (6–18 drops in 30 mL)
Deodorants		1–3% (6–18 drops in 30 mL)
Exfoliants		1–3% (6–18 drops in 30 mL)
HANDS AND FEET		
Creams		1–3% (6–18 drops in 30 mL)
HAIR AND SCALP		
Shampoos and conditioners*		3% (18 drops in 30 mL)
Hair serums		1–2% (6–12 drops in 30 mL)

* Exposing oils to heat and water will cause them to oxidize at a faster rate. (The d-limonene in mandarin essential oil will cause it to oxidize particularly quickly.) Consider packaging shampoos and conditioners in flip-top or pump bottles to help reduce oxidation.

Sweet Marjoram

Botanical name: *Origanum majorana*

Botanical family: Lamiaceae

Habitat: native to North Africa and southwest Asia; cultivated in the United States, Egypt, Hungary and several Mediterranean countries

Aroma: warm, herbaceous, spicy, camphor and woody scent

OXIDATION ALERT

Sweet marjoram essential oil contains a significant amount of linalool, a constituent that absorbs through the skin and helps relieve swelling and inflammation. It is a pain-reliever as well as an antimicrobial. Linalool has a calming floral scent that has many beneficial properties, but at high concentrations it can cause an allergic reaction. Also, when oxidized it can lead to irritation (see page 27). Be particularly conscious of keeping any products containing this essential oil away from heat, water and light.

Description of Plant

This perennial herb reaches a height of just over $1^1/_2$ feet (45 cm). It has small, oval gray-green leaves and pink or purple flowers.

EXTRACTION: steam distillation of the dried herb

Using Sweet Marjoram Oil in Natural Products

In traditional aromatherapy, sweet marjoram is used to help ease pain and tension. It is the perfect essential oil to use in products for those who are feeling stressed and agitated. Sweet marjoram essential oil acts as a sedative that helps calm and soothe the nervous system; it also has strong antibacterial properties. Add it to nighttime moisture creams, lotions and body oils.

CAUTION: In large amounts, sweet marjoram essential oil may make you drowsy. Do not exceed the maximum recommended dilution.

PRECAUTIONS: Sweet marjoram essential oil is non-irritating when applied at or below the maximum recommended dilutions, unless you have a pre-existing sensitivity to any of its components (such as linalool.) Avoid use during pregnancy and while breastfeeding. Properly stored, sweet marjoram essential oil has a shelf life of 2 years.

Main Chemical Constituents of Sweet Marjoram Essential Oil

TERPINEN-4-OL (48–53%) This constituent is a potent antibacterial agent; studies show that it's effective at clearing skin infections and relieving acne. It's also effective against skin mites and yeast infections on the skin. This anti-inflammatory is absorbed easily into the skin.

LINALOOL (18–20%) This constituent absorbs through the skin and helps relieve swelling and inflammation. It is a pain-reliever as well as an antimicrobial. Linalool has many beneficial properties — for instance, it is calming — but at high concentrations it can cause an allergic reaction (see page 31).

ALPHA-TERPINEOL (10–12%) This constituent has strong antibacterial properties, which can help prevent skin infections.

LINALYL ACETATE (8–10%) Combined with linalool, this constituent can help prevent and treat skin inflammation. It absorbs through the skin and has antispasmodic effects, so it can help relax muscles and relieve cramps.

MYRCENE (5%) This non-irritating, non-allergenic constituent is an antioxidant. It has sedative properties that help calm and soothe the nervous system.

TERPINOLENE (5%) There's evidence that this constituent has antioxidant and antiviral properties.

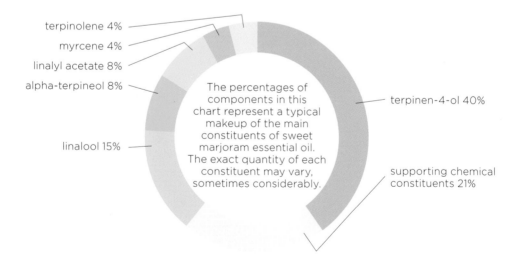

terpinolene 4%
myrcene 4%
linalyl acetate 8%
alpha-terpineol 8%
linalool 15%

terpinen-4-ol 40%

supporting chemical constituents 21%

The percentages of components in this chart represent a typical makeup of the main constituents of sweet marjoram essential oil. The exact quantity of each constituent may vary, sometimes considerably.

Sweet Marjoram Essential Oil in Personal Care Products

SKIN CARE: A dilution of up to 3% can be used in products that are left on the skin.

BENEFITS

- calming and sedating
- antibacterial
- antifungal

CONDITIONS

- acne
- hyperpigmentation
- candida skin infections
- blotchy skin

PRODUCT	SKIN TYPE / CONDITION	QUANTITY
FACE		
Moisture creams	oily skin and acne	2% (12 drops in 30 mL)
Facial masks	oily skin and acne	2% (12 drops in 30 mL)
Toners	oily skin and acne	2–3% (12–18 drops in 30 mL)
Cleansers	oily skin and acne	2–3% (12–18 drops in 30 mL)
Exfoliants	oily skin and acne	2–3% (12–18 drops in 30 mL)
BODY		
Massage oils		2–3% (12–18 drops in 30 mL)
Body lotions		2–3% (12–18 drops in 30 mL)
HANDS AND FEET		
Ointments		2–3% (12–18 drops in 30 mL)
HAIR AND SCALP		
Shampoos and conditioners*		3% (18 drops in 30 mL)
Scalp serums		1% (6 drops in 30 mL)

* Exposing oils to heat and water will cause them to oxidize at a faster rate. Consider packaging shampoos and conditioners in flip-top or pump bottles to help reduce oxidation.

Myrrh

Botanical name: *Commiphora myrrha*

Botanical family: Burseraceae

Habitat: native to northeast Africa and southwest Asia; cultivated in the Red Sea region, including Somalia, Yemen and Ethiopia

Aroma: deep amber resin aroma

Description of the Plant

Typically found in rocky, hilly areas, this shrubby tree grows to more than 10 feet (3 m) tall. Its thorny branches have small green leaves and it blooms with green flowers in the months of August and September. To harvest myrrh, deep incisions are made in the trunk of the tree and small waxy droplets of resin exude from the wounds. The solidified resin is yellow and glossy.

EXTRACTION: steam distillation of the resin

Using Myrrh Oil in Natural Products

Myrrh essential oil is a potent viscous liquid that is known in aromatherapy as one of the leading oils for skin repair. One of its main constituents, curzerene, has been found to have wound-healing properties. Use this oil in cleansers, toners and moisturizers for wounded or inflamed skin and in ointments for dry, chapped hands and feet.

PRECAUTIONS: Myrrh is non-irritating when applied at or below the maximum recommended dilutions, although it may be irritating to sensitive skin. Avoid using during pregnancy and breastfeeding. Properly stored, myrrh essential oil has a shelf life of up to 2 years.

Main Chemical Constituents of Myrrh Essential Oil

FURANOEUDESMA (38–40%) The exact properties of this constituent are unknown at the moment; more studies are required. However, we do know that the chemical group it belongs to is classified as an anti-inflammatory.

CURZERENE (26–30%) This constituent has been found to have wound-healing properties.

FURANODIENE (18–20%) The exact properties of this constituent are unknown at the moment; more studies are required. However, we do know that the chemical group it belongs to is classified as an anti-inflammatory.

LINDESTRENE (12–15%) The exact properties of this constituent are unknown at the moment; more studies are required. However, we do know that the chemical group it belongs to is classified as an anti-inflammatory.

BETA-ELEMENE (1–3%) Research found that this constituent helped stop cancer cells from proliferating.

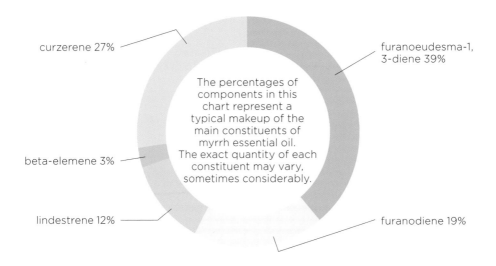

curzerene 27%

furanoeudesma-1, 3-diene 39%

The percentages of components in this chart represent a typical makeup of the main constituents of myrrh essential oil. The exact quantity of each constituent may vary, sometimes considerably.

beta-elemene 3%

lindestrene 12%

furanodiene 19%

GUIDELINES FOR USING

Myrrh Essential Oil
in Personal Care Products

SKIN CARE: A dilution of up to 2% can be used in products that are left on the skin.

BENEFITS

- toning
- antiseptic
- antibacterial
- wound healing

CONDITIONS

- oily and combination skin
- aging skin
- acne
- fine lines

PRODUCT	SKIN TYPE / CONDITION	QUANTITY
FACE		
Moisture gels	acne, wounds and inflamed skin	1% (6–8 drops in 30 mL)
Eye creams	all skin types	0.5% (3 drops in 30 mL)
Facial masks	acne, wounds and inflamed skin	1% (6 drops in 30 mL)
Toners	acne, wounds and inflamed skin	1.5% (9 drops in 30 mL)
Cleansers	acne, wounds and inflamed skin	2% (12 drops in 30 mL)
Lip balms		1–2% (6–12 drops in 30 mL)
BODY		
Massage oils		1–2% (6–12 drops in 30 mL)
Body lotions		1–2% (6–12 drops in 30 mL)
Ointments	various skin conditions	1–2% (6–12 drops in 30 mL)
HANDS AND FEET		
Ointments		2–3% (12–18 drops in 30 mL)
Lotions/butters		2–3% (12–18 drops in 30 mL)
HAIR AND SCALP		
Hair serums		1% (6 drops in 30 mL)

* Exposing oils to heat and water will cause them to oxidize at a faster rate. Consider packaging shampoos and conditioners in flip-top or pump bottles to help reduce oxidation.

Neroli (Orange Blossom)

Botanical name: *Citrus* x *aurantium* subsp. *amara*

Botanical family: Rutaceae

Habitat: native to India and southern China; now cultivated primarily in Italy, Tunisia, Morocco, Egypt, France and the United States

Aroma: soft herbaceous and white floral middle notes

A NICE ALTERNATIVE

Neroli essential oil is expensive. An alternative is petitgrain essential oil, which is more economical but will still add that beautiful herbaceous scent to your personal care products.

SENSITIVITY ALERT

Synthetic linalool is a fragrance that is commonly used in many mainstream products such as detergents, fabric softeners, air fresheners and cosmetics. If you have been overexposed to linalool, you may react to its presence in essential oils such as neroli.

Description of the Plant

The bitter orange tree grows from 10 to 30 feet (3 to 9 m) in height. It yields three types of essential oils that are very different in their chemical components: neroli (from the blossoms), petitgrain (from the leaves) and bitter orange (from the fruit). The tree is in full bloom from November to March; the highly fragrant waxy white flowers develop in clusters, forming "bouquets" around the tree.

EXTRACTION: steam distillation of the freshly picked flowers (orange flower water and an absolute are by-products)

Using Neroli Oil in Natural Products

Despite its being quite expensive, neroli essential oil is used extensively in personal care products because it is a gentle and versatile oil. Neroli's soft, heavenly scent has been shown to have a calming effect on the nervous system. This oil is suitable for all skin types and is ideal for anti-aging facial products, as it has a toning effect on mature skin. The fragrance also makes it a wonderful addition to relaxing massage oils, and it's gentle enough to be used in massage oils for sensitive skin. Neroli essential oil can be used in all morning and evening skin-care products.

PRECAUTIONS: This oil is non-irritating when applied at or below the maximum recommended dilutions, unless you have a pre-existing sensitivity to any of its components (such as linalool, which makes up a large percentage). Use with caution during pregnancy or while breastfeeding. Properly stored, neroli essential oil has a shelf life of up to 2 years.

Main Chemical Constituents of Neroli Essential Oil

LINALOOL (48–50%) This constituent is absorbed through the skin and helps relieve swelling and inflammation. It is a pain-reliever as well as antimicrobial. Linalool has many beneficial properties, but at high concentrations it can cause an allergic reaction (see page 31). When oxidized it can also lead to skin irritation (see Oxidation Alert, page 162).

LINALYL ACETATE (8–10%) This constituent is absorbed through the skin and helps prevent and treat skin inflammation. It also has antispasmodic effects, so it can help relax muscles and relieve cramps.

ALPHA-TERPINEOL (6–8%) This constituent has strong antibacterial properties, which can help prevent skin infections.

GERANIOL (4–7%) This component has strong antifungal and antibacterial activity, meaning that it can prevent or slow the growth of fungi and bacteria. Geraniol has many beneficial properties, but at high concentrations it can be a skin irritant and sensitizer, or even lead to an allergic reaction.

BETA-PINENE (4–6%) This constituent has strong antimicrobial properties and is also very good at preventing skin infections. It carries a low allergy risk. When oxidized it can lead to skin irritation.

FARNESOL (3–5%) This is an antimicrobial that helps prevent and treat skin infections. It's also known for its ability to reduce skin inflammation. As a bonus, farnesol helps smooth fine lines and increases the skin's elasticity.

MYRCENE (1–3%) This is non-irritating, non-allergenic and an antioxidant. It has sedative properties that help calm and soothe the nervous system.

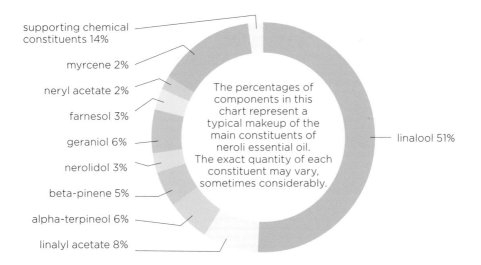

supporting chemical constituents 14%
myrcene 2%
neryl acetate 2%
farnesol 3%
geraniol 6%
nerolidol 3%
beta-pinene 5%
alpha-terpineol 6%
linalyl acetate 8%

The percentages of components in this chart represent a typical makeup of the main constituents of neroli essential oil. The exact quantity of each constituent may vary, sometimes considerably.

linalool 51%

GUIDELINES FOR USING

Neroli Essential Oil in Personal Care Products

SKIN CARE: A dilution of up to 3% can be used in products that are left on the skin.

BENEFITS

- toning
- gentle
- suitable for all skin types

CONDITIONS

- eczema
- psoriasis
- broken capillaries
- acne
- dull or blotchy skin
- fine lines

PRODUCT	SKIN TYPE / CONDITION	QUANTITY
FACE		
Moisture creams	all skin types	1–2% (6–12 drops in 30 mL)
Facial masks	all skin types	1–2% (6–12 drops in 30 mL)
Toners	all skin types	2% (12 drops in 30 mL)
Cleansers	all skin types	2–3% (12–18 drops in 30 mL)
BODY		
Massage oils	all skin types	1–2% (6–12 drops in 30 mL)
Body lotions		1–2% (6–12 drops in 30 mL)
Ointments		1–2% (6–12 drops in 30 mL)
HANDS AND FEET		
Foot balms and butters		2–3% (12–18 drops in 30 mL)
HAIR AND SCALP		
Leave-in conditioning balms for scalp treatment*		1–2% (6–12 drops in 30 mL)

* Exposing oils to heat and water will cause them to oxidize at a faster rate. Consider packaging shampoos and conditioners in flip-top or pump bottles to help reduce oxidation.

Orange

Botanical names: *Citrus* x *aurantium* subsp. *amara* (bitter orange); *Citrus* x *sinensis* (sweet orange)

Botanical family: Rutaceae

Habitat: native to India and southern China

Aroma: full-bodied bitter citrus top notes (bitter orange); light citrus top notes (sweet orange)

Description of the Plant

Both species of orange trees have dark green leaves and fragrant star-shaped white blossoms. Bitter oranges are cultivated primarily in Italy, Tunisia, Morocco, Egypt, France and the United States; sweet oranges are grown in Spain, the West Indies, Italy and Brazil.

EXTRACTION: cold expression of the outer peel of almost ripe fruit.

Using Orange Oil in Natural Products

The delightful radiant fragrance of orange essential oil makes it a terrific addition to many personal care products. The scent of orange is almost universally calming — there's evidence that bitter orange essential oil may have sedative effects, while sweet orange essential oil has been found to relieve anxiety. Use it in cleansers, toners, moisturizers and masks for all skin types, and also in rejuvenating body lotions and massage oils.

CAUTIONS: Orange essential oil contains trace amounts of furocoumarins, which are organic chemical compounds known to promote phototoxicity on the skin. Use products containing this oil sparingly if you will be exposing your skin to the sun or other UV radiation, or avoid sun exposure for 12 hours after regular application.

PRECAUTIONS: Orange essential oil is non-irritating when applied at or below the maximum recommended dilutions. However, the oil should not be applied to damaged or sunburned skin. The high level of d-limonene in this essential oil makes it prone to oxidization, which may cause irritation. Properly stored, orange essential oil has a shelf life of 6 to 8 months.

KNOW THE TYPE

Bitter orange and sweet orange essential oils are produced from the fruit of different subspecies of orange trees. Here they are grouped together as "orange" because they can be used interchangeably when creating personal care products.

OXIDATION ALERT

Orange essential oil contains a significant amount of d-limonene, one of the most commonly found constituents in fruit. However, it oxidizes quite quickly, which can lead to skin irritation. Be particularly conscious of keeping any products containing this essential oil away from heat, water and light.

Main Chemical Constituents of Orange Essential Oils

D-LIMONENE (85–95%) This is one of the most commonly found constituents in fruit, and it's what gives oranges and other citrus fruits their distinctive citrus scent. D-limonene oxidizes quite quickly, which can lead to skin irritation.

MYRCENE (1–3%) This non-irritating, non-allergenic constituent is an antioxidant. It has sedative properties that help calm and soothe the nervous system.

LINALOOL (1–2%) This constituent is absorbed through the skin and helps relieve swelling and inflammation. It is a pain-reliever as well as antimicrobial. Linalool has many beneficial properties — for instance, it is calming and has a pleasant floral scent — but at high concentrations it can cause an allergic reaction (see page 31). When oxidized it can lead to skin irritation.

ALPHA-PINENE (1–2%) This constituent is known for its ability to relieve pain and inflammation, and for being a potent antimicrobial that can help prevent and treat skin infections. When oxidized, it can lead to skin irritation.

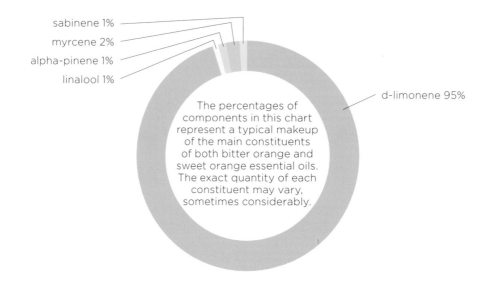

sabinene 1%
myrcene 2%
alpha-pinene 1%
linalool 1%

d-limonene 95%

The percentages of components in this chart represent a typical makeup of the main constituents of both bitter orange and sweet orange essential oils. The exact quantity of each constituent may vary, sometimes considerably.

GUIDELINES FOR USING

Orange Essential Oils in Personal Care Products

SKIN CARE: A dilution of up to 3% can be used in products that are left on the skin.

BENEFITS

- calming
- toning
- suitable for all skin types

CONDITIONS

- acne
- dull, tired-looking skin

PRODUCT	SKIN TYPE / CONDITION	QUANTITY
FACE		
Moisture creams and gels	oily skin	1% (6 drops in 30 mL)
Facial masks	oily skin	1% (6 drops in 30 mL)
Toners	oily skin	1.5% (9 drops in 30 mL)
Cleansers	oily skin	2% (12 drops in 30 mL)
BODY		
Massage oils		1–2% (6–12 drops in 30 mL)
Body lotions		1–2% (6–12 drops in 30 mL)
Deodorants		1–2% (6–12 drops in 30 mL)
Exfoliants		1–2% (6–12 drops in 30 mL)
HANDS AND FEET		
Creams		1–2% (6–12 drops in 30 mL)
HAIR AND SCALP		
Shampoos and conditioners*		3% (18 drops in 30 mL)

* Exposing oils to heat and water will cause them to oxidize at a faster rate. (The d-limonene in orange essential oil will cause it to oxidize particularly quickly.) Consider packaging shampoos and conditioners in flip-top or pump bottles to help reduce oxidation.

Palmarosa

Botanical name: *Cymbopogon martinii*

Botanical family: Poaceae

Habitat: native to India; now grown in Brazil, Indonesia and the Seychelles and Comoro Islands

Aroma: Bold, floral rose middle notes

Description of the Plant

Palmarosa essential oil comes from a species of *Cymbopogon*, better known as lemongrass. This fragrant perennial clumping grass grows to heights of 3 to 10 feet (1 to 3 m). It has long, slender green stems and flowering tops.

EXTRACTION: steam distillation of the fresh or dried grass

Using Palmarosa in Natural Products

Palmarosa essential oil is used in many cosmetic products for its rose-like fragrance. This oil is used to treat conditions such as acne, oily skin and thrush and other fungal infections. Use it in cleansers, toners, creams and gels for oily and acne-prone skin. Palmarosa essential oil also has a deodorizing effect, which makes it a good choice for deodorants, body washes, shampoos and conditioners.

PRECAUTIONS: The high levels of geraniol in this essential oil can lead to skin irritation, particularly with sensitive skin. Avoid using when pregnant or breastfeeding. Properly stored, palmarosa essential oil has a shelf life of 2 years.

Major Chemical Constituents of Palmarosa Essential Oil

GERANIOL (75-80%) This constituent contributes to palmarosa's rose-like scent. Geraniol has strong antifungal and antibacterial activity, meaning that it can prevent or slow the growth of fungi and bacteria. Geraniol has many beneficial properties, but at high concentrations it can be a skin irritant and sensitizer, or even lead to an allergic reaction.

GERANYL ACETATE (8-10%) This constituent has antispasmodic effects, so it can help relax muscles and relieve cramps.

FARNESOL (4-6%) As an antimicrobial, farnesol helps prevent and treat skin infections. It's also known for its ability to reduce skin inflammation. As a bonus, farnesol helps smooth fine lines and increases the skin's elasticity.

LINALOOL (3-5%) This constituent is absorbed through the skin and helps reduce swelling and inflammation. It is a pain-reliever as well as an antimicrobial. Linalool has many beneficial properties, but at high concentrations it can cause an allergic reaction (see page 31).

OCIMENE (1-4%) This constituent has antioxidant properties.

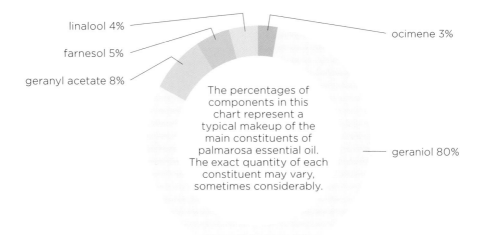

linalool 4%

farnesol 5%

geranyl acetate 8%

ocimene 3%

geraniol 80%

The percentages of components in this chart represent a typical makeup of the main constituents of palmarosa essential oil. The exact quantity of each constituent may vary, sometimes considerably.

Palmarosa Essential Oil in Personal Care Products

SKIN CARE: A dilution of up to 3% can be used in products that are left on the skin.

BENEFITS

- deodorizing
- antibacterial
- antifungal

CONDITIONS

- acne
- oily skin
- dandruff
- body odor
- fungal foot infections

PRODUCT	SKIN TYPE / CONDITION	QUANTITY
FACE		
Moisture creams and gels	oily skin	1% (6 drops in 30 mL)
Facial masks	oily skin	1% (6 drops in 30 mL)
Toners	oily skin and fungal infections	1% (6 drops in 30 mL)
Cleansers	oily skin and fungal infections	1% (6 drops in 30 mL)
Exfoliants	oily skin	1–2% (6–12 drops in 30 mL)
BODY		
Massage oils		1–2% (6–12 drops in 30 mL)
Body lotions		1–2% (6–12 drops in 30 mL)
Deodorants		1–2% (6–12 drops in 30 mL)
Exfoliants		1–2% (6–12 drops in 30 mL)
HANDS AND FEET		
Creams		1–2% (6–12 drops in 30 mL)
HAIR AND SCALP		
Shampoos and conditioners*	dandruff	1–3% (6–18 drops in 30 mL)

* Exposing oils to heat and water will cause them to oxidize at a faster rate. Consider packaging shampoos and conditioners in flip-top or pump bottles to help reduce oxidation.

Patchouli

Botanical names: *Pogostemon cablin*

Botanical Family: Lamiaceae (formerly Labiatae)

Habitat: native to Southeast Asia; cultivated extensively in Indonesia, the Philippines, Malaysia, China, India, West Africa and Vietnam

Aroma: deep, smooth amber, chocolate and wood base notes

Description of the Plant

This aromatic perennial shrub has erect, square stems that grow to a height of about 3 feet (1 m). It has large, egg-shaped green leaves and purple-tinged white flowers.

EXTRACTION: steam distillation of the dried leaves

Using Patchouli in Natural Products

Patchouli is considered one of the safest essential oils to use in aromatherapy. Many studies have been conducted on its potential to calm and relax the mind. It's also effective at treating skin infections, as well as wounds and sores, and there's some evidence that the antioxidant in patchouli oil may prevent skin-aging symptoms caused by UV exposure. These attributes make it a prime oil for all skin types, especially mature skin. It can be used in anti-aging face products as well as in most skin- and hair-care formulations.

PRECAUTIONS: This oil is non-irritating when applied at or below the maximum recommended dilutions. Use with caution during pregnancy and while breastfeeding. Properly stored, patchouli essential oil has a shelf life of up to 2 years.

Main Chemical Constituents of Patchouli Essential Oil

PATCHOULOL (25–30%) This constituent can help prevent many types of skin infections, as it has potent antibacterial, antifungal and antiviral properties. It can also help prevent and soothe skin inflammation.

DELTA-GUAIENE (14–18%) This constituent can help prevent and soothe skin inflammation.

ALPHA-GUAIENE (12–15%) This is an antibacterial agent that can help prevent and treat bacterial skin infections.

ALPHA-PATCHOULENE (8–10%) It can help prevent and soothe skin inflammation.

GAMMA-PATCHOULENE (7–9%) This is an antibacterial agent that can help prevent and treat bacterial skin infections.

SEYCHELLENE (7–9%) Seychellene may have anti-inflammatory and insect-repelling capabilities. More research is needed on this constituent.

BETA-PATCHOULENE (6–8%) This is an antibacterial agent that can help prevent and treat bacterial skin infections.

BETA-CARYOPHYLLENE (3–5%) It is known for its ability to relieve pain and inflammation. It also has potential as a skin-lightening agent.

POGOSTONE (2–5%) Pogostone is an antibacterial and antifungal agent that can help prevent and treat bacterial and fungal skin infections.

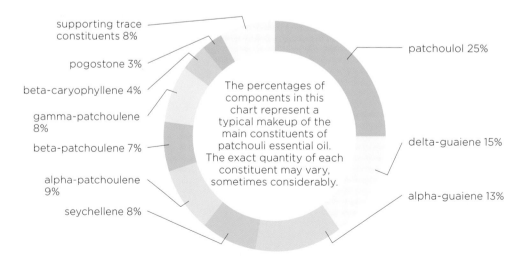

supporting trace constituents 8%

pogostone 3%

beta-caryophyllene 4%

gamma-patchoulene 8%

beta-patchoulene 7%

alpha-patchoulene 9%

seychellene 8%

patchoulol 25%

delta-guaiene 15%

alpha-guaiene 13%

The percentages of components in this chart represent a typical makeup of the main constituents of patchouli essential oil. The exact quantity of each constituent may vary, sometimes considerably.

Patchouli Essential Oil in Personal Care Products

SKIN CARE: A dilution of up to 3% can be used in products that are left on the skin.

BENEFITS

- suitable for all skin types
- antibacterial
- antifungal

CONDITIONS

- eczema
- fungal infections
- scar tissue
- wounds
- dry, scaly or cracked skin

PRODUCT	SKIN TYPE / CONDITION	QUANTITY
FACE		
Moisture creams	all skin types	2% (12 drops in 30 mL)
Facial masks	all skin types	2% (12 drops in 30 mL)
Toners	all skin types	2–3% (12–18 drops in 30 mL)
Cleansers	oily skin and acne	2–3% (12–18 drops in 30 mL)
Exfoliants	all skin types	2–3% (12–18 drops in 30 mL)
BODY		
Massage oils		2–3% (12–18 drops in 30 mL)
Body lotions		2–3% (12–18 drops in 30 mL)
Exfoliants	dry skin	2–3% (12–18 drops in 30 mL)
HANDS AND FEET		
Ointments		2–3% (12–18 drops in 30 mL)
Lotions and butters		2–3% (12–18 drops in 30 mL)
HAIR AND SCALP		
Shampoos and conditioners*		3% (18 drops in 30 mL)
Serums	dry scalp	1% (6 drops in 30 mL)

* Exposing oils to heat and water will cause them to oxidize at a faster rate. Consider packaging shampoos and conditioners in flip-top or pump bottles to help reduce oxidation.

Peppermint

Botanical name: *Mentha x piperita*

Botanical family: Lamiaceae (formerly Labiatae)

Habitat: native to the Mediterranean region; now cultivated all over the world

Aroma: fresh, cooling mint base notes

ALERT

Peppermint products can cause a tingling, cooling sensation on the scalp when they come in contact with water, so be particularly conscious of keeping them away from heat and water.

Description of the Plant

This perennial aromatic herb can grow up to 3 feet (1 m) in height. It has smooth stems, fibrous roots and dark green leaves with red-brown veins. The peppermint plant should be replanted regularly in new fields to produce a good quantity of essential oil. (The plant does not seed; it is reproduced by cuttings.)

EXTRACTION: steam distillation of the leaves, usually harvested before the plant flowers

Using Peppermint Oil in Natural Products

When it comes to skin-care products, peppermint essential oil is a double-edged sword. On the one hand, it has many therapeutic benefits, such as its cooling properties, which make it a great addition to after-sun products. It's also a natural antiseptic that can clear out dead skin and bacteria, so it's well suited for oily and acne-prone skin. And its SPF (sun-protection factor) is rated as 7, making it ideal for use in daytime lotions, gels and lip balms. On the other hand, this is an oil that has to be used very carefully, as it can cause severe skin reactions (see Cautions, below).

CAUTIONS: Peppermint essential oil may enhance the penetration of topical drugs; do not use on skin treated with topical drugs. Overexposure to this oil can cause severe skin reactions. High concentrations of the oil may be toxic; do not exceed the maximum recommended dilution. Products containing peppermint essential oil should not be used around infants.

PRECAUTIONS: Overexposure to peppermint essential oil can lead to sensitization. Do not use while pregnant or breastfeeding. Properly stored, peppermint essential oil has a shelf life of 1 to 2 years.

Main Chemical Constituents of Peppermint Essential Oil

MENTHOL (40-50%) Menthol is a cooling agent known for its natural pain-relieving properties. This constituent is able to enhance the penetration of certain topically applied drugs.

MENTHONE (20-30%) Menthone is an antimicrobial agent that can help prevent and treat skin infections.

EUCALYPTOL (8-10%) This constituent acts as a penetration enhancer (see page 54). It has also been shown to have antimicrobial and antifungal properties. When inhaled, it acts as a decongestant that helps to release phlegm.

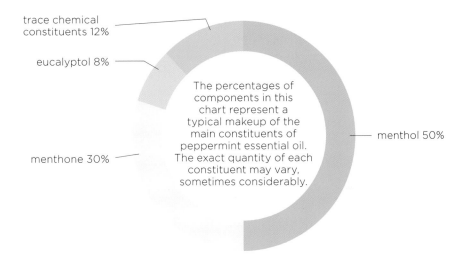

trace chemical constituents 12%

eucalyptol 8%

menthone 30%

menthol 50%

The percentages of components in this chart represent a typical makeup of the main constituents of peppermint essential oil. The exact quantity of each constituent may vary, sometimes considerably.

GUIDELINES FOR USING

Peppermint Essential Oil in Personal Care Products

SKIN CARE: A dilution of up to 1% can be used in products that are left on the skin.

BENEFITS

- cooling
- stimulating
- antibacterial

CONDITIONS

- acne
- dull skin
- candida skin infections
- oily skin
- athlete's foot
- cold sores
- insect bites

PRODUCT	SKIN TYPE / CONDITION	QUANTITY
FACE		
Moisture gels	acne	0.5% (3 drops in 30 mL)
Facial masks	oily skin and acne	0.5% (3 drops in 30 mL)
Toners	oily skin and acne	0.5% (3 drops in 30 mL)
Cleansers	oily skin and acne	0.5% (3 drops in 30 mL)
Exfoliants	oily skin and acne	0.5% (3 drops in 30 mL)
Lip balms		0.5% (3 drops in 30 mL)
BODY		
Massage oils		0.5% (3 drops in 30 mL)
Body lotions		0.5% (3 drops in 30 mL)
Deodorants		0.5% (3 drops in 30 mL)
Exfoliants		0.5% (3 drops in 30 mL)
HANDS AND FEET		
Foot balms and butters		0.5% (3 drops in 30 mL)
HAIR AND SCALP		
Shampoos*	dandruff	1% (6 drops in 30 mL)
Leave-in conditioning balms for scalp treatment*		0.5% (3 drops in 30 mL)

* Exposing oils to heat and water will cause them to oxidize at a faster rate. Consider packaging shampoos and conditioners in flip-top or pump bottles to help reduce oxidation.

Petitgrain

Botanical name: *Citrus aurantium subsp. amara*

Botanical family: Rutaceae

Habitat: native to India and southern China; now cultivated primarily in Italy, Tunisia, Morocco, Egypt, France and the United States

Aroma: sharp, deep herbaceous tobacco/green scent

Description of the Plant

The bitter orange tree grows from 10 to 30 feet (3 to 9 m) in height. It yields three types of essential oils that are very different in their chemical components: neroli (from the blossoms), petitgrain (from the leaves) and orange (from the fruit). The tree is in full bloom from November to March; the highly fragrant waxy white flowers develop in clusters, forming "bouquets" around the tree.

EXTRACTION: steam distillation of the leaves and twigs

Using Petitgrain in Natural Products

Petitgrain and neroli essential oils have similar fragrances, but the former has a bolder tobacco note. Petitgrain can be used in most skin-care formulations. It can also complement products that contain the more expensive neroli essential oil, especially in those with a heavier base, such as shampoos, conditioners, cleansers, balms and butters. The chemical compounds in this essential oil help stave off skin infections. The oil also has a calming effect on the whole being. Use it for skin care during stressful times — it makes a great addition to relaxing massage oils.

CAUTIONS: Although a number of reports indicate that petitgrain does not cause irritation or sensitization, this essential oil is known to dissolve in sweat, and when sweaty skin is exposed to sunlight, the oil can be irritating. For some people, this may even cause an allergic reaction.

PRECAUTIONS: This oil is non-irritating when applied at or below the maximum recommended dilutions, unless you have a pre-existing sensitivity to any of its components (such as linalool, which makes up a large percentage). Do not use during pregnancy or while breastfeeding. Properly stored, petitgrain essential oil has a shelf life of up to 2 years.

OXIDATION ALERT

Petitgrain essential oil contains a significant amount of linalool, a constituent that absorbs through the skin and helps relieve swelling and inflammation. It is a pain-reliever as well as an antimicrobial. Linalool has a calming floral scent that has many beneficial properties, but at high concentrations it can cause an allergic reaction. Also, when oxidized it can lead to irritation (see page 31). Be particularly conscious of keeping any products containing this essential oil away from heat, water and light.

Main Chemical Constituents of Petitgrain Essential Oil

LINALYL ACETATE (40-50%) This constituent is absorbed through the skin and helps to prevent and treat skin inflammation. It also has antispasmodic effects, so it can help relax muscles and relieve cramps.

LINALOOL (20-30%) This constituent is also absorbed through the skin and helps to reduce swelling and inflammation. It is a pain-reliever as well as an antimicrobial. Linalool has many beneficial properties, but at high concentrations it can cause an allergic reaction (see page 31).

NEROL (7-9%) This constituent contributes to the oil's rose-like scent.

ALPHA-TERPINEOL (5-6%) This constituent has antioxidant and antiviral properties.

D-LIMONENE (5%) One of the most commonly found constituents in fruit, d-limonene gives citrus fruits their distinctive scent. It oxidizes quite quickly, which can lead to skin irritation.

GERANYL ACETATE (4-5%) This constituent also contributes to the oil's sweet floral scent. Geranyl acetate has antispasmodic effects, so it can help relax muscles and relieve cramps.

GERANIOL (1-2%) This constituent contributes to the oil's rose-like scent. Geraniol has strong antifungal and antibacterial activity. At high concentrations it can be a skin irritant and sensitizer, or even lead to an allergic reaction.

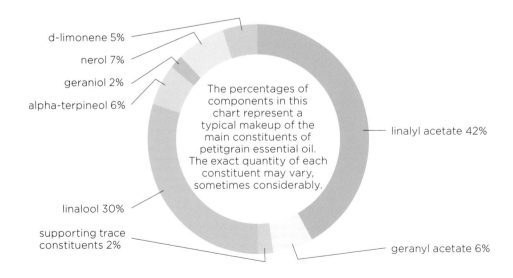

d-limonene 5%

nerol 7%

geraniol 2%

alpha-terpineol 6%

The percentages of components in this chart represent a typical makeup of the main constituents of petitgrain essential oil. The exact quantity of each constituent may vary, sometimes considerably.

linalyl acetate 42%

linalool 30%

supporting trace constituents 2%

geranyl acetate 6%

Petitgrain Essential Oil in Personal Care Products

SKIN CARE: A dilution of up to 3% can be used in products that are left on the skin.

BENEFITS

- deodorizing
- suitable for all types of skin
- anti-inflammatory

CONDITIONS

- acne
- oily skin
- combination skin
- tired-looking skin

PRODUCT	SKIN TYPE / CONDITION	QUANTITY
FACE		
Moisture gels	all skin types	1–2% (6–12 drops in 30 mL)
Facial masks	all skin types	1–2% (6–12 drops in 30 mL)
Toners	all skin types	2% (12 drops in 30 mL)
Cleansers	all skin types	2–3% (12–18 drops in 30 mL)
Exfoliants	all skin types	2–3% (12–18 drops in 30 mL)
Lip balms		2–3% (12–18 drops in 30 mL)
BODY		
Massage oils		1–2% (6–12 drops in 30 mL)
Body lotions		1–2% (6–12 drops in 30 mL)
Deodorants		1–2% (6–12 drops in 30 mL)
Exfoliants		1–2% (6–12 drops in 30 mL)
HANDS AND FEET		
Foot balms and butters		2–3% (12–18 drops in 30 mL)
HAIR AND SCALP		
Shampoos and conditioners*		1–3% (6–18 drops in 30 mL)
Leave-in conditioning balms for scalp treatment*		1% (6 drops in 30 mL)

* Exposing oils to heat and water will cause them to oxidize at a faster rate. Consider packaging shampoos and conditioners in flip-top or pump bottles to help reduce oxidation.

Pine

Botanical name: *Pinus sylvestris*

Botanical family: Pinaceae

Habitat: native to Siberia, eastern Asia and Europe

Aroma: fresh woody, earthy, resinous and camphor-like notes

Description of the Plant

The Scots pine grows up to 150 feet (46 m) in height. It has sharp, narrow needles and plump seed cones. This tree grows in many regions of the world and is the national tree of Scotland.

EXTRACTION: steam distillation of the needles

Using Pine Essentail Oil in Natural Products

Pine essential oil is widely used in aromatherapy to ease respiratory tract infections and symptoms such as shortness of breath. It's also a natural antiseptic that can clear out dead skin and bacteria, so it's well suited for oily and acne-prone skin. Use it in moisture creams and lotions, body cleansers, scrubs, shampoos and conditioners.

CAUTION: Pine essential oil contains a high level of alpha-pinene, a constituent that has a tendency to oxidize quickly, which can lead to skin irritation.

PRECAUTIONS: This oil is non-irritating when applied at or below the maximum recommended dilutions. Do not use when pregnant or breastfeeding. Properly stored, pine essential oil has a shelf life of up to 2 years.

Main Chemical Constituents of Pine Essential Oil

ALPHA-PINENE (45–48%) This constituent, which is absorbed into the skin, is known for its ability to relieve pain and inflammation and for being a potent antimicrobial that can help prevent and treat skin infections. When oxidized, it can lead to skin irritation.

BETA-PINENE (30–34%) This constituent has strong antimicrobial activity that can help prevent skin infections. Beta-pinene carries a low risk of allergy. When oxidized it can lead to skin irritation.

BORNYL ACETATE (10–12%) This constituent has potential anti-inflammatory activity; one study showed that it was able to reduce lung inflammation.

D-LIMONENE (5%) This is one of the most commonly found constituents in fruit, and it gives grapefruit and other citrus fruits their distinctive scent. D-limonene oxidizes quite quickly, which can lead to skin irritation (see page 27).

MYRCENE (3–5%) This non-irritating, non-allergenic constituent is an antioxidant. It has sedative properties that help calm and soothe the nervous system.

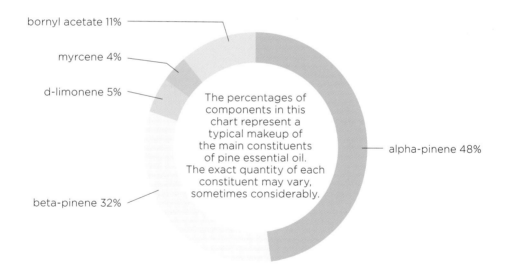

bornyl acetate 11%

myrcene 4%

d-limonene 5%

The percentages of components in this chart represent a typical makeup of the main constituents of pine essential oil. The exact quantity of each constituent may vary, sometimes considerably.

alpha-pinene 48%

beta-pinene 32%

GUIDELINES FOR USING

Pine Essential Oil
in Personal Care Products

SKIN CARE: A dilution of up to 2% can be used in products that are left on the skin.

BENEFITS

- invigorating
- antibacterial

CONDITIONS

- oily skin
- acne
- cuts

PRODUCT	SKIN TYPE / CONDITION	QUANTITY
FACE		
Moisture gels	acne	1% (6 drops in 30 mL)
Facial masks	oily skin and acne	1% (6 drops in 30 mL)
Toners	oily skin and acne	1% (6 drops in 30 mL)
Cleansers	oily skin and acne	1% (6 drops in 30 mL)
BODY		
Massage oils		1–2% (6–12 drops in 30 mL)
Body lotions		1–2% (6–12 drops in 30 mL)
Exfoliants		1% (6 drops in 30 mL)
HANDS AND FEET		
Foot balms		1–2% (6–12 drops in 30 mL)
HAIR AND SCALP		
Shampoos and conditioners*		1–3% (6–18 drops in 30 mL)

* Exposing oils to heat and water will cause them to oxidize at a faster rate. Consider packaging shampoos and conditioners in flip-top or pump bottles to help reduce oxidation.

Rose Otto

Botanical name: *Rosa* x *damascena*

Botanical family: Rosaceae

Habitat: native to Europe and western Asia; cultivated worldwide. The major producers of rose otto (also called rose oil or attar of roses) are France, Bulgaria, Morocco, Turkey, Italy and China.

Aroma: classic floral rose middle notes

Description of the Plant

There are more than 5,000 varieties of rose. They can range in height but they all have thorny, cylindrical stems with ovate dark green leaves. Their colors vary from pure white to almost black, and every color variation in between. Some species and varieties are very aromatic, while some have no aroma whatsoever. Rose otto is made from the Damask rose, a pink to red hybrid known for its lovely fragrance.

EXTRACTION: steam distillation of the whole flowers

Using Rose Otto in Natural Products

Rose otto, which has outstanding therapeutic properties for the mind and the body, is one of the most valued essential oils in aromatherapy and in the cosmetic industry. Studies show that it can reduce levels of adrenalin in the body; it can also help combat stress, anxiety, insomnia and inflammation. Rose otto contains citronellol and geraniol, which help ward off bacterial and fungal infections. They are also antioxidants that can balance skin tone and smooth and prevent fine lines in mature skin, making this oil ideal for use in anti-aging products. Rose otto essential oil benefits all skin types, especially mature and sensitive skin. Use it in face cleansers, toners and masks and in skin-balancing body lotions and massage oils. It also makes a lovely moisturizing hair serum.

CAUTION: Overexposure to rose essential oil may cause an allergic reaction to one of its major chemical constituents, geraniol (see page 31).

PRECAUTIONS: At high concentrations, this oil is a skin irritant and sensitizer; do not exceed the maximum recommended dilutions. Use cautiously when pregnant or breastfeeding. Properly stored, rose otto essential oil has a shelf life of up to 2 years.

A NICE ALTERNATIVE

Rose otto essential oil is expensive, and therefore not recommended for wash-off products such as shampoos, conditioners or body washes. An alternative to rose otto is geranium essential oil.

Main Chemical Constituents of Rose Otto Essential Oil

CITRONELLOL (35–45%) This constituent has proven antibacterial abilities, and it also has antioxidant properties. Citronellol contributes to rose otto's scent.

GERANIOL (20–25%) This constituent also contributes to the oil's scent. Geraniol has strong antifungal and antibacterial activity, meaning that it can prevent or slow the growth of fungi and bacteria. Geraniol has many beneficial properties, but at high concentrations it can be a skin irritant and sensitizer, or even lead to an allergic reaction (see page 31).

NEROL (7–8%) This constituent also contributes to the oil's rose-like scent.

FARNESOL (2%) Farnesol is an antimicrobial that helps prevent and treat skin infections. It's also known for its ability to reduce skin inflammation. As a bonus, farnesol helps smooth fine lines and increases the skin's elasticity.

PHENYLETHYL ALCOHOL (2%) Studies show that this constituent has calming and relaxing properties. It also contributes to the scent.

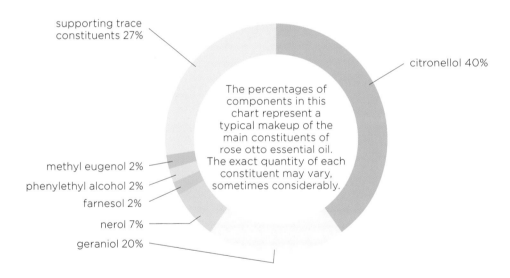

supporting trace constituents 27%

citronellol 40%

The percentages of components in this chart represent a typical makeup of the main constituents of rose otto essential oil. The exact quantity of each constituent may vary, sometimes considerably.

methyl eugenol 2%
phenylethyl alcohol 2%
farnesol 2%
nerol 7%
geraniol 20%

Rose Otto Essential Oil in Personal Care Products

SKIN CARE: A dilution of up to 2% can be used in products that are left on the skin.

BENEFITS

- calming and relaxing
- suitable for all skin types
- antibacterial

CONDITIONS

- dry or aging skin
- broken capillaries
- dull or blotchy skin
- fine lines

PRODUCT	SKIN TYPE / CONDITION	QUANTITY
FACE		
Moisture creams	mature skin	0.5–1% (3–6 drops in 30 mL)
Facial masks	mature and sensitive skin	0.5–1% (3–6 drops in 30 mL)
Toners	mature and sensitive skin	0.5–1% (3–6 drops in 30 mL)
Cleansers	mature and sensitive skin	1–2% (6–12 drops in 30 mL)
BODY		
Massage oils		1% (6 drops in 30 mL)
Body lotions		1% (6 drops in 30 mL)
HANDS AND FEET		
Creams		1% (6 drops in 30 mL)
HAIR AND SCALP		
Hair serum		1% (6 drops in 30 mL)

* Exposing oils to heat and water will cause them to oxidize at a faster rate. Consider packaging shampoos and conditioners in flip-top or pump bottles to help reduce oxidation.

Rosemary

Botanical name: *Rosmarinus officinalis*

Botanical family: Lamiaceae

Habitat: native to the Mediterranean region; cultivated worldwide

Aroma: herbaceous, with camphor middle and top notes

Description of the Plant

Rosemary is a shrubby perennial herb with short, stiff, needle-like leaves. The flowers can be pink, purple, deep blue or occasionally white. This aromatic herb can grow up to 6 feet (2 m) in height.

EXTRACTION: steam distillation of the entire herb

Using Rosemary Oil in Natural Products

Rosemary has been used for centuries in culinary applications, practical home remedies and ritualistic ceremonies. Rosemary-leaf infusions have been used historically to treat dry scalp, dandruff and hair loss. Today rosemary essential oil is a wonderful addition to shampoos, conditioners and scalp tonics to help strengthen hair and prevent hair loss. It's also a natural preservative that can be used in cleansers, toners, face creams and body lotions.

CAUTIONS: Because of its highly stimulating effects, rosemary essential oil should not be used by people with high blood pressure or epilepsy.

PRECAUTIONS: This oil is non-irritating when applied at or below the maximum recommended dilutions. Overuse of the oil can cause skin irritation in some individuals. Do not use when pregnant or breastfeeding. Rosemary essential oil can oxidize quite quickly, which can lead to skin irritation. Properly stored, it has a shelf life of up to 2 years.

Main Chemical Constituents of Rosemary Essential Oil

EUCALYPTOL (35–48%) This constituent acts as a penetration enhancer (see page 54). It has also been shown to have antimicrobial and antifungal properties. When inhaled, it acts as a decongestant that helps to release phlegm.

CAMPHOR (16–18%) Camphor is an analgesic that can help relieve pain. However, in excessive quantities it can be a neurotoxin.

ALPHA-PINENE (12–15%) This constituent, which is absorbed into the skin, is known for its ability to relieve pain and inflammation and for being a potent antimicrobial that can help prevent and treat skin infections. When oxidized, it can lead to skin irritation.

BETA-PINENE (10–15%) This constituent has strong antimicrobial activity that can help prevent skin infections. Beta-pinene carries a low risk of allergy, but when oxidized can irritate skin.

MYRCENE (2%) This non-irritating, non-allergenic constituent is an antioxidant. It has sedative properties that help calm and soothe the nervous system.

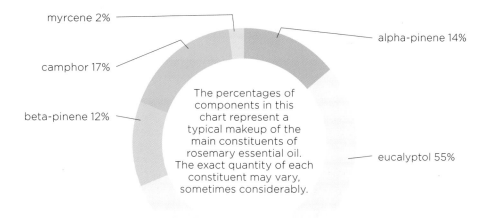

myrcene 2%

camphor 17%

beta-pinene 12%

alpha-pinene 14%

eucalyptol 55%

The percentages of components in this chart represent a typical makeup of the main constituents of rosemary essential oil. The exact quantity of each constituent may vary, sometimes considerably.

GUIDELINES FOR USING

Rosemary Essential Oil in Personal Care Products

SKIN CARE: A dilution of up to 2% can be used in products that are left on the skin.

BENEFITS

- stimulating and invigorating
- antibacterial

CONDITIONS

- acne
- oily skin
- blotchy skin
- dandruff

PRODUCT	SKIN TYPE / CONDITION	QUANTITY
FACE		
Moisture creams	oily skin and acne	1–2% (6–12 drops in 30 mL)
Facial masks	oily skin and acne	1–2% (6–12 drops in 30 mL)
Toners	oily skin and acne	1–2% (6–12 drops in 30 mL)
Cleansers	oily skin and acne	1–2% (6–12 drops in 30 mL)
Exfoliants	oily skin and acne	1–2% (6–12 drops in 30 mL)
BODY		
Massage oils		1–2% (6–12 drops in 30 mL)
Body lotions		1–2% (6–12 drops in 30 mL)
HANDS AND FEET		
Ointments		1–2% (6–12 drops in 30 mL)
Lotions and butters		1–2% (6–12 drops in 30 mL)
HAIR AND SCALP		
Shampoos and conditioners*		1–3% (18 drops in 30 mL)
Scalp serums		1% (6 drops in 30 mL)

* Exposing oils to heat and water will cause them to oxidize at a faster rate. Consider packaging shampoos and conditioners in flip-top or pump bottles to help reduce oxidation.

Australian Sandalwood

Botanical name: *Santalum austrocaledonicum*

Botanical Family: Santalaceae

Habitat: the islands of New Caledonia and Vanuatu, in the southwest Pacific Ocean

Aroma: soft woody base notes

Description of the Plant

Drought-tolerant Australian sandalwood — officially named New Caledonia sandalwood — is a bushy multi-stemmed tree that grows 16 to 40 feet (5 to 12 m) high. The leaves are bluish green and shiny on top and a dull light green underneath. The bark of the tree is slightly rough, with grayish or reddish brown patches.

EXTRACTION: steam distillation of the heartwood (the inner part of the tree trunk)

Using Australian Sandalwood Oil in Natural Products

Sandalwood essential oil is a luxurious addition to skin-care products. Research shows that alpha-santalol, a major constituent of the oil, is able to permeate the skin and lower blood pressure. Both alpha- and beta-santalol are good candidates for treating inflamed skin. This oil is also used to lighten — it's one of the top essential oils for enhancing skin radiance. And it has potent antifungal properties, making it beneficial in the treatment of conditions such as acne and athlete's foot. Use this essential oil in skin-lightening cleansers, toners and creams, and in balms and butters for fungal foot infections.

PRECAUTIONS: This oil is non-irritating when applied at or below the maximum recommended dilutions. Overuse can cause skin irritation in individuals with sensitive skin. Use cautiously when pregnant or breastfeeding. Properly stored, sandalwood essential oil has a shelf life of up to 2 years.

KNOW THE VARIETY

The sandalwoods are a good reminder of why we need to take our natural resources into consideration when purchasing and using essential oils. There are 19 different species in the sandalwood family. Historically, Indian sandalwood (*Santalum album*) essential oil was used in cosmetics, as well as in spiritual practices. However, today Indian sandalwood is classified as an endangered species and its use is heavily regulated. Australian sandalwood has now become the alternative to Indian sandalwood — their constituents are very similar. When purchasing sandalwood essential oil, make sure the label says "*Santalum austrocaledonicum.*"

Main Chemical Constituents of Australian Sandalwood Essential Oil

ALPHA-SANTALOL (40–53%) This constituent is absorbed through the skin and can lower blood pressure. It's an antibacterial and antifungal that can help prevent and treat skin infections. Studies have found alpha-santalol to be a skin-lightening agent, and there's also evidence that it's toxic to skin cancers and can slow down growths in oral cancers.

BETA-SANTALOL (20–25%) This constituent contributes to the sedative effect of Australian sandalwood essential oil.

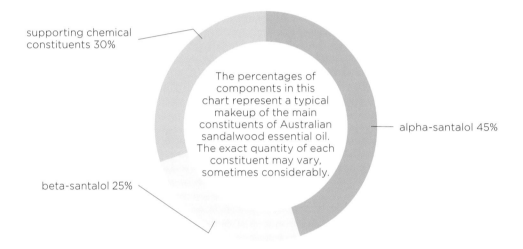

supporting chemical constituents 30%

alpha-santalol 45%

beta-santalol 25%

The percentages of components in this chart represent a typical makeup of the main constituents of Australian sandalwood essential oil. The exact quantity of each constituent may vary, sometimes considerably.

Australian Sandalwood Essential Oil in Personal Care Products

SKIN CARE: A dilution of up to 3% can be used in products that are left on the skin.

BENEFITS

- antibacterial
- calming
- skin brightening
- antifungal

CONDITIONS

- hyperpigmentation
- acne
- aging skin
- sunburn

PRODUCT	SKIN TYPE / CONDITION	QUANTITY
FACE		
Moisture creams	all skin types, mature skin	1–2% (6–12 drops in 30 mL)
Facial masks	all skin types, mature skin	1–2% (6–12 drops in 30 mL)
Toners	all skin types, mature skin	2% (12 drops in 30 mL)
Cleansers	all skin types, mature skin	2–3% (12–18 drops in 30 mL)
BODY		
Massage oils		1–2% (6–12 drops in 30 mL)
Body lotions		1–2% (6–12 drops in 30 mL)
HANDS AND FEET		
Foot balms and butters		2–3% (12–18 drops in 30 mL)
HAIR AND SCALP		
Leave-in conditioning balms for scalp treatment*		1% (6 drops in 30 mL)

* Exposing oils to heat and water will cause them to oxidize at a faster rate. Consider packaging shampoos and conditioners in flip-top or pump bottles to help reduce oxidation.

Tea Tree

Botanical name: *Melaleuca alternifolia*

Botanical Family: Myrtaceae

Habitat: native to Australia, mainly New South Wales

Aroma: fresh, pungent notes

Description of the Plant

Melaleuca shrubs and trees, also known as paperbarks, grow from 6 to 100 feet (2 to 30 m) tall, depending on the species. They have flaky white bark and oval dark green to gray-green leaves. Flowers develop in dense clusters along the stems, each with small, fine petals that can be white, pink, red, pale yellow or green. The tree's fruit is a small capsule containing numerous minute seeds.

EXTRACTION: steam distillation of the leaves and twigs

Using Tea Tree in Natural Products

In aromatherapy, tea tree essential oil is used for treating fungal, bacterial and viral infections. This essential oil has been extensively researched and is proven to help sunburn, boils, acne, thrush, rashes, insect bites and cold sores. It's also a common addition to anti-dandruff shampoos. Use this oil in creams, cleansers and exfoliants for oily and acne-prone skin, as well as in shampoos, conditioners and scalp serums.

CAUTION: Tea tree oil is widely used in natural skin-care formulations. Recently it has been overused, as many companies have now turned to tea tree to give their products a "natural" appeal. Overexposure to tea tree oil can cause skin irritation and sensitization.

PRECAUTIONS: This oil is non-irritating when applied at or below the maximum recommended dilutions. Pregnant or breastfeeding women should use it with caution. Tea tree oil can oxidize quite quickly, which can lead to skin irritation. Properly stored, tea tree essential oil has a shelf life of up to 2 years.

Main Chemical Constituents of Tea Tree Essential Oil

GAMMA-TERPINENE (30–33%) This constituent has strong antibacterial properties that can help prevent skin infections. It also slows the oxidation of linoleic acid, so it can act as a preservative when added to most carrier oils.

TERPINEN-4-OL (19–22%) This constituent is a potent antibacterial agent; studies show that it's effective at clearing skin infections and relieving acne. It's also effective against skin mites and yeast infections on the skin. An anti-inflammatory as well, it is easily absorbed into the skin.

CYMENE (18–20%) This constituent is an antioxidant.

EUCALYPTOL (16–20%) This constituent acts as a penetration enhancer (see page 54). It has also been shown to have antimicrobial and antifungal properties. When inhaled, it acts as a decongestant that helps to release phlegm.

ALPHA-TERPINENE (7–9%) This constituent has strong antifungal and antibacterial activity, meaning that it can prevent or slow the growth of fungi and bacteria.

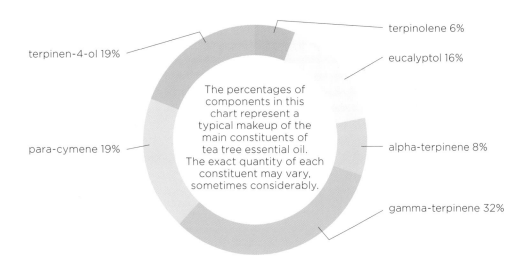

terpinolene 6%

eucalyptol 16%

terpinen-4-ol 19%

para-cymene 19%

alpha-terpinene 8%

gamma-terpinene 32%

The percentages of components in this chart represent a typical makeup of the main constituents of tea tree essential oil. The exact quantity of each constituent may vary, sometimes considerably.

Tea Tree Essential Oil in Personal Care Products

SKIN CARE: A dilution of up to 3% can be used in products that are left on the skin.

BENEFITS

- antibacterial
- antifungal

RECOMMENDED TO USE

- candida skin infections
- acne
- oily skin
- blotchy skin
- hyperpigmentation

PRODUCT	SKIN TYPE / CONDITION	QUANTITY
FACE		
Moisture creams	oily skin and acne	2% (12 drops in 30 mL)
Facial masks	oily skin and acne	2% (12 drops in 30 mL)
Toners	oily skin and acne	2–3% (12–18 drops in 30 mL)
Cleansers	oily skin and acne	2–3% (12–18 drops in 30 mL)
Exfoliants	oily skin and acne	2–3% (12–18 drops in 30 mL)
BODY		
Massage oils		2–3% (12–18 drops in 30 mL)
Body lotions		2–3% (12–18 drops in 30 mL)
HANDS AND FEET		
Ointments		2–3% (12–18 drops in 30 mL)
Lotions and butters		2–3% (12–18 drops in 30 mL)
HAIR AND SCALP		
Shampoos and conditioners*		3% (18 drops in 30 mL)
Scalp serums		1% (6 drops in 30 mL)

* Exposing oils to heat and water will cause them to oxidize at a faster rate. Consider packaging shampoos and conditioners in flip-top or pump bottles to help reduce oxidation.

Ylang-Ylang

Botanical name: *Cananga odorata*

Botanical family: Annonaceae

Habitat: native to tropical Asia; the oil is produced in Madagascar, Réunion and the Comoros Islands.

Aroma: sweet floral and herbaceous notes

Description of the Plant

Cananga odorata is a tree that grows to a height of about 40 feet (12 m). It has glossy green leaves and large yellow flowers with elongated petals that are very fragrant, especially at night.

EXTRACTION: steam distillation of the flower petals in stages. This yields three different grades of essential oil: Extra, produced in the first few hours of distillation; Grade 1, produced after 5 or 6 hours; and Complete, produced once distillation is complete. The entire extraction process takes about 8 to 12 hours.

Using Ylang-Ylang in Natural Products

You don't need to add much ylang-ylang essential oil to a formulation to experience its beautiful uplifting and sensual fragrance. Ylang-ylang is a potent antiseptic that helps to improve oily and acne-prone skin. It also helps tone skin and increase its suppleness, making this an ideal oil to use in anti-aging formulations. Ylang-ylang essential oil can be used in most skin- and hair-care formulations.

PRECAUTIONS: This oil is non-irritating when applied at or below the maximum recommended dilutions. Overexposure to ylang-ylang essential oil can cause skin sensitization; it can also provoke headaches. Pregnant or breastfeeding women should use it with caution. Properly stored, ylang-ylang essential oil has a shelf life of up to 2 years.

KNOW THE GRADE

Three grades of ylang-ylang essential oil are available on the market. Ylang-Ylang Extra has a bold, sweet floral scent and is most often used in perfumes. Ylang-Ylang 1 has a lighter floral scent; it is used in perfumes and also in skin care, since the second extraction yields more therapeutic constituents. Ylang-Ylang Complete has a floral, herbaceous bouquet and is also used in both perfumes and skin care.

Major Chemical Constituents of Ylang-Ylang Essential Oil

BETA-CARYOPHYLLENE (10-21%) It is known for its ability to relieve pain and inflammation. It also has potential as a skin-lightening agent.

GERMACRENE D (15-24%) This constituent, found in many plant species, can act as an insecticide against mosquitoes, aphids and ticks.

BENZYL BENZOATE (10-15%) This constituent is known for its disinfectant properties, which are useful in formulations that target germs and viruses. It's also been shown to stop the spread of scabies, a contagious skin disease that causes itching and raised red spots. Benzyl benzoate has many beneficial properties, but it is sensitizing (see page 27).

METHYL BENZOATE (6%) This constituent is used in the perfume industry because of its pleasant smell. High levels of this compound can be a skin irritant.

FARNESENE (8-10%) Farnesene is an antimicrobial that helps prevent and treat skin infections. It's also known for its ability to reduce skin inflammation.

LINALOOL (4-15%) This constituent is absorbed through the skin and helps relieve swelling and inflammation. It is a pain-reliever as well as an antimicrobial. Linalool has many beneficial properties, but at high concentrations it can cause an allergic reaction (see page 31) and when oxidized is a skin irritant.

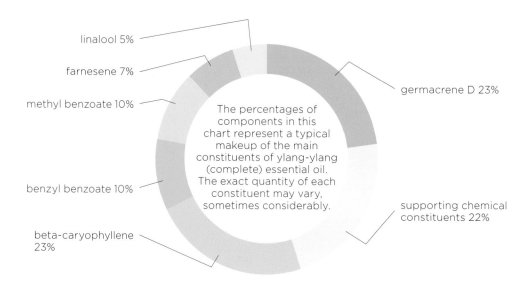

linalool 5%

farnesene 7%

methyl benzoate 10%

benzyl benzoate 10%

beta-caryophyllene 23%

germacrene D 23%

supporting chemical constituents 22%

The percentages of components in this chart represent a typical makeup of the main constituents of ylang-ylang (complete) essential oil. The exact quantity of each constituent may vary, sometimes considerably.

Ylang-Ylang Essential Oil in Personal Care Products

SKIN CARE: A dilution of up to 3% can be used in products that are left on the skin.

BENEFITS

- antibacterial
- insect repellant
- calming and relaxing

CONDITIONS

- dry skin
- oily skin
- combination skin
- fine lines
- tense muscles

PRODUCT	SKIN TYPE / CONDITION	QUANTITY
FACE		
Moisture gels	all skin types	1% (6 drops in 30 mL)
Facial masks	all skin types	1% (6 drops in 30 mL)
Toners	all skin types	1% (6 drops in 30 mL)
Cleansers	all skin types	1% (6 drops in 30 mL)
Exfoliants	all skin types	1% (6 drops in 30 mL)
Lip balms		1% (6 drops in 30 mL)
BODY		
Massage oils		1% (6 drops in 30 mL)
Body lotions		1% (6 drops in 30 mL)
Deodorants		1% (6 drops in 30 mL)
HANDS AND FEET		
Foot balms and butters		1% (6 drops in 30 mL)
HAIR AND SCALP		
Shampoos and conditioners*		1–3% (6–18 drops in 30 mL)
Leave-in conditioning balms for scalp treatment*		1–2% (6–12 drops in 30 mL)

* Exposing oils to heat and water will cause them to oxidize at a faster rate. Consider packaging shampoos and conditioners in flip-top or pump bottles to help reduce oxidation.

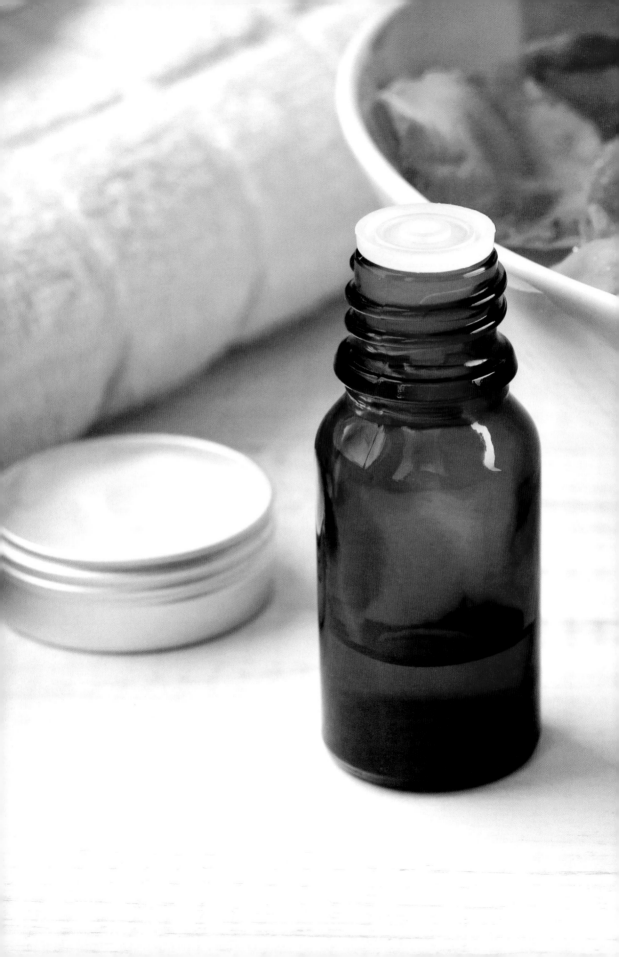

PART 4

Formulations

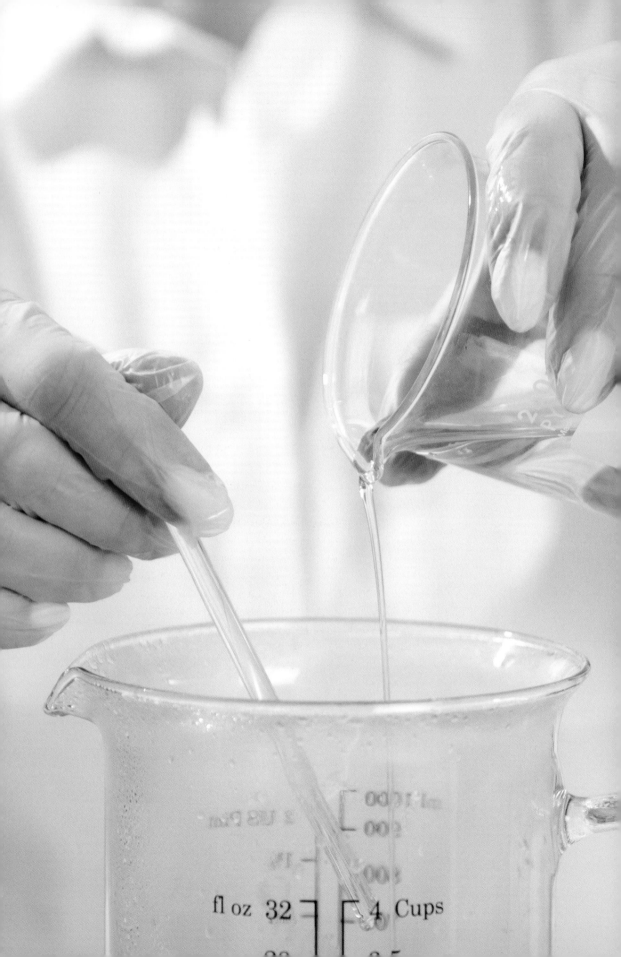

Making Skin-Care Products: A Step-by-Step Guide

Making skin-care products at home is not complicated. Moisturizers, lotions, butters, creams, balms and ointments — all these products are made by the same basic method but with different raw ingredients. Once you learn the basic techniques, you can make an almost infinite variety of products to suit a myriad of skin-care needs.

Moisturizers and lotions tend to be lighter and more fluid in texture, whereas creams and butters have a heavier texture. This is because lotions and moisturizers contain more water and less emulsifier, which makes them suitable for the face and torso. Butters and creams contain less water and more emulsifier, which makes them suitable for hands, feet and legs. On the other hand, ointments and balms do not contain any water, which results in an oilier, thicker base that is perfect for body-specific care products such as lip balms, deodorants and salves.

I have created three basic skin-care formulations — a moisturizing cream, a lotion and a lip balm — each of which can be personalized to suit your specific needs. Before getting to the actual formulations, I have broken them down step by step in a diagram, then in words, to guide you through the universal methods for making personal skin-care products. Once you master the basic techniques, you should be able to make any of the formulations in this book with confidence. While the directions for making specific products in this book may vary slightly, their processes share these common steps.

Steps for Making a Natural Skin-Care Formulation

When it comes to the ingredients in natural skin-care products, the options are almost limitless. Every day, new natural ingredients become trendsetters. See pages 44 to 203 for an overview of those most commonly used at the time of this writing. Always research the ingredients you are using and know the recommended maximum amount you can add to products.

1. CREATE AN EMULSION

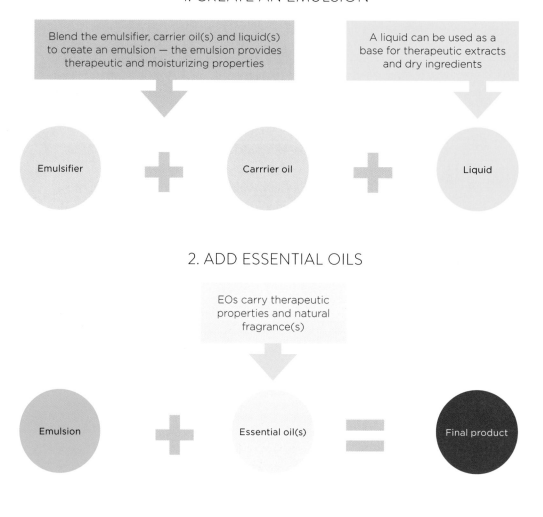

Blend the emulsifier, carrier oil(s) and liquid(s) to create an emulsion — the emulsion provides therapeutic and moisturizing properties

A liquid can be used as a base for therapeutic extracts and dry ingredients

Emulsifier + Carrrier oil + Liquid

2. ADD ESSENTIAL OILS

EOs carry therapeutic properties and natural fragrance(s)

Emulsion + Essential oil(s) = Final product

A TYPICAL FORMULA: NOURISHING ROSE-SCENTED MOISTURIZER

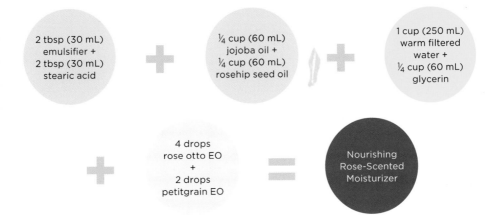

2 tbsp (30 mL) emulsifier + 2 tbsp (30 mL) stearic acid **+** ¼ cup (60 mL) jojoba oil + ¼ cup (60 mL) rosehip seed oil **+** 1 cup (250 mL) warm filtered water + ¼ cup (60 mL) glycerin

+ 4 drops rose otto EO + 2 drops petitgrain EO **=** Nourishing Rose-Scented Moisturizer

STEP 1: MELT EMULSIFIER

This is one of the most important steps when making a cream or lotion. The emulsifier — for example, emulsifying wax or stearic acid — is the substance in your formulation that binds together the water and lipids (fats). If you do not include an emulsifier or the correct quantity of a specific emulsifier in your formula, the liquids and lipids will separate. This is an invitation for mold and bacteria to develop at a very fast rate.

STEP 2: ADD CARRIER OIL(S)

The carrier oil — for example, sweet almond oil or rosehip seed oil — is what gives your product its desired emollient and therapeutic value. Choose an oil that is suitable for your skin type or skin condition and that is not likely to cause an allergic response (see pages 57 to 73).

STEP 3: ADD LIQUID

The liquid gives your product a cooler, lighter feel and helps to add volume to the final result. You can enhance the therapeutic properties of your products by dissolving extracts in or infusing the liquid with teas, gels, preservatives or powdered ingredients (see pages 77 to 85).

STEP 4: ADD ESSENTIAL OIL(S)

Essential oils provide your products with natural fragrance and also influence their therapeutic properties, such as calming, antiseptic, antibacterial, antiviral, anti-inflammatory or antifungal (see pages 88 to 203).

CHOOSING YOUR OILS

The following charts will guide you in selecting carrier and esential oils that best suit your skin type and price range.

Selecting Carrier Oils

CARRIER OIL	SKIN TYPE					PRICE RANGE
	DRY	OILY	COMBINATION	SENSITIVE	AGING	
Almond, sweet	*				*	$$
Apricot kernel	*	*	*	*	*	$$
Argan	*	*	*	*	*	$$$
Avocado (crude)	*			*	*	$$
Borage	*	*	*		*	$$$
Camellia seed	*	*	*	*	*	$
Cocoa butter	*				*	$$
Coconut, extra virgin	*	*	*	*	*	$
Coconut, fractionated	*				*	$
Evening primrose	*	*	*	*	*	$$$
Grapeseed	*	*	*	*	*	$
Hazelnut		*	*			$$
Hempseed	*	*	*	*	*	$$$
Jojoba	*	*	*	*	*	$$$
Marula	*	*	*	*	*	$$$
Rosehip seed	*		*	*	*	$$$
Sesame seed	*				*	$$$
Shea butter	*			*	*	$$
Sunflower seed	*			*	*	$

Key: $ = inexpensive; $$ = moderate price; $$$ = expensive

NUT ALLERGY ALERT

If you are sensitive to nuts, use carrier oils such as grapeseed oil, fractionated coconut oil or apricot kernel oil instead of a nut oil such as sweet almond oil. These oils also result in a light-textured base.

Selecting Essential Oils

ESSENTIAL OILS	SKIN TYPE					PRICE RANGE
	DRY	OILY	COMBINATION	AGING	SENSITIVE	
Benzoin	*			*		$
Bergamot		*	*			$$
Cajuput		*				$
Cardamom		*				$$
Carrot seed		*	*	*		$$
Chamomile, German	*	*	*	*	*	$$$
Chamomile, Roman	*	*	*	*	*	$$$
Citronella		*				$$
Clary sage	*		*	*		$
Frankincense	*	*	*	*	*	$$
Geranium	*	*		*		$$
Ginger		*	*			$$
Grapefruit		*				$
Helichrysum	*	*	*	*	*	$$$
Jasmine	*			*		$$$
Juniper berry		*	*	*		$$
Lavender	*	*	*	*	*	$$
Lemon		*				$
Lemongrass		*				$
Lime		*	*			$
Mandarin	*	*	*			$
Myrrh		*	*	*		$$$
Neroli	*	*	*	*	*	$$$
Orange		*				$
Palmarosa		*				$
Patchouli	*	*	*	*		$
Peppermint		*				$
Petitgrain		*	*	*		$
Pine		*				$
Rose otto	*		*	*	*	$$$
Rosemary		*	*			$
Sandalwood (Australian)	*	*	*	*		$$$
Sweet basil		*				$
Sweet marjoram		*	*	*		$$$
Tea tree		*	*			$
Ylang-ylang	*		*	*		$$

Key: $ = inexpensive; $$ = moderate price; $$$ = expensive

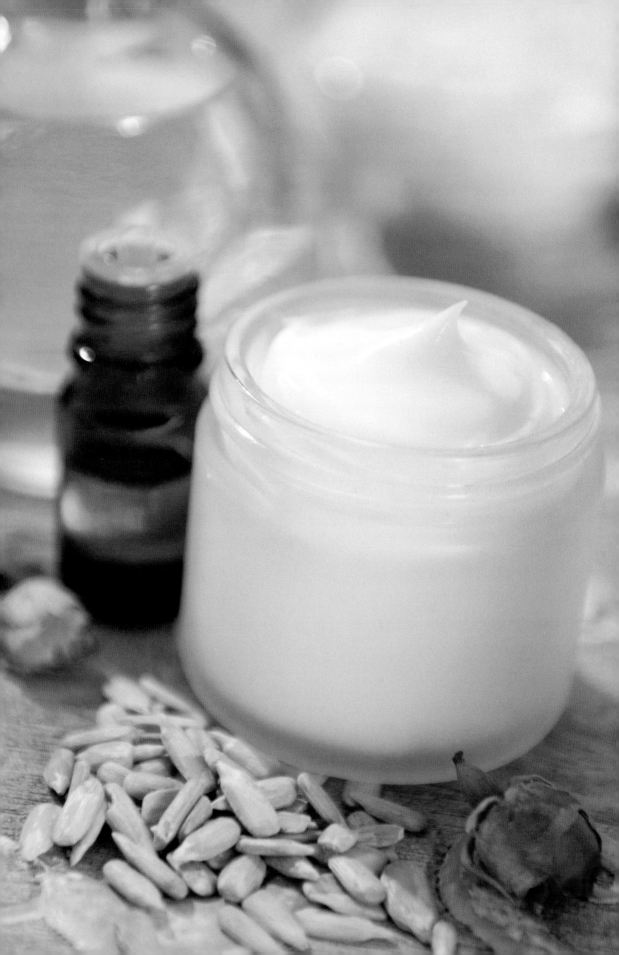

Basic Moisturizing Cream

Making a basic moisturizing cream is quite simple, but you do need to follow a specific procedure to ensure good results. This formulation outlines, step by step, the techniques for making a facial cream using basic ingredients.

**Makes about
18 oz (530 mL)**

TIPS

Always start the mixer at a low speed. Mix patiently, without stopping, to ensure that the wax and oil do not cool off before they are emulsified. Otherwise they can separate.

Always research the ingredients you are using and know the recommended maximum amount you can add to products.

Your final product relies on proper storage and packaging. Always sanitize the jar before using, seal it properly and store it in a cool, dark place.

Label your finished product with the dates of manufacture and expiry.

- Bowl-style double boiler
- Glass stir stick
- Electric mixer
- Glass jar (14 oz/400 mL) sprayed with 70% ethyl alcohol

3 tbsp (45 mL)	emulsifying wax NF
½ cup (125 mL)	sunflower seed oil
¾ cup (175 mL)	warm (86°F/30°C) filtered water
20 drops (1 mL)	essential oil of your choice (see page 211)

Variations

For an alcohol-free moisturizer, substitute an equal amount of beeswax or shea butter for the emulsifying wax.

If desired, use an eco-certified emulsifying wax (see Resources, page 371).

You can use an equal amount of any carrier oil you prefer (see pages 57 to 76).

BASIC DAY CREAM: Use carrier oils with a lighter texture that are rich in monounsaturated and polyunsaturated fatty acids, and essential oils that are balancing and stimulating (see pages 94 to 203).

BASIC NIGHT CREAM: Use carrier oils that are rich in saturated and unsaturated fatty acids, along with calming and relaxing essential oils (see pages 94 to 203).

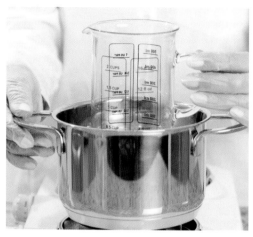

1 Set a heatproof glass measuring cup with spout over a saucepan of hot (not boiling) water (86°F/30°C) and heat until warm to the touch.

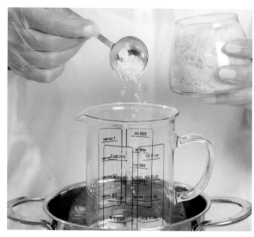

2 Add emulsifying wax and let melt completely.

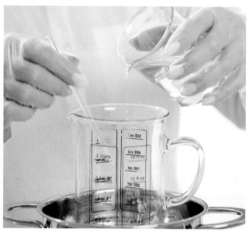

3 Add sunflower oil and stir gently until completely incorporated. Remove from heat.

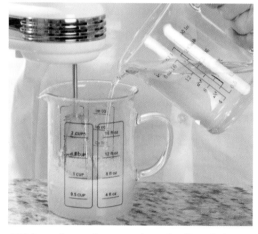

4 Using mixer at low speed, gradually mix in warm water. Continue to mix until emulsified (thick and creamy), 5 to 10 minutes.

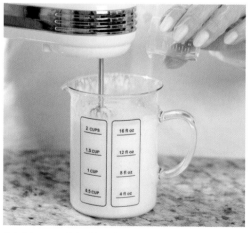

5 Add essential oil and mix until completely incorporated.

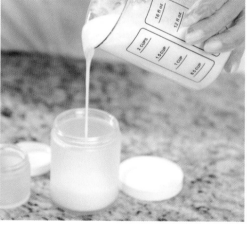

6 Transfer mixture to prepared jars and seal tightly. Properly stored, the cream will keep for up to 3 months.

Different Carrier Oils

You can use up to four different carrier oils in one formulation, as long as the total doesn't exceed the specified quantity. Consider the properties of each carrier oil and choose oils that are compatible with your skin type and the type of product you are making. See pages 57 to 76 for a complete list of options, or try these variations:

- **Oily skin:** argan, grapeseed or borage oil
- **Sensitive skin:** sweet almond, hempseed or jojoba oil
- **Combination and acne-prone skin:** evening primrose or rosehip seed oil
- **Dry and aging skin:** argan, sesame seed or borage oil

Choosing Essential Oils for Your Skin Type

The essential oils in this book have been specifically selected for making natural skin-care products. Consider the following when selecting oils:

- Is the oil is suitable and safe to use for your skin type? See pages 94 to 203.
- What effect do you want the fragrance to have (for example, to relax or stimulate)? Fragrance plays a huge role in how your product will make you feel (see page 92).
- What is your budget? Essential oils are available in a range of prices, and some can be quite expensive. Consult the variations for each formulation as well as the table on page 211 for recommended oils that can be substituted if needed.

Shelf Life and Storage

When you make your own personal care products, they do not include strong chemical preservatives, and they often call for ingredients such as water and grains, in which bacteria tend to flourish. Therefore, I recommend a shelf life of 3 months for most of the formulations in this book. To reduce the potential for bacterial growth, store your products in tightly sealed containers in a cool, dry area or in the refrigerator. Decant small portions into glass containers for day-to-day use and refill as needed.

Caution: If a product separates, discolors or develops an unpleasant odor, discard immediately.

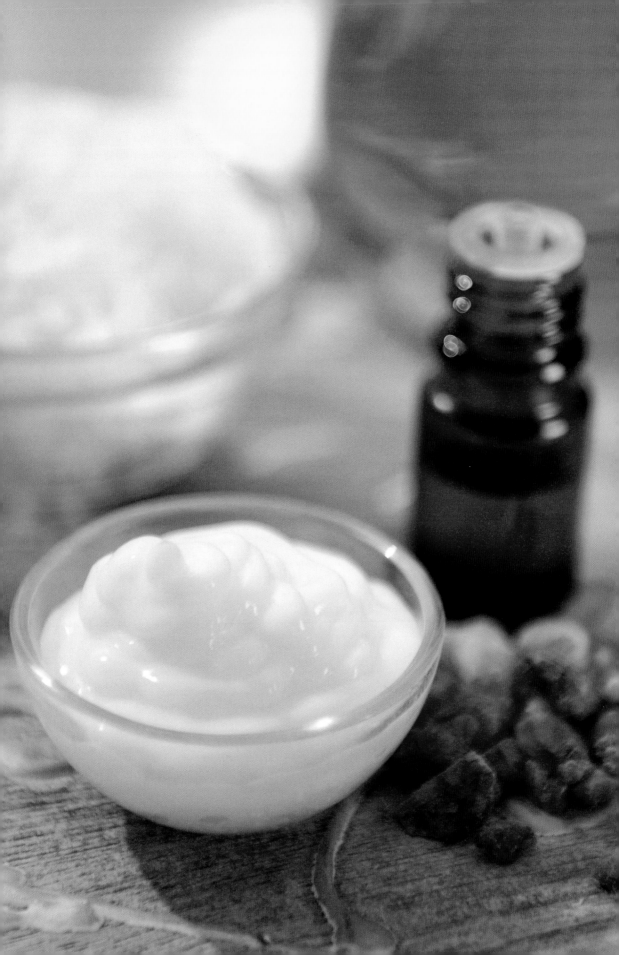

Basic Body Lotion

Making a basic lotion is quite simple, but you do need to follow a specific procedure to ensure good results. This formulation outlines, step by step, the techniques for making a basic lotion with basic ingredients.

SKIN TYPE

All (see Variations, below right)

WHEN TO USE

Morning

Makes about 29 oz (870 mL)

TIPS

Always start the mixer at a low speed. Mix patiently, without stopping, so the wax and oils do not cool off before they are emulsified. Otherwise they may separate.

Always research the ingredients you are using and know the recommended maximum amount you can add to products.

Label the finished product with the dates of manufacture and expiry.

- Bowl-style double boiler
- Glass stir stick
- Electric mixer
- PET flip-top bottle (30 oz/900 mL) sprayed with 70% ethyl alcohol

¼ cup (60 mL)	emulsifying wax NF
¼ cup (60 mL)	extra virgin coconut oil
½ cup (125 mL)	grapeseed oil
2 cups (500 mL)	warm (86°F/30°C) filtered water
30 drops (1.5 mL)	essential oil of your choice (see page 211)

Variations

For an alcohol-free moisturizer, substitute $1^1/_2$ tbsp (22 mL) beeswax and 2 tbsp (30 mL) shea butter for the emulsifying wax.

If desired, use an eco-certified emulsifying wax (see Resources, page 371).

You can use equal amounts of any carrier oil you prefer (see pages 57 to 66).

RICH BODY LOTION: Use a portion of carrier oils that are rich in saturated and polyunsaturated fatty acids. Use essential oils that are balancing and stimulating, see pages 94 to 203.

Managing Yields

This formulation, like many in this book, produces a large yield. I recommend storing larger yields in the fridge and transferring smaller quantities to a clean container for day-to-day use. If you prefer, you can also halve these formulations.

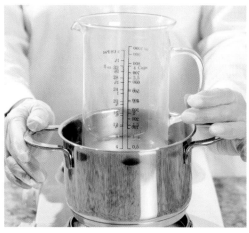

1 Set a heatproof glass measuring cup with spout over a saucepan of hot (not boiling) water (86°F/30°C) and heat until warm to the touch.

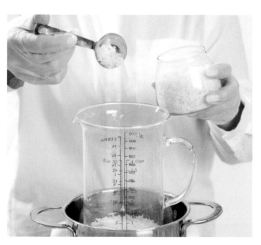

2 Add emulsifying wax and let melt completely.

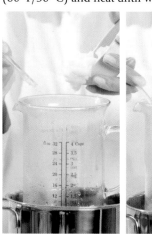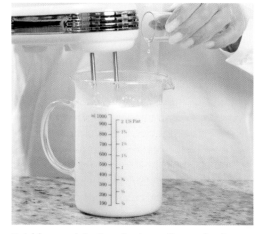

3 Add coconut oil and stir gently until completely incorporated. Add grapeseed oil and stir until completely incorporated. Remove from heat.

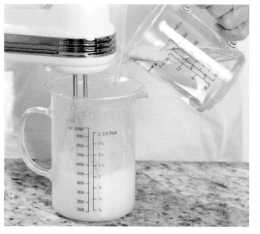

4 Using mixer at low speed, gradually mix in warm water. Continue to mix until emulsified (thick and creamy), 5 to 10 minutes.

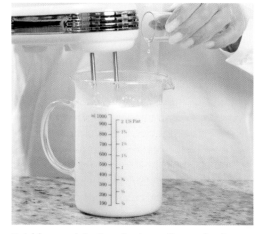

5 Add essential oil and mix until completely incorporated.

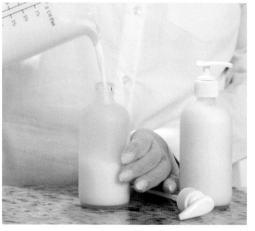

6 Transfer mixture to prepared bottles and seal tightly. Properly stored, the lotion will keep for up to 3 months.

Different Carrier Oils

You can use up to four different carrier oils in one formulation, as long as the total doesn't exceed the specified quantity. Consider the properties of each carrier oil and choose oils that are compatible with your skin type and the type of product you are making. See pages 56 to 76 for a complete list of options, or try these variations:

- **Oily skin:** apricot kernel or grapeseed oil
- **Sensitive skin:** sweet almond, hempseed or jojoba oil
- **Combination and acne-prone skin:** evening primrose or rosehip seed oil
- **Dry and aging skin:** argan, sesame seed or borage oil

Storage

Your final product relies on proper storage and packaging. Always sanitize the container before using, seal it properly and store it in a cool, dark place.

Sanitization

Sanitization of equipment is one of the most important parts of making your own skin-care products. Always use equipment that is dedicated to your skin-care apothecary. Wash it with soap and water, then dry with paper towels. Spray the equipment with 70% ethyl alcohol, rinse thoroughly and then dry. Use immediately or store in an airtight plastic bin.

Saturated Fats

Oils high in saturated fats — for example, extra virgin coconut oil, cocoa butter and shea butter — are solid at room temperature. If you decide to double the amount of saturated fat in your lotion, it will have a thicker consistency, becoming more of a cream than a lotion. It will also be more suitable for storage in a jar rather than a bottle.

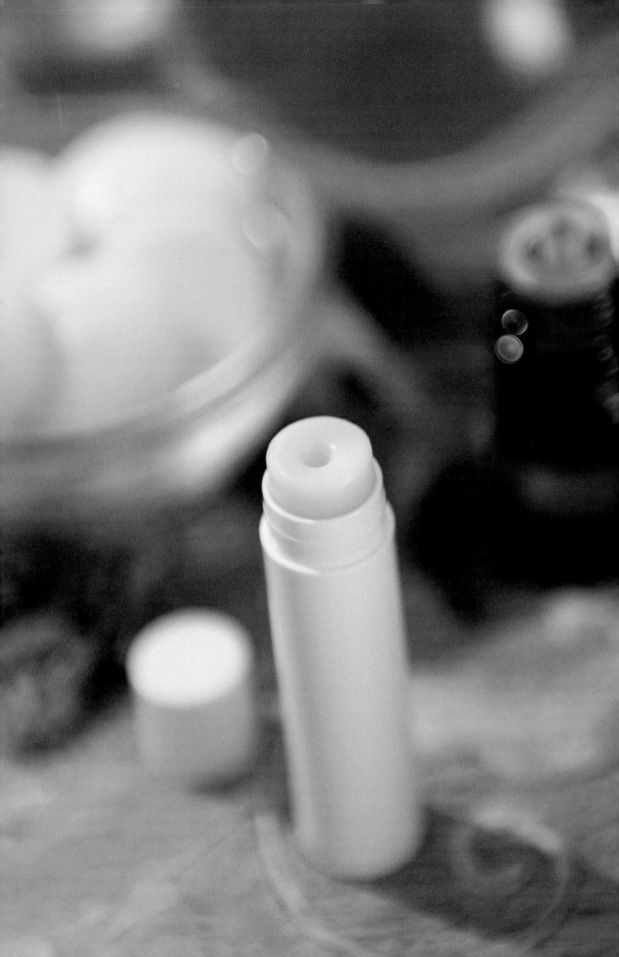

Basic Lip Balm

Making your own lip balm is quite simple, but you do need to follow a specific procedure to ensure good results. This formulation outlines, step by step, the techniques for making a basic lip balm with basic ingredients.

- Bowl-style double boiler (see Tips, left)
- Glass stir stick
- 10 to 12 lip balm tubes (0.15 oz/10 mL each) sprayed with 70% ethyl alcohol

2 tbsp (30 mL)	candelilla wax
2 tbsp (30 mL)	cocoa butter
¼ cup (60 mL)	calendula-infused oil
20 drops (1 mL)	essential oil of your choice (see page 211)

Variations

For dry, chapped lips: Substitute an equal amount of any carrier oil high in saturated fat — for example, sweet almond or carrot root–infused sunflower or sesame seed oil — for the calendula-infused oil.

You can use up to four different carrier oils in one formulation, as long as the total doesn't exceed the specified quantity. Consider the properties of each carrier oil and choose oils that are compatible with your skin type and the type of product you are making. See pages 57 to 76 for a complete list of options.

Substitute an equal amount of emulsifying wax, beeswax or carnauba wax for the candelilla wax.

If desired, use an eco-certified emulsifying wax (see Resources, page 371).

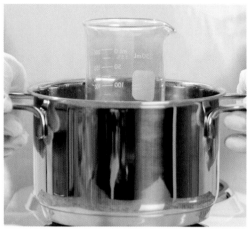

1 Set a heatproof glass measuring cup with spout over a saucepan of hot (not boiling) water (86°F/30°C) and heat until warm to the touch.

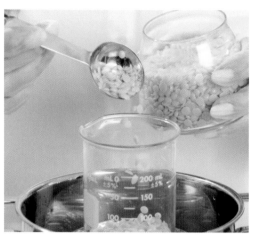

2 Add candelilla wax and let melt completely.

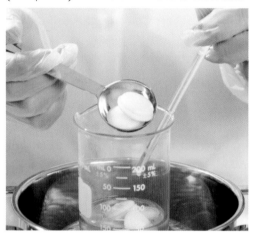

3 Add cocoa butter and stir gently until completely incorporated.

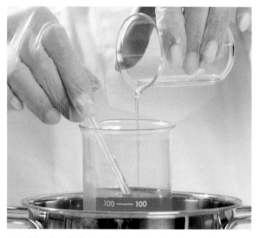

4 Add calendula-infused oil and stir gently until incorporated.

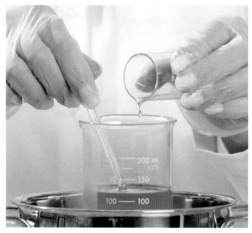

5 Add essential oil and mix until completely incorporated. Remove from heat.

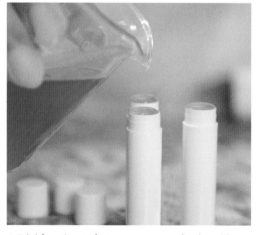

6 Divide mixture between prepared tubes (there will be extra). Let set for 5 minutes, top off with remaining mixture. Let cool for 20 minutes; then cover with caps.

Troubleshooting Lip Balms

To ensure that your lip balm will set correctly in the tubes, check before pouring to make sure that your formulation has reached the correct consistency:

1. Dip a wooden stir stick into the wax and oil mixture and let a few drops fall onto a piece of parchment paper. Set aside for about 1 minute, until dry.
2. Rub a little onto your fingertips to feel the texture.

- If it is hard and does not melt easily on your finger, there is too much emulsifier. You may need to add another 1 tbsp (15 mL) oil.
- If it is soft and smudgy, your lip balm will not set properly in the tube. Add another ¼ tsp (1 mL) candelilla wax.

Tips for Making Lip Balms

- Work quickly and keep the formula as warm as possible, for easy pouring. If it cools and becomes difficult to pour, just re-melt the mixture in the double boiler.
- Once the lip balm sets, it will shrink a bit in the tube. You can top it off with any remaining mixture.
- Your final product relies on proper storage and packaging. Always sanitize the tubes before using, seal them properly and store them in a cool, dark place.
- Label finished products with the dates of manufacture and expiry.

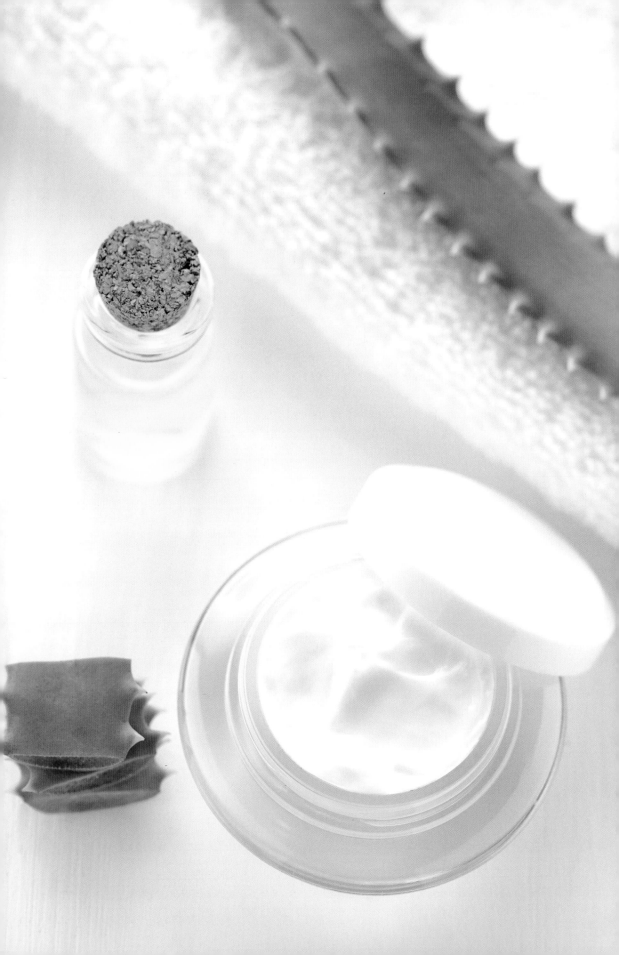

Facial Cleansers

Cleansing your face is an important part of any skin-care routine. The main reason for cleansing is to remove sweat, makeup and dirt without drying your skin. It should also be a pleasing, mindful experience. Choose cleansers that are suitable to your skin type (see "The Art of Skin Care," pages 21 to 25).

Rejuvenating Facial Cleanser

If you have been experiencing undue stress or sleepless nights, it is important to give your skin a rejuvenating boost. Your body has a crucial need for sleep and repair; when it is under any form of stress, it is likely to have an inflammatory response. The first symptoms of inflammation may appear on your face — your eyes may be puffy, your skin may seem swollen and clammy, and your complexion may look pale and grayish. The aromatherapy approach to resolving these symptoms is to formulate products with essential oils that calm the nervous system and stimulate circulation.

SKIN TYPE

All

WHEN TO USE

Morning

**Makes
9 oz (280 mL)**

TIPS

In Step 4, if your refrigerated base is too firm to mix, place the bowl on top of a pan filled with warm water for about 30 seconds, just until pliable.

I prefer to use carrot root-infused sesame oil in this formulation, but other carrier oils, such as extra virgin olive oil, are also fine. You can purchase carrot root-infused sesame seed oil from reliable suppliers (see page 371). For this formulation, whatever the carrier, be sure you are getting an infusion of carrot root, not carrot seed essential oil.

- Bowl-style double boiler
- Glass stir stick
- Small beaker
- Electric mixer
- Glass jar (9 oz/280 mL) sprayed with 70% ethyl alcohol (see Tip, right)

BASE

1 cup (250 mL)	extra virgin coconut oil
1 tbsp (15 mL)	carrot root-infused oil (see Tips, left)
1 tbsp (15 mL)	sodium laurel sulfate (SLS)–free liquid soap (see page 34)

ESSENTIAL OIL SYNERGY

20 drops (1 mL)	mandarin EO
5 drops (0.25 mL)	cardamom EO
5 drops (0.25 mL)	tea tree EO

1. *Base:* Set a heatproof glass bowl over a saucepan of hot (not boiling) water (86°F/30°C) and heat until warm to the touch. Add coconut oil and let melt completely. Add carrot root-infused oil and warm until mixture is perfectly clear, 1 to 2 minutes. Stir gently to ensure that ingredients are dissolved and evenly combined.
2. Remove bowl from heat and set aside to cool slightly. Place cooled bowl in the refrigerator for 30 minutes, until mixture has slightly solidified.
3. *Essential Oil Synergy:* Meanwhile, in beaker, combine mandarin, cardamom and tea tree essential oils. Cover with foil or plastic wrap and set aside.
4. Once cooled mixture has solidified, add liquid soap and, using electric mixer at low speed, beat until mixture is white and fluffy (see Tips, left).

You can use two 5-ounce (150 mL) jars to store this cleanser. Keep one for daily use and store the other in the refrigerator.

KNOW THE BENEFITS

Coconut oil contains lauric acid, which is found in mother's milk and has antibacterial and antifungal properties. The gentle infusion of carrot root provides beta-carotene, which nourishes the skin with antioxidants and protects from sun damage.

The dominant essential oil in the blend is mandarin. Its scent calms the nervous system while stimulating the circulatory system, thanks to its d-limonene content. Cardamom strengthens the scent of the synergy. Its two major constituents — eucalyptol (which is decongesting and antimicrobial) and terpinyl acetate (which is antispasmodic) — will help open pores and calm facial muscles. Tea tree oil has skin-protective qualities, as well as being antimicrobial and antifungal.

5. Add prepared synergy blend and mix until combined.
6. Transfer to prepared jar and seal tightly. Properly stored (see page 219), the cleanser will keep for up to 6 months.

Variations

Substitute an equal amount of castile soap for the SLS-free soap.

If you have sensitive skin, reduce the quantities of essential oils by half.

HOW TO USE

Begin your morning cleanse by wiping your face with a cloth soaked in warm water. Using your fingers, scoop out ¼ tsp (1 mL) of the cleanser and apply to your slightly moist skin. Massage for 30 seconds, then gently rinse off with warm water. Follow with toner and moisturizer, if needed.

Essential Oil Synergies

Combining essential oils that have similar therapeutic properties creates synergy among the components, which means that the blend is more powerful than the sum of its individual parts. In addition, when adding essential oils to skin-care products, it is important to blend the oils together before adding them to the base; otherwise the oils will not disperse properly.

Soothing Facial Cleanser

When you are exposed to allergens in foods, harsh chemicals or environmental pollutants, your body releases histamine. This can make your skin red, sore and itchy. The aromatherapy approach to resolving these symptoms is topical use of essential oils that have anti-inflammatory properties and support your body's immune response. To bolster their therapeutic properties, they are delivered in a base of carrier oils that acts as a protective barrier.

SKIN TYPE
Sensitive

WHEN TO USE
Morning and night

Makes about 7 oz (200 mL)

TIP

Avoid using arnica-infused oil on broken skin (see Variation).

KNOW THE BENEFITS

The shea butter, jojoba and arnica oil are very gentle and known for their anti-inflammatory properties. German chamomile essential oil is also well-known for its anti-inflammatory properties; it is often used to alleviate symptoms associated with eczema, dermatitis and other pronounced skin conditions.

- Bowl-style double boiler
- Glass stir stick
- Flip-top or pump bottle (7 oz/200 mL) sprayed with 70% ethyl alcohol

1 tbsp (15 mL)	shea butter
¾ cup (175 mL)	jojoba oil
1 tbsp (15 mL)	arnica-infused oil (see Tip, left)
5 drops (0.25 mL)	German chamomile EO

1. Set a heatproof glass bowl over a saucepan of hot (not boiling) water (86°F/30°C) and heat until warm to the touch. Add shea butter and let melt completely. Add jojoba and arnica-infused oils and warm until mixture is completely clear, 1 to 2 minutes. Stir gently to ensure that ingredients are dissolved and evenly combined. Remove bowl from heat.
2. Add German chamomile essential oil and stir until cool.
3. Transfer to prepared bottle and seal tightly. Properly stored (see page 219), the cleanser will keep for up to 6 months.

Variation
Substitute an equal quantity of calendula-infused oil (see page 78) for the arnica-infused oil.

HOW TO USE
Wipe your face with a cloth soaked in warm water. Squeeze about ¼ tsp (1 mL) of the cleanser onto your fingertips and apply to your slightly moist skin. Massage for 30 seconds, then gently rinse off with warm water. Follow with toner and moisturizer, if needed.

Skin-Lightening Facial Cleanser

Dull skin and hyperpigmentation may be caused by overexposure to sun and environmental pollution, adding years to your appearance. This formulation gently lightens your complexion, helping it to feel rejuvenated and youthful. Use twice a week for one month, substituting it for your regular cleanser.

SKIN TYPE

All

WHEN TO USE

Night

Makes 2¾ oz (80 mL)

TIPS

If your honey has crystallized, heat it in a double boiler until softened before adding the borage oil.

Do not use this cleanser more than twice a week. Avoid overexposure to direct sunlight when using.

KNOW THE BENEFITS

Honey is an age-old remedy for naturally glowing skin. Not only is it loaded with antioxidants, it also has antibacterial properties that support your skin's immunity and help to slow down aging.

- Glass stir stick
- Glass jar (3 oz/80 mL) sprayed with 70% ethyl alcohol

¼ cup (60 mL)	unpasteurized raw honey
1 tbsp (15 mL)	borage or evening primrose oil
20 drops (1 mL)	lemon EO

1. In a bowl, stir together honey, borage oil and lemon essential oil.
2. Transfer to prepared glass jar and seal tightly. Properly stored (see page 219), the cleanser will keep for up to 6 weeks.

Variations

To enhance the skin-lightening properties of this formula, add 5 drops (0.25 mL) German chamomile EO, which contains about 50% alpha-bisabolol, a skin-lightening agent.

If you do not have lemon essential oil, you may substitute an equal quantity of grapefruit or mandarin EO.

HOW TO USE

Begin by wiping your face with a cloth soaked in warm water. Using your fingers, scoop out ¼ tsp (1 mL) of the cleanser and apply to your slightly moist skin. Massage for 30 seconds, then leave on for 5 minutes. Gently rinse off with warm water. Follow with toner and moisturizer, if needed.

Penetrating Evening Facial Cleanser

When your skin is dry, it is prone to flaking and forming fine lines. It may feel tight and itchy, especially after washing. It is important to use gentle cleansers when caring for dry skin, especially at night, when the skin is much more dehydrated and needs more moisture. The right combination of oils will help to nourish your skin while you sleep.

SKIN TYPE

Dry

WHEN TO USE

Night

Makes 8 oz (240 mL)

TIPS

If you find the scent of ylang-ylang too floral or the patchouli too strong, reduce the quantity to 3 drops each.

When cleaning utensils and equipment, always wipe them down with dry paper towels before rinsing. This will prevent drains from becoming clogged by oil residue and keep scum from accumulating in the sink.

- Small beaker
- Bowl-style double boiler
- Glass stir stick
- Flip-top or pump bottle (8 oz/240 mL) sprayed with 70% ethyl alcohol

ESSENTIAL OIL SYNERGY

5 drops (0.25 mL)	ylang-ylang EO
10 drops (0.5 mL)	patchouli EO

BASE

1 tsp (5 mL)	unscented cocoa butter
¾ cup (175 mL)	sweet almond oil
¼ cup (60 mL)	rosehip seed oil

1. *Essential Oil Synergy:* In beaker, combine ylang-ylang and patchouli essential oils. Cover with foil or plastic wrap and set aside.

2. *Base:* Set a heatproof glass bowl over a saucepan of hot (not boiling) water (86°F/30°C) and heat until warm to the touch. Add cocoa butter and let melt completely. Add sweet almond and rosehip seed oils and warm until mixture is perfectly clear, 1 to 2 minutes. Stir gently to ensure that the ingredients are dissolved and evenly combined. Remove bowl from heat.

3. Add prepared synergy blend and stir until cool. Transfer to prepared bottle and seal tightly. Properly stored (see page 219), the cleanser will keep for up to 6 months.

Cleansing dry skin with water and any detergent-based soap may dry it out even further and affect its natural pH. This will be especially noticeable if your water contains high levels of chlorine. That is why it is especially important to use a cleanser that also provides a rich protective barrier to prevent moisture from escaping. Sweet almond oil is rich in oleic acid (its average content is 60 to 65%), which makes it an excellent emollient. Rosehip seed oil adds omega-3, -6 and -9 fatty acids, beta-carotene and vitamin E. These nutrients nurture dry, damaged and aging skin. Floral-scented ylang-ylang is chemically made up of a variety of constituents that have a balancing effect and antibacterial properties. Musky patchouli oil delivers anti-inflammatory benefits.

Variations

Rosehip seed oil can be expensive and is sometimes hard to find. Substitute an equal quantity of hempseed oil, which contains similar amounts of omega-3, -6 and -9 essential fatty acids.

For sensitive skin, substitute an equal amount of Roman chamomile essential oil for the ylang-ylang.

HOW TO USE

Before going to bed, wipe your face with a cloth soaked in warm water. Squeeze out about ¼ tsp (1 mL) of the cleanser and apply to your slightly moist skin. Massage for 30 seconds, then gently rinse with warm water. Follow with toner and moisturizer, if needed.

NUT
ALLERGY ALERT

If you are sensitive to nuts, you can use alternative carrier oils. Substitute an equal amount of grapeseed, fractionated coconut or apricot kernel oil for the sweet almond oil. These oils also result in a light-textured base.

Facial Cleanser for Oily Skin

Overproductive sebaceous glands create oily skin, mainly on the face and scalp. To keep oily skin refreshed, regular cleansing is particularly important. However, you need to be careful that you don't cleanse too aggressively. Over-cleansing can lead to an imbalance in the natural oils (sebum) your body produces, which help to protect your skin.

SKIN TYPE

Oily

WHEN TO USE

Morning and night (see Variation, page 233)

Makes about 8 oz (235 mL)

TIPS

If you have very sensitive skin, reduce the quantity of each essential oil by half.

When cleaning utensils and equipment, always wipe them down with dry paper towels before rinsing. This will prevent drains from becoming clogged by oil residue and keep scum from accumulating in the sink.

- Bowl-style double boiler
- Small beaker
- Glass stir stick
- Glass jar (8 oz/250 mL) sprayed with 70% ethyl alcohol

BASE

¼ cup (60 mL)	shea butter
¼ cup (60 mL)	aloe vera gel

ESSENTIAL OIL SYNERGY

10 drops (0.5 mL)	cajuput EO
10 drops (0.5 mL)	tea tree EO
10 drops (0.5 mL)	grapefruit EO

1. *Base:* Set a heatproof glass bowl over a saucepan of hot (not boiling) water (86°F/30°C) and heat until warm to the touch. Add shea butter and let melt completely.

2. Remove bowl from heat and set aside to cool slightly. Place cooled bowl in the refrigerator for 10 minutes, until mixture is completely cooled but still liquid.

3. *Essential Oil Synergy:* Meanwhile, in beaker, combine cajuput, tea tree and grapefruit essential oils. Cover with foil or plastic wrap and set aside.

4. Add aloe vera to cooled shea butter, stirring constantly until ingredients have emulsified. Add reserved essential oil synergy and stir until well blended. Transfer to prepared jar and seal tightly. Properly stored, the mixture will keep for up to 6 months.

Oily skin is prone to acne. This formula contains two potent ingredients, aloe vera and shea butter, that help balance sebum production. Shea butter also moisturizes, reduces inflammation and repairs skin. Aloe vera is astringent, helping to maintain moisture while cleansing the skin of impurities.

Variation

Cajuput, grapefruit and tea tree essential oils are stimulating. You may substitute an equal quantity of calming and relaxing essential oils that are suitable for sensitive skin — such as sweet marjoram, lavender and mandarin — for evening application.

HOW TO USE

Wipe your face with a cloth soaked in warm water. Scoop out about ¼ tsp (1 mL) of the cleanser and apply to your slightly moist skin. Massage for 30 seconds, then gently rinse with warm water. Follow with toner and moisturizer, if needed.

SENSITIVITY ALERT

While the components of grapefruit EO have not been researched in this regard, there are substances (furocoumarins) in grapefruit juice that may undermine the performance of certain prescription drugs. So if you are taking prescription drugs and have been advised to avoid grapefruit, I recommend substituting an equal amount of bergamot FCF (furocoumarin-free) or lime essential oil (distilled) instead.

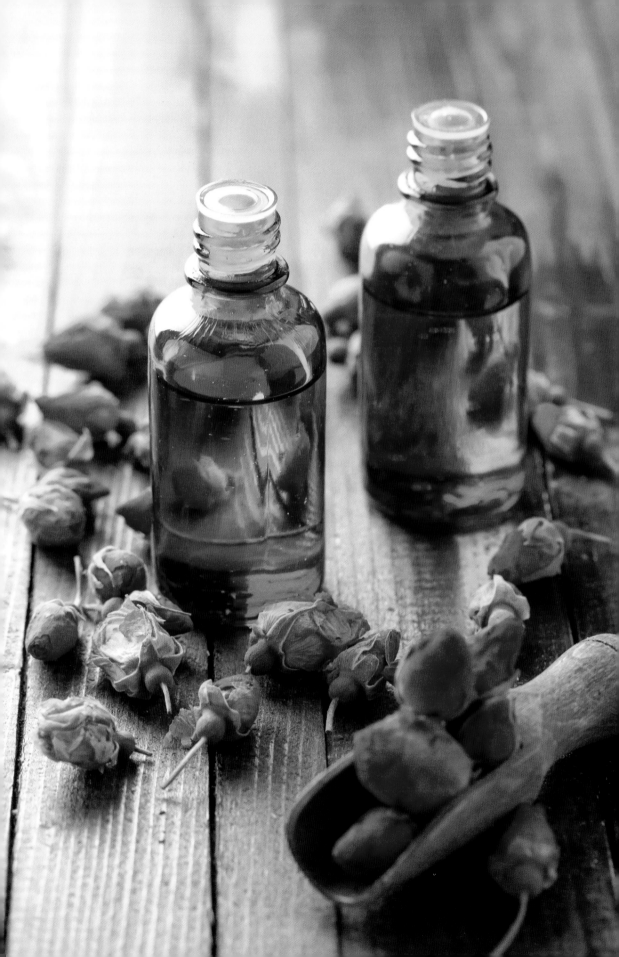

Skin Toners

Toners are a very important part of a skin-care routine. They remove excess oil and help close pores, leaving a smooth appearance. Toners also play an important role in balancing the skin's pH level — how alkaline or acidic it is. Most skin has an average pH of 4.5 to 6 (slightly acidic), which helps it protect itself from germs and environmental pollution and prevents dehydration. When skin is alkaline (a pH of 7 to 8), it has a tendency to be dry, sensitive and susceptible to inflammation; it also loses its elasticity, which can lead to premature aging.

A toner should be refreshing and have humectant properties that help the skin retain its moisture. Regular tap water usually has a pH of 9 to 10 (alkaline), which disrupts the skin's ability to protect itself. A toner suited to your skin type will help to balance excessive exposure to alkaline water.

Flower Power Toner

When selecting a toner for sensitive skin, to avoid potential irritation, look for one that contains a few simple but effective ingredients. This toner pairs calendula and water with a low dilution of essential oils to soothe and hydrate the skin.

SKIN TYPE

All, especially sensitive

WHEN TO USE

Morning and night, after cleansing

Makes about 3 oz (100 mL)

TIP

Toners should feel refreshing and leave the skin feeling slightly tightened, thanks to their mild astringent properties. If you feel a burning sensation, immediately rinse your face with water and discontinue use.

KNOW THE BENEFITS

Calendula glycerin infusion has anti-inflammatory properties that soothe the skin and humectant properties that help restore moisture. Helichrysum helps to ease symptoms of rosacea and other inflammatory skin conditions.

- Small beaker
- Glass spray bottle (3 oz/100 mL) sprayed with 70% alcohol

1 tsp (5 mL)	calendula infusion in glycerin
5 drops (0.25 mL)	Floral Antimicrobial Synergy (page 37)
5 drops (0.25 mL)	helichrysum EO
¾ cup (175 mL)	warm (86°F/30°C) filtered water

1. In beaker, combine calendula infusion, floral antimicrobial synergy and helichrysum essential oil. Add water and whisk well.
2. Transfer to prepared bottle and seal tightly. Properly stored, the toner will keep for up to 8 weeks.

Variation

Substitute an equal amount of German chamomile essential oil for the helichrysum.

HOW TO USE

Shake well before using. After cleansing your skin, spray toner onto two cotton pads. With one pad in each hand, starting at the chin and working upward to the forehead, pat toner evenly over both sides of your face. Avoid vigorous stroking, which will agitate the skin. Let skin absorb toner for 5 to 10 seconds, then apply Flower Power Moisturizing Cream (page 252).

Saffron Nights Skin-Lightening Toner

Thanks to apple cider vinegar, this mild toner firms skin and reduces the size of pores — wonderful for aging skin.

SKIN TYPE

Dry, aging skin

WHEN TO USE

Morning and night

Makes about 3 oz (100 mL)

TIP

You can also use this toner as a deodorant or body mist.

KNOW THE BENEFITS

Saffron gives the skin a radiant glow, while apple cider vinegar softens and brightens it. Rose hydrolat delicately enhances the moisturizing effects of this toner. Sandalwood lightens the skin, and its earthy scent relaxes the nervous system. The exotic fragrance of jasmine is sensual and uplifting.

- Small beaker
- Glass spray bottle (3 oz/100 mL) sprayed with 70% ethyl alcohol (see page 219)

¼ cup (60 mL)	warm (86°F/30°C) filtered water
3 threads	saffron
1 tsp (5 mL)	apple cider vinegar
2 tbsp (30 mL)	rose hydrolat
5 drops (0.25 mL)	jasmine absolute
5 drops (0.25 mL)	sandalwood EO

1. In beaker, combine water and saffron; set aside for 15 minutes to soak.
2. Add apple cider vinegar and rose hydrolat and whisk well. Add jasmine absolute and sandalwood essential oil and whisk until well incorporated.
3. Transfer to prepared bottle and seal tightly. Properly stored (see page 219), the toner will keep for up to 8 weeks.

Variation

Substitute an equal amount of neroli hydrolat for the rose hydrolat.

HOW TO USE

Shake well before using. After cleansing your skin, spray toner onto two cotton pads. With one pad in each hand, starting at the chin and working upward to the forehead, pat toner evenly over both sides of your face. Avoid vigorous stroking, which will agitate the skin. Let skin absorb toner for 5 to 10 seconds, then apply Saffron Night Repair Moisturizing Cream (page 254).

Orange Blossom Floral Water Toner

Oily and sensitive skin can take on a blotchy appearance. This formulation has mild astringent properties that disinfect and tone, leaving the skin feeling soft and smooth.

SKIN TYPE

Sensitive, oily

WHEN TO USE

After cleansing

Makes about 3 oz (100 mL)

TIP

Toners should feel cool and refreshing on the skin and leave it feeling slightly tightened, thanks to their mild astringent properties. If you feel a burning sensation, immediately rinse your face with water and discontinue use.

KNOW THE BENEFITS

Neroli hydrolat has antiseptic and antibacterial properties that work to prevent breakouts and clear the skin. The antibacterial properties of petitgrain (the leaf of the bitter orange tree) also help to clear up breakouts.

- Small beaker
- Glass spray bottle (3 oz/100 mL) sprayed with 70% ethyl alcohol (see page 219)

¼ cup (60 mL)	neroli hydrolat
2 tbsp (30 mL)	witch hazel hydrolat
1 tsp (5 mL)	aloe vera gel
5 drops (0.25 mL)	neroli EO
5 drops (0.25 mL)	petitgrain EO

1. In beaker, combine neroli and witch hazel hydrolats and aloe vera gel. Add neroli and petitgrain essential oils and whisk well.
2. Transfer to prepared bottle and seal tightly. Properly stored (see page 219), the toner will keep for up to 8 weeks.

Variations

To treat severe acne breakouts, add 5 drops (0.25 mL) tea tree essential oil at the end of Step 1.

For a more cost-effective blend, you can substitute an equal amount of lavender or bergamot FCF essential oil for the neroli. Both lavender and bergamot deliver the same calming, antiseptic and antibacterial qualities as neroli.

HOW TO USE

Shake well before using. After cleansing your skin, spray toner onto two cotton pads. With one pad in each hand, starting at the chin and working upward to the forehead, pat toner evenly over both sides of your face. Avoid vigorous stroking, which will agitate the skin. Let skin absorb toner for 5 to 10 seconds, then apply Orange Blossom Moisturizing Cream (page 264).

Pomegranate Hibiscus Face-Lifting Toner

This gentle toner leaves the skin feeling firm and uplifted — perfect for those times when it can look tired and worn, especially if you have dry, aging skin.

SKIN TYPE
All

WHEN TO USE
Morning and night

Makes 4 oz (125 mL)

TIP

Refrain from using facial hair removers for at least 48 hours before and after using a toner. Toners often contain substances that will mildly exfoliate the skin.

KNOW THE BENEFITS

Rose hydrolat and aloe vera gel are cooling agents that also help repair sun-damaged skin. Hibiscus glycerin infusion contains quercetin, an antioxidant that protects the elastin in your skin, keeping it supple and resistant. Pomegranate extract has antioxidant properties and reduces the effects of sun damage.

- Small beaker
- Glass spray bottle (4 oz/125 mL) sprayed with 70% ethyl alcohol (see page 219)

¼ cup (60 mL)	hibiscus infusion in glycerin
¼ cup (60 mL)	rose hydrolat
1 tsp (5 mL)	aloe vera gel
5 drops (0.25 mL)	pomegranate extract
5 drops (0.25 mL)	lime EO (distilled)

1. In beaker, combine hibiscus infusion, rose hydrolat and aloe vera gel. Add pomegranate extract and lime essential oil and whisk well.
2. Transfer to prepared bottle and seal tightly. Properly stored (see page 219), the toner will keep for up to 8 weeks.

Variations

For a cooling and calming effect, substitute an equal amount of Roman chamomile hydrolat for the rose hydrolat.

For a calming anti-inflammatory effect, substitute an equal amount of Roman chamomile essential oil for the lime.

HOW TO USE

Shake well before using. After cleansing skin, spray toner onto two cotton pads. With one pad in each hand, starting at the chin and working upward to the forehead, pat toner evenly over both sides of your face. Avoid vigorous stroking, which will agitate the skin. Let skin absorb toner for 5 to 10 seconds, then apply Hibiscus Astringent Moisturizing Cream (page 262).

Rejuvenating Toner

Sometimes the skin needs a wakeup. This toner is designed to leave you feeling more alert and stimulated, thanks to the synergy of mandarin, tea tree and cardamom essential oils. It is especially beneficial in the middle of the day, when you may be feeling tired. A light spray of this toner is very refreshing.

SKIN TYPE

Dry, mature skin

WHEN TO USE

Morning or midday

**Makes
3 oz (90 mL)**

TIP

Toners should feel cool and refreshing and leave your skin feeling slightly tightened, thanks to their mild astringent properties. If you feel a burning sensation, immediately rinse your face with water and discontinue use.

KNOW THE BENEFITS

Carrot root infusion in glycerin is rich in carotenoids and nutrients that help to regenerate and repair skin. Combined with aloe vera gel, it leaves the skin feeling cool and refreshed. Rosemary extract preserves the toner and also delivers a fresh scent.

- Small beaker
- Glass spray bottle (3 oz/100 mL) sprayed with 70% ethyl alcohol (see page 219)

¼ cup (60 mL)	warm (86°F/30°C) filtered water
1 tbsp (15 mL)	carrot root infusion in glycerin
1 tbsp (15 mL)	aloe vera gel
20 drops (1 mL)	mandarin EO
1 drop	tea tree EO
1 drop	cardamom EO
5 drops (0.25 mL)	rosemary extract

1. In beaker, combine water, carrot root infusion and aloe vera gel. Add mandarin, tea tree and cardamom essential oils and rosemary extract and whisk well.
2. Transfer to prepared bottle and seal tightly. Properly stored (see page 219), the toner will keep for up to 8 weeks.

Variation

Substitute an equal amount of bergamot FCF or lime essential oil for the mandarin.

HOW TO USE

Shake well before using. After cleansing skin, spray toner onto two cotton pads. With one pad in each hand, starting at the chin and working upward to the forehead, pat toner evenly over both sides of your face. Avoid vigorous stroking, which will agitate the skin. Let skin absorb toner for 5 to 10 seconds, then apply Anti-Aging Moisturizing Day Cream (page 266).

Lavender and Green Tea Antioxidant Toner

Acne breakouts can occur at any time and for many reasons, no matter what the age. This toner soothes the skin, relieving redness and inflammation.

SKIN TYPE

Acne-prone, oily

WHEN TO USE

Morning or night

Makes 3½ oz (105 mL)

TIP

Refrain from using facial hair removers for at least 48 hours before and after using a toner. Aloe vera gel contains a small amount of salicylic acid, making it a mild exfoliant. Waxing in conjunction with using aloe vera gel may wound the skin.

KNOW THE BENEFITS

This toner is rich in antioxidants that help repair and protect the skin from premature aging. Witch hazel and aloe vera are both astringent; they help to reduce the size of pores and leave the skin looking supple. Lavender heals damaged skin.

- Small beaker
- Glass spray bottle (4 oz/125 mL) sprayed with 70% ethyl alcohol (see page 219)

¼ cup (60 mL)	warm (86°F/30°C) filtered water
1 tbsp (15 mL)	witch hazel hydrolat
1 tbsp (15 mL)	aloe vera gel
1 tbsp (15 mL)	green tea infusion in glycerin
20 drops (1 mL)	lavender EO

1. In beaker, combine water, witch hazel hydrolat, aloe vera gel and green tea infusion. Add lavender essential oil and whisk well.
2. Transfer to prepared bottle and seal tightly. Properly stored (see page 219), the toner will keep for up to 8 weeks.

Variations

Substitute 10 drops (0.5 mL) Roman chamomile essential oil for the lavender.

For a morning toner, substitute an equal quantity of bergamot FCF essential oil for the lavender.

HOW TO USE

Shake well before using. After cleansing skin, spray toner onto two cotton pads. With one pad in each hand, starting at the chin and working upward to the forehead, pat toner evenly over both sides of your face. Avoid vigorous stroking, which will agitate the skin. Let skin absorb toner for 5 to 10 seconds, then apply Green Beauty Moisturizing Cream (page 258).

Soothing Toner

The cooling agents in this toner — aloe vera gel and Roman chamomile infusion — soothe damaged skin, helping to reduce redness and inflammation.

- Small beaker
- Glass spray bottle (3 oz/100 mL) sprayed with 70% ethyl alcohol (see page 219)

¼ cup (60 mL)	warm (86°F/30°C) filtered water
1 tbsp (15 mL)	chamomile infusion in glycerin
1 tbsp (15 mL)	aloe vera gel
5 drops (0.25 mL)	Roman chamomile EO
5 drops (0.25 mL)	German chamomile EO

1. In beaker, combine water, chamomile infusion and aloe vera gel. Add Roman and German chamomile essential oils and whisk well.
2. Transfer to prepared bottle and seal tightly. Properly stored (see page 219), the toner will keep for up to 8 weeks.

Variation

If you have a sensitivity to any plant in the chamomile family (Asteraceae), substitute an equal amount of green tea infusion for the chamomile infusion. Use 3 drops of patchouli EO and 3 drops of Australian sandalwood EO instead of the Roman and German chamomile essential oils.

HOW TO USE

Shake well before using. After cleansing skin, spray toner onto two cotton pads. With one pad in each hand, starting at the chin and working upward to the forehead, pat toner evenly over both sides of your face. Avoid vigorous stroking, which will agitate the skin. Let skin absorb toner for 5 to 10 seconds, then apply Everyday Facial Moisturizing Cream (page 256).

Rose-Enriched Floral Hydrolat Toner

Turn to this toner when you feel like you need a little pampering. Rose has a luxurious floral scent that is both calming and relaxing.

All

WHEN TO USE

After cleansing

**Makes
3 oz (90 mL)**

TIP

Aloe vera gel can be purchased in health food stores. It should be stored in an airtight container in the refrigerator.

KNOW THE BENEFITS

The combination of aloe vera gel and rose water is both refreshing and moisturizing. If you suffer from extra-dry skin or flushing caused by hormonal fluctuations, rose otto essential oil is especially healing.

- Small beaker
- Glass spray bottle (3 oz/100 mL) sprayed with 70% ethyl alcohol (see page 219)

¼ cup (60 mL)	rose hydrolat
2 tbsp (30 mL)	aloe vera gel
1 drop (0.5 mL)	rose otto EO

1. In beaker, combine rose hydrolat and aloe vera gel. Add rose otto essential oil and whisk well.
2. Transfer to prepared bottle and seal tightly. Properly stored (see page 219), the toner will keep for up to 8 weeks.

Variation

For a more cost-effective blend, substitute an equal amount of geranium essential oil for the rose otto.

HOW TO USE

Shake well before using. After cleansing skin, hold bottle 6 to 8 inches (15 to 20 cm) from your face and gently mist toner onto your face for a few seconds. Using your fingertips, gently tap face all over until toner has dried — the tapping motion helps the ingredients penetrate the skin and promotes blood circulation, making the skin look plush. If applying to aggravated skin, simply pat your face dry with a cotton ball.

Refreshing Green Toner

When you are uncomfortably warm and flushed, this toner will leave you feeling cool and refreshed. It's also perfect for when you may have been overexposed to the sun and need to soothe damaged skin.

SKIN TYPE

All, especially oily

WHEN TO USE

After cleansing

**Makes
3 oz (90 mL)**

TIP

Toners should feel cool and refreshing and leave your skin feeling slightly tightened, thanks to their mild astringent properties. If you feel a burning sensation, immediately rinse your face with water and discontinue use.

KNOW THE BENEFITS

The combination of aloe vera gel and chlorophyll delivers powerful antioxidants, helping the skin repair itself and leaving you feeling cool and refreshed. This bouquet of floral, citrus and mint essential oils makes a pleasant pick-me-up with antiseptic and antibacterial properties.

- Small beaker
- Glass spray bottle (3 oz/100 mL) sprayed with 70% ethyl alcohol (see page 219)

¼ cup (60 mL)	warm (86°F/30°C) filtered water
2 tbsp (30 mL)	aloe vera gel
10 drops (0.5 mL)	liquid chlorophyll
5 drops (0.25 mL)	bamboo extract
5 drops (0.25 mL)	neroli EO
5 drops (0.25 mL)	jasmine EO
5 drops (0.25 mL)	grapefruit EO
1 drop	peppermint EO

1. In beaker, combine water and aloe vera gel. Add chlorophyll, bamboo extract, and neroli, jasmine, grapefruit and pepper mint essential oils. Whisk well.
2. Transfer to prepared bottle and seal tightly. Properly stored (see page 219), the toner will keep for up to 8 weeks.

Variations

For an herbaceous rose scent, substitute 5 drops of rose otto and 3 drops of petitgrain for the essential oils called for in this formulation.

For a more cost-effective blend, substitute an equal amount of lavender or bergamot FCF essential oil for the neroli. Both deliver the same calming, antiseptic and antibacterial effects as neroli.

HOW TO USE

Shake well before using. After cleansing skin, spray toner onto two cotton pads. With one pad in each hand, starting at the chin and working upward to the forehead, pat toner evenly over both sides of your face. Avoid vigorous stroking, which will agitate the skin. Let skin absorb toner for 5 to 10 seconds, then apply Green Beauty Moisturizing Cream (page 258).

HYDROLATS

Hydrolats (also referred to as hydrosols, floral waters or distillates) are produced via steam distillation. Plants or flowers are put into a distillation tank and exposed to boiling water and steam. The steam bursts the cell walls of the plant, which contain the aromatic essences, and these essences blend with the steam. Once the steam cools and becomes liquid again, the molecules of essential oil separate and float to the surface, forming two layers: the essential oil floating on top and the hydrolat beneath it. The hydrolat contains a small amount (1 to 2%) of the chemical constituents found in the essential oil, and it also contains the same nonvolatile compounds as the plant.

Hydrolats can be used on their own as toners and are versatile enough to use as aftershave mists, perfumed body sprays or bath fragrances. The following are some common hydrolats that can be used in place of toners. (See also page 22.)

ROMAN CHAMOMILE (*Chamaemelum nobile*) HYDROLAT

Shelf life . . . . 1–12 months
pH . . . . 3.0–3.3 (astringent)
Skin type . . . . oily, acne-prone, sensitive

This herbal, fruit-scented mist has antiseptic qualities, is calming to the skin and helps relieve bruising. It can be used on oily and sensitive skin and skin that has acne. It can also be applied after blackhead extractions or even after facial acupuncture.

continued on next page

Know the pH of Your Hydrolats

Like your skin, hydrolats have an acidic pH, ranging from 3.5 to 6. Any change from the hydrolat's normal pH range can indicate contamination. Contamination can occur for many reasons, including poor storage, cross-contamination during the distillation process, or simply age (using past the expiry date). Measure the acidity of your hydrolats with pH strips to make sure that they haven't become alkaline (above 7). Alkalinity indicates that a hydrolat may be contaminated by microbes and could cause adverse effects on the skin or shorten the shelf life of your formulation.

LAVENDER (*Lavandula angustifolium*) HYDROLAT

Shelf life . . . . 1–12 months
pH . . . . 5.6–5.9 (slightly astringent)
Skin type . . . . all

Lavender hydrolat smells very herbaceous rather than like lavender essential oil, so I usually add a drop of lavender EO to give it that scent. Its pH is more or less balanced (close to neutral), which makes it suitable for all types of skin. It makes an excellent toner and also helps heal wounds and insect bites and calms down skin rashes and sunburn.

NEROLI (ORANGE BLOSSOM) HYDROLAT

Shelf life . . . . 1–12 months
pH . . . . 3.8–4.5 (astringent)
Skin type . . . . oily, acne-prone, sensitive

I call the soft, floral, gentle aroma of neroli hydrolat "the scent of the heavens," perhaps from my childhood memories, when this perfumed water was used in celebrations to symbolize the fragrance beyond this earth. Both the essential oil and the hydrolat of this plant calm the nervous system. Its pH is slightly acidic, making it very suitable for oily skin and sensitive skin that is prone to infection and inflammation.

ROSE (*Rosa x damascena*) HYDROLAT

Shelf life . . . . 1–12 months
pH . . . . 4.1–4.4 (astringent)
Skin type . . . . all

The subtle rose aroma of this hydrolat is captivating. It will pamper all types of skin and is particularly helpful for dry, aging skin because of its humectant properties. It is antiseptic and antibacterial and also has a cooling effect. Rose hydrolat is ideal to use as a natural perfume or deodorant.

WITCH HAZEL (*Hamamelis virginiana*) HYDROLAT

Shelf life . . . . 1–12 months
pH . . . . 4.0–4.2 (astringent)
Skin type . . . . oily, sensitive

Witch hazel has a slightly dry, herbaceous scent. It reduces inflammation and redness and helps to relieve scaly, dry, sensitive patches, as well as acne breakouts.

How to Check pH

It is easy to check the pH of liquids such as hydrolats, infused teas or tap water by using pH strips, which you can find at health food stores and other suppliers (see page 371). Simply dip the pH strip into the liquid, shake off the excess and wait 15 seconds. Then compare the color to the chart provided to determine the pH.

Neroli-Enriched Floral Hydrolat Toner

This toner is extremely gentle, making it a good match for people who have oily and/or sensitive skin or skin that is prone to infection, inflammation or allergies.

SKIN TYPE

All

WHEN TO USE

After cleansing, morning and night

**Makes
3 oz (90 mL)**

TIP

Aloe vera gel can be purchased in health food stores. It should be stored in an airtight container in the refrigerator.

KNOW THE BENEFITS

The combination of aloe vera gel and neroli EO is gentle and refreshing while delivering antiseptic and antibacterial effects.

- Small beaker
- Glass spray bottle (3 oz/100 mL) sprayed with 70% ethyl alcohol (see page 219)

¼ cup (60 mL)	neroli hydrolat
2 tbsp (30 mL)	aloe vera gel
1 drop	neroli EO

1. In beaker, combine neroli hydrolat and aloe vera gel. Add neroli essential oil and whisk well.
2. Transfer to prepared bottle and seal tightly. Properly stored (see page 219), the toner will keep for up to 8 weeks.

Variation

For a more cost-effective blend, substitute an equal amount of petitgrain essential oil for the neroli.

HOW TO USE

Shake well before using. After cleansing skin, hold bottle 6 to 8 inches (15 to 20 cm) from your face and gently mist toner onto your face for a few seconds. Using your fingertips, gently tap face all over until toner has dried — the tapping motion helps the ingredients penetrate the skin and promotes blood circulation, making the skin look plush. If applying to aggravated skin, simply pat your face dry with a cotton ball.

Lavender-Enriched Floral Hydrolat Toner

Because of its therapeutic and calming properties, lavender is considered an effective first-aid treatment. Turn to this toner when your skin is in need of some extra attention as a result of inflammation or breakouts.

SKIN TYPE

All

WHEN TO USE

After cleansing

Makes
3 oz (90 mL)

TIP

Aloe vera gel can be purchased in heath food stores. It should be stored in an airtight container in the refrigerator.

KNOW THE BENEFITS

The combination of aloe vera gel and lavender hydrolat is cooling, soothing, antiseptic and antibacterial. Lavender essential oil helps to heal wounds and insect bites and soothes rashes and sunburn.

- Small beaker
- Glass spray bottle (3 oz/100mL) sprayed with 70% ethyl alcohol (see page 219)

¼ cup (60 mL)	lavender hydrolat
2 tbsp (30 mL)	aloe vera gel
1 drop	lavender EO

1. In beaker, combine lavender hydrolat and aloe vera gel. Add lavender essential oil and whisk well.
2. Transfer to prepared bottle and seal tightly. Properly stored (see page 219), the toner will keep for up to 8 weeks.

Variation

Substitute an equal amount of benzoin essential oil for the lavender.

HOW TO USE

Shake well before using. After cleansing skin, hold bottle 6 to 8 inches (15 to 20 cm) from your face and gently mist toner onto your face for a few seconds. Using your fingertips, gently tap face all over until toner has dried — the tapping motion helps the ingredients penetrate the skin and promotes blood circulation, making the skin look plush. If applying to aggravated skin, simply pat your face dry with a cotton ball.

Chamomile-Enriched Floral Hydrolat Toner

When skin has been bruised and abraded by trauma, this toner can help cool and soothe the wounds. When applied topically, chamomile has been shown to help bruises heal at a much faster pace.

SKIN TYPE

All

WHEN TO USE

After cleansing

**Makes
3 oz (90 mL)**

TIP
. . . .

Aloe vera gel can be purchased in health food stores. It should be stored in an airtight container in the refrigerator.

KNOW THE BENEFITS
. . . .

Not only are aloe vera gel and chamomile hydrolat antiseptic and antibacterial, they work together to cool and calm damaged skin. Roman chamomile essential oil is an effective treatment for bruises, wounds, insect bites, rashes and sunburn.

- Small beaker
- Glass spray bottle (3 oz/100 mL) sprayed with 70% ethyl alcohol (see page 219)

¼ cup (60 mL)	chamomile hydrolat
2 tbsp (30 mL)	aloe vera gel
1 drop	Roman chamomile EO

1. In beaker, combine chamomile hydrolat and aloe vera gel. Add Roman chamomile essential oil and whisk well.
2. Transfer to prepared bottle and seal tightly. Properly stored (see page 219), the toner will keep for up to 8 weeks.

Variation
Substitute an equal amount of German chamomile essential oil for the Roman chamomile.

HOW TO USE
Shake well before using. After cleansing skin, hold bottle 6 to 8 inches (15 to 20 cm) from your face and gently mist toner onto your face for a few seconds. Using your fingertips, gently tap face all over until has dried — the tapping motion helps the ingredients penetrate the skin and promotes blood circulation, making the skin look plush. If applying to aggravated skin, simply pat your face dry with a cotton ball.

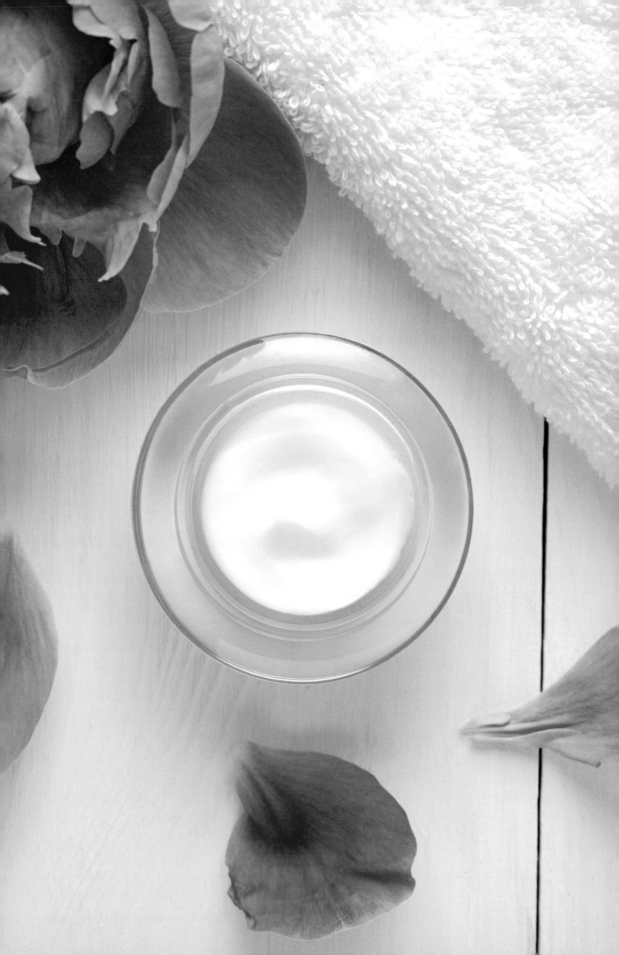

Facial
Moisturizing Creams

Moisturizers help protect, tone and nourish the skin. Facial moisturizers should have a velvety texture and a light (not overbearing) scent. Selecting a moisturizer that suits your skin type is crucial to supporting a normal balance in the skin. (See "The Art of Skin Care," pages 21 to 25.)

Flower Power Moisturizing Cream

Redness, a burning sensation and itchiness are all symptoms that people with sensitive skin may suffer because of environmental stresses. A daytime moisturizer rich in fatty acids and antioxidant properties can help to protect the skin from irritants.

SKIN TYPE

All, especially sensitive

WHEN TO USE

Morning and night

Makes about 15 oz (450 mL)

TIPS

Always start the mixer at a low speed. Mix patiently, without stopping, so the waxes and oils do not cool off before they are emulsified, which can cause separation of the components.

This makes a fairly large quantity. If you prefer, reduce the yield to produce half or even one quarter of the amount.

- 2 small beakers
- Glass stir stick
- Bowl-style double boiler
- Electric mixer
- Glass jar (15 oz/500 mL) sprayed with 70% ethyl alcohol (see page 219)

1 cup (250 mL)	warm (86°F/30°C) filtered water
20 drops (1 mL)	Floral Antimicrobial Synergy (page 37)
2 tbsp (30 mL)	glycerin
2 tbsp (30 mL)	emulsifying wax NF
1 tbsp (15 mL)	stearic acid
¼ cup (60 mL)	sunflower seed oil
¼ cup (60 mL)	calendula-infused oil
5 drops (0.25 mL)	helichrysum EO

1. In a beaker, combine warm water, antimicrobial synergy and glycerin. Cover with foil or plastic wrap and set aside. Keep warm.
2. Set a heatproof glass bowl over a saucepan of hot (not boiling) water (86°F/30°C) and heat until warm to the touch. Add emulsifying wax and let melt completely. Add stearic acid and stir gently until completely incorporated.
3. In second beaker, combine sunflower seed and calendula-infused oils. Add to melted wax and stir until completely incorporated. Remove bowl from heat.
4. Using electric mixer at low speed, gradually add prepared antimicrobial synergy mixture. Continue to mix until emulsified (thick and creamy), 5 to 10 minutes.
5. Add helichrysum essential oil and mix until completely incorporated.

Sunflower seed oil, calendula-infused oil and helichrysum essential oil all belong to the Asteraceae family, which has powerful healing properties. When used in a moisture cream, this combination is considered very soothing to inflamed skin. Sunflower seed oil is high in linoleic acid (70 to 75%) and rich in vitamin E, which makes it a good emollient for dry, patchy skin; it is also antimicrobial. Calendula-infused oil also helps to relieve dry, scaly skin and itchiness. Helichrysum essential oil is high in curcumins and is anti-inflammatory and antibacterial; it also helps to soothe burns and chapped skin, treat rosacea and help repair scar tissue.

6. Transfer mixture to prepared jar and seal tightly. Properly stored (see page 219), the cream will keep for up to 3 months.

Variations

Substitute an equal amount of Earthy Antimicrobial Synergy (page 38) for the Floral Antimicrobial Synergy.

For an anti-inflammatory boost, add 2 drops German chamomile essential oil in Step 5.

If you prefer an alcohol-free moisturizer, reduce the quantity of water to $1/2$ cup (125 mL). Substitute $1^1/_2$ tbsp (22 mL) yellow or cosmetic-grade beeswax for the emulsifying wax and 2 tbsp (30 mL) shea butter for the stearic acid. This will reduce the yield to about 11 oz (325 mL), so select your jar accordingly.

HOW TO USE

Cleanse face and pat dry with a towel. Apply toner, if using. Using your fingertips, apply small dollops of the cream to your forehead, cheeks and chin. Gently massage into skin.

Saffron Night Repair Moisturizing Cream

The natural rhythms of sleep are nature's way of repairing the mind and body. Lack of sleep can place stress on the body and cause premature aging. The scents of sandalwood and jasmine essential oils can have calming and soothing effects, promoting relaxation and sleep; they are also known for their skin-repairing and skin-lightening properties. Using a moisturizer enriched with these oils is a simple way to nurture your skin while helping yourself unwind and fall asleep at night.

SKIN TYPE

Dry, aging

WHEN TO USE

Night

Makes about 4 oz (110 mL)

TIPS

Always start the mixer at a low speed. Mix patiently, without stopping, so the wax and oils do not cool off before they are emulsified, which can cause separation of the components.

When borage oil is called for in a formulation, you can always substitute an equal amount of evening primrose oil. It, too, contains a significant amount of gamma-linolenic acid (GLA).

- Small beaker
- Glass stir stick
- Bowl-style double boiler
- Electric mixer
- Glass jar (4 oz/125 mL) sprayed with 70% ethyl alcohol (see page 219)

ESSENTIAL OIL SYNERGY

10 drops (0.5 mL)	sandalwood EO
5 drops (0.25 mL)	jasmine absolute

BASE

2 tbsp (30 mL)	warm (86°F/30°C) filtered water
5 threads	saffron
¼ cup (60 mL)	sweet almond oil
1 tsp (5 mL)	borage or evening primrose oil
1 tbsp (15 mL)	unscented white beeswax
10 drops (0.5 mL)	vitamin E oil

1. *Essential Oil Synergy:* In beaker, combine sandalwood and jasmine essential oils. Cover with foil or plastic wrap and set aside.
2. *Base:* In a small bowl, cover saffron with the warm water and set aside for 10 to 15 minutes. Using a fine-mesh sieve, strain saffron water into a clean bowl and set aside; discard solids. Keep warm.
3. In another small bowl, combine sweet almond oil and borage oil. Set aside.

KNOW THE BENEFITS

. . . .

Borage oil has therapeutic properties that encourage skin regeneration and, along with sweet almond oil, nourish dehydrated skin. Both vitamin E oil and beeswax have antioxidant properties. Saffron hydrates and lightens skin, both of which help to combat the signs of aging.

4. Set a heatproof glass bowl over a saucepan of hot (not boiling) water (86°F/30°C) and heat until warm to the touch. Add beeswax and let melt completely. Add almond oil mixture and stir until completely incorporated. While stirring, add prepared saffron water and stir gently until completely incorporated. Remove bowl from heat.

5. Using electric mixer at low speed, gradually add vitamin E oil. Continue to mix until emulsified (thick and creamy), 5 to 10 minutes.

6. Add prepared synergy blend and mix until completely incorporated.

7. Transfer to prepared jar and seal tightly. Properly stored (see page 219), the cream will keep for up to 3 months.

Variations

If you are sensitive to nuts, you can use an alternative carrier oil. Substitute an equal amount of grapeseed, fractionated coconut or apricot kernel oil for the sweet almond oil. These oils will also result in a light-textured base.

If you are sensitive to bee products, substitute an equal quantity of emulsifying wax for the beeswax.

For sensitive skin, substitute an equal amount of patchouli essential oil for the sandalwood and an equal amount of neroli essential oil for the jasmine.

HOW TO USE

Cleanse face and pat dry with a towel. Apply toner, if using. Using your fingertips, apply small dollops of the cream to your forehead, cheeks and chin. Gently massage into skin.

Everyday Facial Moisturizing Cream

The power of simplicity goes a long way when it comes to skin moisturizing. Jojoba oil is a light, gentle moisturizer suitable for all skin types. Evening primrose oil contains gamma-linolenic acid and vitamin E, both of which help to rejuvenate the skin. The Citrus Antimicrobial Synergy not only gives this cream an uplifting and refreshing natural scent, it also helps preserve it.

SKIN TYPE

All

WHEN TO USE

Morning

Makes about 17 oz (520 mL)

TIPS

Always start the mixer at a low speed. Mix patiently, without stopping, so the wax and oils do not cool off before they are emulsified, which can cause separation of the components.

When evening primrose oil is called for in a formulation, unless you have sensitive skin, you can always substitute an equal amount of borage oil. It, too, contains a significant amount of gamma-linolenic acid (GLA).

- Small beaker
- Glass stir stick
- Bowl-style double boiler
- Electric mixer
- Glass jar (18 oz/550 mL) sprayed with 70% ethyl alcohol

1 cup (250 mL)	warm (86°F/30°C) filtered water
20 drops (1 mL)	Citrus Antimicrobial Synergy (page 36)
3 tbsp (45 mL)	emulsifying wax NF
¾ cup (175 mL)	jojoba oil
¼ cup (60 mL)	evening primrose oil
20 drops (1 mL)	vitamin E oil

1. In beaker, combine warm water and antimicrobial synergy. Cover with foil or plastic wrap and set aside. Keep warm.
2. Set a heatproof glass bowl over a saucepan of hot (not boiling) water (86°F/30°C) and heat until warm to the touch. Add emulsifying wax and let melt completely.
3. In a small bowl, combine jojoba and evening primrose oils. Add to melted wax and stir until completely incorporated. Remove bowl from heat.
4. Using electric mixer at low speed, gradually add prepared antimicrobial synergy mixture. Continue to mix until emulsified (thick and creamy), 5 to 10 minutes. Add vitamin E oil and mix until completely incorporated.
5. Transfer to prepared jar and seal tightly. Properly stored (see page 219), the cream will keep for up to 3 months.

Variations

EVERYDAY FACIAL MOISTURIZING CREAM FOR HIM: Substitute an equal amount of Minted Camphor Antimicrobial Synergy (page 37) for the Citrus Antimicrobial Synergy.

If you prefer an alcohol–free moisturizer, reduce the quantity of water to $^1/_2$ cup (125 mL). Substitute $1^1/_2$ tbsp (22 mL) yellow or cosmetic-grade beeswax and 2 tbsp (30 mL) shea butter for the emulsifying wax. Melt the beeswax thoroughly in Step 2, then add the shea butter and stir until melted. This will reduce the yield to about 14 oz (420 mL), so select your jar accordingly.

HOW TO USE

Cleanse face and pat dry with a towel. Apply toner, if using. Using your fingertips, apply small dollops of the cream to your forehead, cheeks and chin. Gently massage into skin.

Green Beauty Moisturizing Cream

This powerful yet gentle formulation is enriched with antioxidants (vitamin E and beta-carotene), phytosterols and a range of minerals that will help maintain and nourish the skin. The chlorophyll in the carrier oils promotes healthy skin growth and can help to heal wounds and infections on the skin. Neroli and frankincense oils both have calming scents and antimicrobial and skin-repairing properties.

SKIN TYPE

All, especially dry and sensitive; skin that is sun-damaged or prone to psoriasis and eczema

WHEN TO USE

Night

Makes 8 oz (240 mL)

TIPS

Always start the mixer at a low speed. Mix patiently, without stopping, so the waxes and oils do not cool off before they are emulsified, which can cause separation of the components.

This formulation produces a substantial yield. If you prefer, you can divide it and any other formulations in half.

- 2 small beakers
- Glass stir stick
- Bowl-style double boiler
- Electric mixer
- Glass jar (8 oz/250 mL) sprayed with 70% ethyl alcohol

10 drops (0.5 mL)	Citrus Antimicrobial Synergy (page 36)
½ cup (125 mL)	warm (86°F/30°C) filtered water
10 drops (0.5 mL)	neroli EO
10 drops (0.5 mL)	frankincense EO
1 tsp (5 mL)	emulsifying wax NF
1 tsp (5 mL)	stearic acid
¼ cup (60 mL)	grapeseed oil
1 tbsp (15 mL)	hempseed oil
1 tbsp (15 mL)	avocado oil
1 tbsp (15 mL)	aloe vera gel

1. In a beaker, combine antimicrobial synergy and warm water. Cover with foil or plastic wrap and set aside. Keep warm.
2. In second beaker, combine neroli and frankincense essential oils. Cover with foil or plastic wrap and set aside.
3. Set a heatproof glass bowl over a saucepan of hot (not boiling) water (86°F/30°C) and heat until warm to the touch. Add emulsifying wax and stearic acid and let melt completely.

Grapeseed oil is high in vitamin E, which is beneficial for oily skin. Hempseed and avocado oils contain high levels of chlorophyll, which helps to repair skin. They are also high in omega-3, -6 and -9 essential fatty acids, which help to rejuvenate and repair skin and reduce fine lines caused by stress and aging. Aloe vera is rich in vitamins A, B_{12}, folic acid and choline, which have antioxidant properties. It also contains calcium, chromium, copper, selenium, magnesium, potassium, sodium and zinc, which, along with saponins, contribute to the cleansing and antiseptic effect of the gel. Aloe vera also helps the skin absorb nutrients.

4. Meanwhile, in a small bowl, combine grapeseed, hempseed and avocado oils. Add to melted wax and stir until completely incorporated. Remove bowl from heat.

5. Using electric mixer at low speed, gradually add prepared antimicrobial synergy mixture. Continue to mix until emulsified (thick and creamy). Add aloe vera gel and mix until completely incorporated.

6. Add prepared neroli and frankincense essential oil synergy and mix until completely incorporated.

7. Transfer to prepared jar and seal tightly. Properly stored (see page 219), the cream will keep for up to 3 months.

Variations

For a more cost-effective blend, substitute an equal amount of lavender or bergamot FCF essential oil for the neroli. Both lavender and bergamot deliver the same calming, antiseptic and antibacterial qualities as neroli.

If you prefer an alcohol–free moisturizer, substitute 2 tbsp (30 mL) yellow or cosmetic-grade beeswax for the emulsifying wax and stearic acid.

HOW TO USE

Cleanse face and pat dry with a towel. Apply toner, if using. Using your fingertips, apply small dollops of the cream to your forehead, cheeks and chin. Gently massage into skin.

Silky Rose Omega Moisturizing Cream

This classic moisturizing cream relies on rose essential oil for its soothing and anti-aging properties. Rosehip seed and apricot kernel oils moisturize and nourish the skin with a balance of omega-3, -6 and -9 essential fatty acids.

SKIN TYPE

All, especially dry or aging

WHEN TO USE

Night

Makes 18 oz (525 mL)

TIPS

This formulation makes a large quantity. For day-to-day use, decant into a small jar (2 oz/50 mL). Store the remainder in the refrigerator until ready to use. Alternatively, this recipe can be halved.

Always start the mixer at a low speed. Mix patiently, without stopping, so the waxes and oils do not cool off before they are emulsified, which can cause separation of the components.

- 2 small beakers
- Glass stir stick
- Bowl-style double boiler
- Electric mixer
- Glass jar (18 oz/550 mL) sprayed with 70% ethyl alcohol (see Tips, left)

1 cup (250 mL)	warm (86°F/30°C) filtered water
20 drops (1 mL)	Earthy Antimicrobial Synergy (page 38)
5 drops (0.25 mL)	rose otto EO
5 drops (0.25 mL)	clary sage EO
1 tbsp (15 mL)	emulsifying wax NF
1 tbsp (15 mL)	stearic acid
½ cup (125 mL)	apricot kernel oil
¼ cup (60 mL)	evening primrose oil
¼ cup (60 mL)	rosehip seed oil

1. In a beaker, combine warm water and antimicrobial synergy. Cover with foil or plastic wrap and set aside. Keep warm.

2. In another beaker, combine rose otto and clary sage essential oils. Cover with foil or plastic wrap and set aside. Keep warm.

3. Set a heatproof glass bowl over a saucepan of hot (not boiling) water (86°F/30°C) and heat until warm to the touch. Add emulsifying wax and stearic acid and let melt completely.

4. Meanwhile, in a small bowl, combine apricot kernel, evening primrose and rosehip seed oils. Add to melted wax and stir until completely incorporated. Remove bowl from heat.

Apricot kernel oil has anti-inflammatory and antioxidant properties. Rosehip seed oil is rich in bioactive carotenoids, which help to reduce the signs of aging as well as hyperpigmentation (dark discoloration of the skin) due to sun damage. Evening primrose oil is abundant in gamma-linolenic acid (GLA), which has been found to be key to skin rejuvenation and repair. The rose otto and clary sage synergy balances skin tone, smoothing and preventing fine lines in mature skin.

5. Using electric mixer at low speed, gradually add prepared antimicrobial synergy mixture. Continue to mix until emulsified (thick and creamy), 5 to 10 minutes.

6. Add prepared rose and clary sage essential oil synergy and mix until completely incorporated.

7. Transfer to prepared jar and seal tightly. Properly stored (see page 219), the cream will keep for up to 3 months.

Variation

For a richer base, you can replace the combination of apricot kernel, evening primrose and rosehip seed oil with 1 cup (250 mL) sweet almond oil.

HOW TO USE

Cleanse face and pat dry with a towel. Apply toner, if using. Using your fingertips, apply small dollops of the cream to your forehead, cheeks and chin. Gently massage into skin.

Hibiscus Astringent Moisturizing Cream

During youth, our skin is in constant flux from changes in our hormone levels, as well as environmental and emotional stresses. This astringent-based formulation, which contains hazelnut and borage oils, helps to balance oily skin and reduce redness. The addition of hibiscus, which contains quercetin (a powerful antioxidant), helps to improve skin's elasticity and even skin tone, as well as the appearance of scars. Not only are bergamot and lime essential oils antiseptic and antibacterial, their scent is also uplifting.

SKIN TYPE

All, especially oily or combination

WHEN TO USE

Night

Makes about 17 oz (505 mL)

TIPS

To avoid phototoxicity, be sure to use bergapten-free bergamot and distilled lime essential oils (see page 156).

This makes a fairly large quantity. If you prefer, reduce the yield to produce half or even one quarter of the amount.

Always start the mixer at a low speed. Mix patiently, without stopping, so the waxes and oils do not cool off before they are emulsified, which can cause separation of the components.

- 2 small beakers
- Glass stir stick
- Bowl-style double boiler
- Electric mixer
- Glass jar (17 oz/510 mL) sprayed with 70% ethyl alcohol

5 drops (0.25 mL)	lime (distilled) EO
5 drops (0.25 mL)	bergamot FCF EO (see page 102)
10 drops (0.5 mL)	Rose-Scented Antimicrobial Synergy (page 36)
2 tbsp (30 mL)	hibiscus infusion in glycerin
1 cup (250 mL)	warm (86°F/30°C) filtered water
1 tbsp (15 mL)	emulsifying wax NF
2 tbsp (30 mL)	stearic acid
¼ cup (60 mL)	hazelnut oil
¼ cup (60 mL)	carrot root–infused oil
¼ cup (60 mL)	borage oil
10 drops (0.5 mL)	pomegranate extract

1. In a beaker, combine lime and bergamot FCF essential oils. Cover with foil or plastic wrap and set aside.

2. In second beaker, combine antimicrobial synergy, hibiscus infusion and warm water. Cover with foil or plastic wrap and set aside. Keep warm.

3. Set a heatproof glass bowl over a saucepan of hot (not boiling) water (86°F/30°C) and heat until warm to the touch. Add emulsifying wax and stearic acid and let melt completely.

TIP

I prefer to use carrot-infused sesame oil in this formulation, but carrot root infused in other carrier oils, such as extra virgin olive oil, will be fine. You can purchase carrot root–infused sesame oil from reliable suppliers (see page 371). Whatever the carrier, for this formulation, be sure you are getting an infusion of carrot root, not carrot seed essential oil.

KNOW THE BENEFITS

Hazelnut oil is an astringent base oil that benefits oily or combination skin. It is enriched with oleic acid and improves the absorption of other nutrients in the formulation. The GLA in the borage oil and the beta-carotene in the carrot root–infused oil help to repair and rejuvenate the skin. Lime and bergamot essential oils have antiseptic and antibacterial properties. The hibiscus infusion is an antioxidant.

4. In a small bowl, combine hazelnut oil, carrot root–infused oil and borage oil. Add to melted wax and stir until completely incorporated. Remove bowl from heat.

5. Using electric mixer at low speed, gradually add prepared antimicrobial synergy mixture. Continue to mix until emulsified (thick and creamy), 5 to 10 minutes.

6. Add prepared line and bergamot essential oil synergy and mix until completely incorporated.

7. Transfer to prepared jar and seal tightly. Properly stored (see page 219), the cream will keep for up to 3 months.

Variations

Substitute an equal amount of Citrus Antimicrobial Synergy (page 36) for the Rose-Scented Antimicrobial Synergy.

Substitute an equal amount of evening primrose oil for the borage oil if you have sensitive skin. Evening primrose oil also contains a significant amount of gamma-linolenic acid (GLA).

HOW TO USE

Cleanse face and pat dry with a towel. Apply toner, if using. Using your fingertips, apply small dollops of the cream to your forehead, cheeks and chin. Gently massage into skin.

NUT ALLERGY ALERT

If you are sensitive to nuts you can use alternative carrier oils. Substitute an equal amount of grapeseed, fractionated coconut or apricot kernel oil for the hazelnut oil. These oils will also produce a light-textured base.

Orange Blossom Moisturizing Cream

This cream is particularly beneficial for skin that tends toward inflammation. The light-textured apricot kernel oil acts as a carrier for the neroli essential oil. The cream has a soft, vibrant scent. Used morning and night, it will provide an all-round moisturizing and nurturing effect.

SKIN TYPE

Sensitive, oily, combination

WHEN TO USE

Morning and night

Makes 11½ oz (345 mL)

TIPS

Always start the mixer at a low speed. Mix patiently, without stopping, so the waxes and oils do not cool off before they are emulsified, which can cause separation of the components.

This formulation produces a substantial yield. If you prefer, you can divide it and any other formulations in half.

- Small beaker
- Glass stir stick
- Bowl-style double boiler
- Electric mixer
- Glass jar (12 oz/350 mL) sprayed with 70% ethyl alcohol

20 drops (1 mL)	Floral Antimicrobial Synergy (see page 37)
5 drops (0.25 mL)	bamboo extract
1 tbsp (15 mL)	glycerin
¾ cup (175 mL)	warm (86°F/30°C) filtered water
1 tbsp (15 mL)	emulsifying wax NF
1 tbsp (15 mL)	stearic acid
½ cup (125 mL)	apricot kernel oil
5 drops (0.25 mL)	neroli EO

1. In beaker, combine antimicrobial synergy, bamboo extract, glycerin and warm water. Cover with foil or plastic wrap and set aside. Keep warm.
2. Set a heatproof glass bowl over a saucepan of hot (not boiling) water (86°F/30°C) and heat until warm to the touch. Add emulsifying wax and stearic acid and let melt completely. Add apricot kernel oil and stir until completely incorporated. Remove bowl from heat.
3. Using electric mixer at low speed, gradually add prepared antimicrobial synergy mixture. Continue to mix until emulsified (thick and creamy), 5 to 10 minutes.
4. Add neroli essential oil and mix well.
5. Transfer to prepared jar and seal tightly. Properly stored (see page 219), the cream will keep for up to 3 months.

∙∙∙∙∙∙∙∙∙∙∙∙∙∙∙∙∙∙∙∙∙

Apricot kernel oil, a light-textured oil high in vitamin E, helps to repair damaged skin. Neroli has a calming and relaxing scent. In addition, farnesol, a natural compound found in neroli, helps maintain skin's elasticity; it is also antibacterial and antifungal.

Variations

You can substitute an equal amount of Earthy Antimicrobial Synergy (page 38) for the Floral Antimicrobial Synergy.

For a more cost-effective blend, substitute an equal amount of petitgrain essential oil for the neroli.

HOW TO USE

Cleanse face and pat dry with a towel. Apply toner, if using. Using your fingertips, apply small dollops of the cream to your forehead, cheeks and chin. Gently massage into skin.

Anti-Aging Moisturizing Day Cream

Every woman is a goddess, especially if she accepts the natural process of aging with grace. Adopting a supportive approach to aging allows women to feel comfortable within their bodies and minds. Limiting your skin's exposure to the sun is the most important thing you can do to protect it from the signs of aging. The carrier oils in this cream contain fatty acids and have antioxidant properties that work to moisturize and repair skin that has been overexposed to environmental pollutants and sunlight.

SKIN TYPE

Normal, dry, aging

WHEN TO USE

Morning

**Makes
9 oz (270 mL)**

TIPS

Grapefruit and ginger essential oils may be phototoxic when used in high concentrations. Even though this blend does not exceed the maximum recommended amount, it is advisable to limit exposure to direct sunlight when using this cream.

Always start the mixer at a low speed. Mix patiently, without stopping, so the waxes and oils do not cool off before they are emulsified, which can cause separation of the components.

- Small beaker
- Glass stir stick
- Bowl-style double boiler
- Electric mixer
- Glass jar (10 oz/300 mL) sprayed with 70% ethyl alcohol

20 drops (1 mL)	Floral Antimicrobial Synergy (page 37)
5 drops (0.25 mL)	bamboo extract
1 tbsp (15 mL)	glycerin
¾ cup (175 mL)	warm (86°F/30°C) filtered water
1 tbsp (15 mL)	emulsifying wax NF
1 tbsp (15 mL)	stearic acid
¼ cup (60 mL)	jojoba oil
¼ cup (60 mL)	rosehip seed oil
¼ cup (60 mL)	carrot root–infused oil (see Tip, right)
¼ cup (60 mL)	evening primrose oil
5 drops (0.25 mL)	pomegranate extract
10 drops (0.5 mL)	grapefruit EO
5 drops (0.25 mL)	ylang-ylang EO
2 drops	rosemary EO
2 drops	ginger EO

1. In beaker, combine antimicrobial synergy, bamboo extract, glycerin and warm water. Cover with foil or plastic wrap and set aside. Keep warm.

TIP

I prefer to use carrot root–infused sesame oil in this formulation, but carrot root infused into other carrier oils, such as extra virgin olive oil, will be fine. You can purchase carrot root–infused sesame oil from reliable suppliers (see page 371). Whatever the carrier, for this formulation be sure you are getting an infusion of carrot root, not carrot seed essential oil.

KNOW THE BENEFITS

Jojoba oil is a balanced emollient that works well for all skin types. Thanks to its omega-3, -6 and -9 fatty acids, as well as the beta-carotene in rosehip, evening primrose and carrot root–infused oils, this cream has antioxidant properties that help to repair damaged skin, as well as reduce the appearance of fine lines and hyperpigmentation due to sun damage. The essential oil synergy has an uplifting and stimulating scent; it also works to improve circulation, giving the skin a plump and youthful appearance.

2. Set a heatproof glass bowl over a saucepan of hot (not boiling) water (86°F/30°C) and heat until warm to the touch. Add emulsifying wax and stearic acid and let melt completely. Add jojoba, rosehip seed, carrot root–infused and evening primrose oils. Warm until mixture is completely clear, 1 to 2 minutes. Stir gently to ensure that ingredients are dissolved and evenly combined. Remove bowl from heat.

3. Using electric mixer at low speed, gradually add prepared antimicrobial synergy mixture. Continue to mix until emulsified (thick and creamy), 5 to 10 minutes.

4. Add pomegranate extract and grapefruit, ylang-ylang, rosemary and ginger essential oils. Mix until evenly distributed.

5. Transfer to prepared jar and seal tightly. Properly stored (see page 219), the cream will keep for up to 3 months.

Variations

Substitute an equal amount of bergamot FCF essential oil for the grapefruit, and helichrysum essential oil for the ginger.

For sensitive skin, substitute an equal amount of Roman chamomile essential oil for the ylang-ylang.

ANTI-AGING MOISTURIZING NIGHT CREAM: To make a richer version of this moisturizer for nighttime use, reduce the amount of jojoba oil to 2 tbsp (30 mL) and increase the amount of rosehip seed oil to 6 tbsp (90 mL).

HOW TO USE

Cleanse face and pat dry with a towel. Apply toner, if using. Using your fingertips, apply small dollops of the cream to your forehead, cheeks and chin. Gently massage into skin.

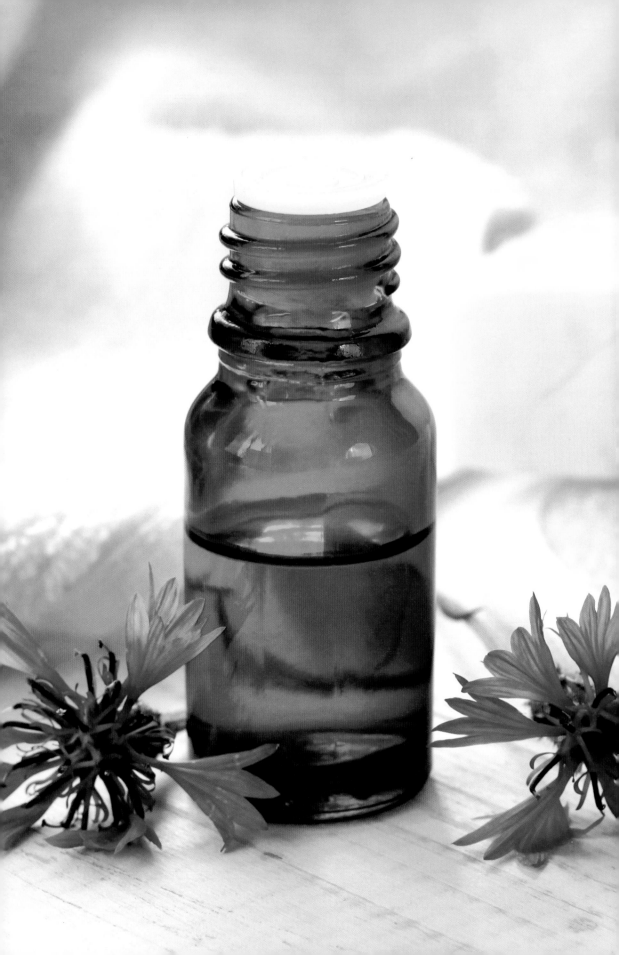

Serums

Serums are used to repair specific skin conditions. They contain high concentrations of active ingredients, targeting what your skin currently needs to help improve certain conditions. For example, serums can provide extra hydration for dry skin, antioxidant and firming agents for sagging skin, and astringent and antimicrobial agents for oily and acne-prone skin.

Serums can also be used to target specific internal imbalances and help to restore balance if required. Most serums should be used on an as-needed basis until the skin or your system recaptures its normal balance. Some gentle serums, such as Sensitive Skin Serum (page 276) and Antioxidant Serum (page 277), can be used daily for extra hydration.

Facial Serums

Serums to Support Body Systems

Emerald Dynasty Serum

Sometimes your skin doesn't appear as vibrant as you'd like. Massaging a nutrient-rich serum onto your face can help restore your skin's vitality.

SKIN TYPE

All

WHEN TO USE

Morning and night

**Makes
6 oz (180 mL)**

TIP

This formulation makes a large quantity. For day-to-day use, decant some into a smaller pump bottle (2 oz/50 mL). Store the remainder in the refrigerator until ready to use.

KNOW THE BENEFITS

Camellia seed, hempseed and apricot kernel oils are lovely moisturizers for all skin types, but especially combination skin. The synergy of neroli, grapefruit and jasmine essential oils is warming and stimulating, encouraging blood flow to the surface of the skin when applied with gentle massage.

- 2 small beakers
- Glass pump bottle (6 oz/200 mL) sprayed with 70% ethyl alcohol (see Tips, left)

ESSENTIAL OIL SYNERGY

5 drops (0.25 mL)	neroli EO
5 drops (0.25 mL)	grapefruit EO
5 drops (0.25 mL)	jasmine absolute

BASE

¼ cup (60 mL)	hempseed oil
¼ cup (60 mL)	camellia seed oil
¼ cup (60 mL)	apricot kernel oil

1. *Essential Oil Synergy:* In a beaker, combine neroli, grapefruit and jasmine essential oils. Cover with foil or plastic wrap and set aside.
2. *Base:* In second beaker, combine hempseed, camellia seed, and apricot kernel oil. Whisk well.
3. Add prepared synergy blend and whisk to combine. Transfer to prepared bottle and seal tightly. Properly stored the serum will keep for up to 6 months.

Variations

Substitute an equal quantity of grapeseed oil for the apricot kernel oil.

For a more cost-effective blend you can substitute an equal amount of lavender or bergamot FCF essential oil for the neroli. Both will deliver the same calming, antiseptic and antibacterial effects as neroli.

HOW TO USE

Wipe your face with a cloth soaked in warm water. Pump 5 to 10 drops of the serum onto your fingertips and apply to your slightly moist skin. Massage for 30 seconds. Follow with toner and moisturizer, if needed.

Enriching Ruby-Red Serum

This firming and anti-aging serum is rich in essential fatty acids that will leave your skin feeling hydrated and looking vibrant.

SKIN TYPE

All

WHEN TO USE

Night

Makes about 4 oz (125 mL)

TIP

Use after an exfoliant such as Tunisian Marmalade Exfoliant (page 295).

KNOW THE BENEFITS

Cocoa butter, rosehip seed oil and sweet almond oil are rich in saturated fats, providing a protective layer that helps repair and moisturize damaged skin. Cocoa butter and almond oil are effective emollients, protecting the skin from dehydration and improving elasticity. Almond oil, with its high levels of vitamin E, is also an antioxidant. Rosehip seed oil, which contains omega-3, -6 and -9 fatty acids, is nurturing. The essential oil synergy balances the skin.

- 2 small beakers
- Glass stir stick
- Glass pump bottle (5 oz/125 mL) sprayed with 70% ethyl alcohol (see page 219)

ESSENTIAL OIL SYNERGY

5 drops (0.25 mL)	each rose otto, petitgrain and bergamot FCF EO

BASE

1 tsp (5 mL)	cocoa butter
¼ cup (60 mL)	each rosehip seed oil and sweet almond oil (see page 263)
5 drops (0.25 mL)	bamboo extract

1. *Essential Oil Synergy:* In a beaker, combine essential oils. Cover and set aside.
2. *Base:* Set a heatproof glass bowl over a saucepan of hot (not boiling) water (86°F/30°C) and heat until warm to the touch. Add cocoa butter and let melt completely. Remove bowl from heat.
3. In second beaker, whisk together rosehip seed oil and sweet almond oil. Add to melted cocoa butter. Stir until completely incorporated and mixture begins to thicken.
4. Add prepared essential oil synergy and stir well.
5. Transfer to prepared bottle and seal tightly. Properly stored, the serum will keep for up to 6 months.

Variations

Substitute an equal amount of shea butter or coconut oil for the cocoa butter, and/or apricot kernel or grapeseed oil for the sweet almond oil.

HOW TO USE

Pump 5 to 10 drops of serum onto fingertips and gently pat onto clean, toned skin. Gently massage with your fingertips. If desired, follow with Anti-Aging Moisturizing Night Cream (see variation, page 267), You may not need additional moisturizer, thanks to the cocoa butter in this formulation.

Anti-Aging Serum

This serum, which contains oils rich in fatty acids, can be used on a daily basis to revive dehydrated or aging skin. When applying this in the morning, it is a good idea to follow it with a moisturizer for extra protection against environmental pollutants. When using this serum at night, you may find that additional moisturizer is not necessary. Experiment and see what works best for you.

SKIN TYPE

All, especially dry or aging

WHEN TO USE

Day and night

Makes about 7 oz (220 mL)

TIP

I prefer to use carrot-infused sesame oil in this formulation, but other carrier oils infused with carrot, such as extra virgin olive oil, will be fine. You can purchase carrot root–infused sesame oil from reliable suppliers (see page 371). Whatever the carrier, for this formulation, be sure you are getting an infusion of carrot root, not carrot seed essential oil.

- 2 small beakers
- Glass stir stick
- Glass pump bottle (8 oz/250 mL) sprayed with 70% ethyl alcohol (see Tips, right)

ESSENTIAL OIL SYNERGY

10 drops (0.5 mL)	grapefruit EO
5 drops (0.25 mL)	ylang-ylang EO
2 drops	rosemary EO
2 drops	ginger EO

BASE

¼ cup (60 mL)	jojoba oil
¼ cup (60 mL)	rosehip seed oil
¼ cup (60 mL)	carrot root-infused oil
¼ cup (60 mL)	evening primrose oil
5 drops (0.25 mL)	bamboo extract
5 drops (0.25 mL)	pomegranate extract

1. *Essential Oil Synergy:* In a beaker, combine grapefruit, ylang-ylang, rosemary and ginger essential oils. Cover with foil or plastic wrap and set aside.
2. *Base:* In second beaker, whisk together jojoba, rosehip seed, carrot root-infused oil and evening primrose oils. Stir well. Add bamboo and pomegranate extracts and stir well.
3. Add prepared synergy blend and stir until combined. Transfer to prepared bottle and seal tightly. Properly stored (see page 219), the serum will keep for up to 6 months.

This formulation makes a large quantity. For day-to-day use, decant some into a smaller pump bottle (2 oz/50 mL). Store the remainder in the refrigerator until ready to use.

When cleaning utensils and equipment, always wipe them down with dry paper towels before rinsing. This will prevent drains from becoming clogged by oil residue and keep scum from accumulating in the sink.

KNOW THE BENEFITS

This formulation is high in fatty acids, which nourish the skin, keeping it hydrated and rejuvenated. Pomegranate extract has antioxidant properties and helps skin repair itself. The essential oil synergy has a stimulating effect on skin that promotes circulation, giving it a healthier, youthful appearance.

Variations

Substitute an equal amount of borage oil for the evening primrose oil. It contains a significant amount of gamma-linolenic acid (GLA), which is an essential fatty acid.

For sensitive skin, substitute an equal amount of Roman chamomile essential oil for the ylang-ylang.

You can substitute an equal amount of lime (distilled) or bergamot FCF essential oil for the grapefruit.

HOW TO USE

Apply after thoroughly cleansing and toning your face. Pump 5 to 10 drops of serum onto fingertips and gently pat onto forehead, cheeks and chin. Gently massage and tap your entire face with your fingertips. Follow with Anti-Aging Moisturizing Day Cream (page 266).

SENSITIVITY ALERT

While the components of grapefruit EO have not been researched in this regard, there are substances (furocoumarins) in grapefruit juice that may undermine the performance of certain prescription drugs. So if you are taking prescription drugs and have been advised to avoid grapefruit, I recommend substituting an equal amount of bergamot FCF or lime (distilled) essential oil instead.

Vitamin C Serum

An immune system compromised by illness, stress or an imbalance in the body is reflected on the skin. Vitamin C works to prevent the decline of collagen, which gives our skin its resiliency and structure. Eating an abundance of fruits and vegetables is one way to replenish our collagen stores. Applying vitamin C topically is another; it can rejuvenate the surface of the skin, resulting in a toned and hydrated complexion.

SKIN TYPE

All

WHEN TO USE

Night
(see "How to Use,"
page 275)

Makes 10½ oz (315 mL)

TIP

I prefer to use carrot-infused sesame oil in this formulation, but other carrier oils, such as extra virgin olive oil, will be fine. You can purchase carrot root–infused sesame oil from reliable suppliers (see page 371). Whatever the carrier, for this formulation, be sure you are getting an infusion of carrot root, not carrot seed essential oil.

- Small beaker
- Glass stir stick
- Glass bottle (12 oz/350 mL) sprayed with 70% ethyl alcohol (see page 219)

ESSENTIAL OIL SYNERGY

5 drops (0.25 mL)	mandarin EO
5 drops (0.25 mL)	orange EO
5 drops (0.25 mL)	grapefruit EO

BASE

1 tsp (5 mL)	emulsifying wax NF
¼ cup (60 mL)	carrot root-infused oil
½ cup (125 mL)	warm (86°F/30°C) filtered water
½ cup (125 mL)	glycerin
½ tsp (2.5 mL)	ascorbic acid (vitamin C; see Tips, right)
5 drops (0.25 mL)	Citrus Antimicrobial Synergy (page 36)
10 drops (0.5 mL)	vitamin E oil

1. *Essential Oil Synergy:* In beaker, combine mandarin, orange and grapefruit essential oils. Cover with foil or plastic wrap and set aside.
2. *Base:* Set a heatproof glass bowl over a saucepan of hot (not boiling) water (86°F/30°C) and heat until warm to the touch. Add emulsifying wax and let melt completely. Add carrot root-infused oil and stir to combine.
3. In a small bowl, combine warm water, glycerin, ascorbic acid, antimicrobial synergy and vitamin E oil. Add to melted wax and stir until completely incorporated. Remove bowl from heat. Stir until mixture begins to thicken.

There are many forms of vitamin C in the marketplace. It is preferable to use the non-synthetic powder, derived from berries and fruits. The product may come in either capsule form (you will need to open the capsules) or as a loose powder.

When cleaning utensils and equipment, always wipe them down with dry paper towels before rinsing. This will prevent drains from becoming clogged by oil residue and keep scum from accumulating in the sink.

KNOW THE BENEFITS

This formulation is rich in vitamins C and E and beta-carotene, whose potent antioxidant properties prevent the free radicals that can speed the effects of aging. Vitamin C also aids with collagen production in the skin, promoting a firm texture and a youthful appearance. The citrus synergy blend leaves the skin feeling clean and fresh.

4. While stirring, gradually add prepared essential oil synergy and stir until well incorporated.
5. Transfer mixture to prepared bottle and seal tightly. Properly stored (see page 219), the serum will keep for up to 3 months.

Variations

Substitute an equal amount of Emulsimulse, an eco-certified wax, for the National Formulary wax.

Substitute 2 tbsp (30 mL) sesame seed oil and 2 tbsp (30 mL) rosehip seed oil for the carrot root–infused oil.

HOW TO USE

Apply after thoroughly cleansing and toning your face. Pump 5 to 10 drops of serum onto fingertips and gently pat onto forehead, cheeks and chin. Gently massage and tap your entire face with your fingertips. Ideally, follow with Saffron Night Moisturizing Cream (page 254).

Because of the ascorbic acid in this serum, it is recommended for use only over a 21-day period — to prevent overexposure, which may lead to sensitivity — breaking for 2 to 3 months in between. If your skin starts feeling like it needs a little extra support, start using the serum again.

SENSITIVITY ALERT

While the components of grapefruit EO have not been researched in this regard, there are substances (furocoumarins) in grapefruit juice that may undermine the performance of certain prescription drugs. So if you are taking prescription drugs and have been advised to avoid grapefruit, I recommend substituting an equal amount of bergamot FCF or lime (distilled) essential oil instead.

Sensitive Skin Serum

This serum is an exotic combination of oils from three different regions of the world: argan oil from Morocco, camellia seed oil from China and marula oil from South Africa. The threesome are powerful antioxidants, protecting all skin types from the free radicals that can speed the effects of aging.

SKIN TYPE

Sensitive

WHEN TO USE

Night and day

Makes 6 oz (180 mL)

TIP

When cleaning utensils and equipment, always wipe them down with dry paper towels before rinsing. This will prevent drains from becoming clogged by oil residue and scum from accumulating in the sink.

KNOW THE BENEFITS

This formula contains a high level of oleic acid, which nourishes, moisturizes and protects the skin. Cornflower extract, a light astringent, has a cooling effect. Neroli essential oil gives this formulation a pleasing exotic scent.

- Small beaker
- Glass pump bottle (6 oz/180 mL) sprayed with 70% ethyl alcohol (see page 219)

¼ cup (60 mL)	argan oil
¼ cup (60 mL)	camellia seed oil
¼ cup (60 mL)	marula oil
10 drops (0.5 mL)	vitamin E oil
10 drops (0.5 mL)	cornflower extract
5 drops (0.25 mL)	neroli EO

1. In beaker, whisk together argan, camellia and marula oils. Add vitamin E oil and cornflower extract and whisk until combined. Add neroli essential oil and whisk well.
2. Transfer to prepared bottle and seal tightly. Properly stored (see page 219), the serum will keep for up to 6 months.

Variations

The three carrier oils (argan, camellia seed and marula) used in this formula are quite expensive and may be hard to find. You can substitute an equal amount of jojoba oil for any of the three. It is a good all-purpose oil for sensitive skin.

For a more cost-effective blend, substitute 3 drops of lavender or petitgrain essential oil for the neroli. Both deliver the same calming, antiseptic and antibacterial effects as neroli.

HOW TO USE

Apply after thoroughly cleansing and toning your face. Pump 5 to 10 drops of serum onto fingertips and gently pat onto forehead, cheeks and chin. Gently massage and tap your entire face with your fingertips. Ideally, follow up with Orange Blossom Moisturizing Cream (page 264).

Antioxidant Serum

Use this serum when you need to focus on skin repair because of overexposure to the sun or other skin damage caused by injury or medication.

SKIN TYPE

All, especially sensitive

WHEN TO USE

Morning and night

Makes about 4 oz (125 mL)

TIP

Orange Blossom Moisturizing Cream (page 264) makes a nice follow-up to this serum.

KNOW THE BENEFITS

As well as being a powerful moisturizer, argan oil has anti-aging and wound-healing properties. It also reduces sebum production, making it beneficial for people who suffer from hormonal breakouts. Apricot kernel oil leaves the skin feeling silky. Cornflower extract is a light astringent that has a cooling effect on the skin.

- 2 small beakers
- Glass stir stick
- Glass pump bottle (5 oz/125 mL) sprayed with 70% ethyl alcohol (see page 219)

ESSENTIAL OIL SYNERGY

5 drops (0.25 mL)	rose otto EO
5 drops (0.25 mL)	neroli EO
1 drop	ylang-ylang EO

BASE

¼ cup (60 mL)	argan oil
¼ cup (60 mL)	apricot kernel oil
20 drops (1 mL)	vitamin E oil
10 drops (0.5 mL)	cornflower extract

1. *Essential Oil Synergy:* In a beaker, combine rose otto, neroli and ylang-ylang essential oils. Cover with foil or plastic wrap and set aside.
2. In second beaker, whisk together argan and apricot kernel oils. Add vitamin E oil and cornflower extract and stir well.
3. Add prepared synergy blend and stir well. Transfer to prepared bottle and seal tightly. Properly stored (see page 219), the serum will keep for up to 6 months.

Variations

For a richer base, substitute an equal amount of sweet almond, sesame or sunflower oil for the apricot kernel.

For a more cost-effective blend, substitute half as much lavender and geranium essential oils for the neroli and rose otto.

For sensitive skin, substitute an equal amount of Roman chamomile essential oil for the ylang-ylang.

HOW TO USE

Apply after thoroughly cleansing and toning your face. Pump 5 to 10 drops of serum onto fingertips and gently pat onto forehead, cheeks and chin.

USING FACIAL DIAGNOSIS TO SELECT ESSENTIAL OILS

In traditional Chinese and Ayurvedic medicine, the face is considered a diagnostic tool that reflects the overall health and well-being of an individual. Each area of the face correlates to an internal organ — if there is an imbalance in any organ, it will be reflected in a person's complexion and facial lines. Certain essential oils can be used to target and help heal an imbalanced system.

BODY SYSTEM	ESSENTIAL OILS
Cardiovascular system	Lavender, rose otto, neroli
Colon	Cardamom, basil, carrot seed
Digestive system	Rose otto, juniper berry, bergamot, orange, lemon, mandarin, cardamom, sweet basil, neroli, ginger, lime
Immune system	Frankincense, lavender, pine, sweet marjoram, lemongrass
Liver and gallbladder	Grapefruit, ginger, peppermint, bergamot, orange, lemon, mandarin, neroli, ginger, lime
Renal and reproductive systems	Geranium, rose otto, juniper berry, sandalwood, clary sage
Respiratory system	Tea tree, cajuput, rosemary, frankincense, pine

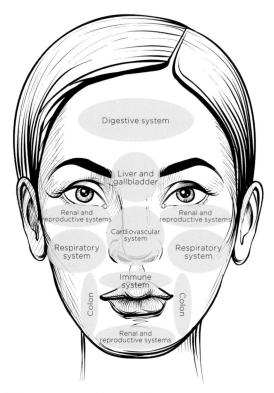

Digestive Detox Serum

Breakouts or redness in the forehead area and dark, congested-looking skin may be signs of digestive stagnation. This can be accompanied by constipation, headaches and nausea. Eliminate caffeine, alcohol, cigarettes, rich fatty foods and dairy products. Use this serum for 3 to 6 weeks, under a moisturizing cream or on its own, to support a cleansing diet and exercise program.

SKIN TYPE
All

WHEN TO USE
Morning and night

**Makes
1 oz (30 mL)**

TIP

If you have sensitive skin, reduce the amounts of essential oils to 2 drops each.

KNOW THE BENEFITS

The combination of rose otto, juniper berry and bergamot essential oils is rejuvenating and balancing. When gently massaged onto the face, the scent relaxes the mind and removes tension throughout the body, including the digestive tract, allowing gastric juices to flow. This will aid in digestion and prevent bloating and gas.

- 2 small beakers
- Glass stir stick
- Glass pump or dropper bottle (1 oz/30 mL) sprayed with 70% ethyl alcohol

ESSENTIAL OIL SYNERGY

5 drops (0.25 mL)	each rose otto EO, juniper berry EO and bergamot FCF EO

BASE

4 tsp (20 mL)	sesame seed oil
2 tsp (10 mL)	carrot root–infused oil

1. *Essential Oil Synergy:* In a beaker, combine essential oils. Cover with foil or plastic wrap and set aside.
2. *Base:* In second beaker, combine sesame seed and carrot root–infused oils. Stir well.
3. Add prepared synergy blend and whisk to combine. Transfer to prepared bottle and seal tightly. Properly stored (see page 219), the serum will keep for up to 6 months.

Variation

DIGESTIVE DETOX FACIAL MASK: In a bowl, combine 6 drops serum, 2 tbsp (30 mL) white (kaolin) clay and 3 tbsp (45 mL) water. Mix until a smooth paste forms. Apply to clean face and let dry for 10 to 15 minutes. Rinse off with warm water. Makes 1 application.

HOW TO USE

Fill a clean basin with warm water. Add 6 drops serum and agitate. Soak a facecloth in the solution. Drape wet cloth over your face for 30 seconds, then remove slowly. Repeat 3 to 6 times. Follow by massaging 3 or 4 drops of serum into skin.

Liver and Gallbladder Support Serum

Breakouts and deep lines between the eyebrows indicate potential issues with the liver; thinner lines suggest issues with the gallbladder. This can be accompanied by nausea, headaches and feelings of frustration. Eliminate fatty foods, alcohol and cigarettes. Use this serum for 3 to 6 weeks to support a cleansing diet and exercise program. See page 279 for how to use.

SKIN TYPE

All

WHEN TO USE

Morning and night

Makes 1 oz (30 mL)

TIP

This serum may be used underneath a moisturizing cream or on its own. Use twice a day, morning and night.

KNOW THE BENEFITS

Grapefruit, ginger and peppermint are invigorating essential oils. When gently massaged onto the face, they increase blood circulation and open up congested pores.

- 2 small beakers
- Glass stir stick
- Glass pump or dropper bottle (1 oz/30 mL) sprayed with 70% ethyl alcohol

ESSENTIAL OIL SYNERGY

10 drops (0.5 mL)	grapefruit EO (see Sensitivity Alert, page 275)
2 drops	ginger EO
2 drops	peppermint EO

BASE

4 tsp (20 mL)	sesame seed oil
2 tsp (10 mL)	carrot root–infused oil (see Tips, page 272)

1. *Essential Oil Synergy:* In a beaker, combine essential oils. Cover with foil and set aside.
2. *Base:* In second beaker, combine sesame seed and carrot root–infused oils. Stir well.
3. Add prepared synergy blend and whisk to combine. Transfer to prepared bottle and seal tightly. Properly stored (see page 219), the serum will keep for up to 6 months.

Variations

If you have sensitive skin, reduce the amount of each essential oil by half.

LIVER AND GALLBLADDER FACIAL MASK: In a bowl, combine 6 drops serum, 2 tbsp (30 mL) white (kaolin) clay and 3 tbsp (45 mL) water. Mix until a smooth paste forms. Apply to clean face and let dry for 10 to 15 minutes. Rinse off with warm water. Makes 1 application.

Lung Support Serum

Breakouts and grayish, clammy skin in the cheek area indicate a potential imbalance in the respiratory system. Eliminate dairy products and create a clean environment by using a diffuser to release negative ions into the air. Use this serum during hay fever season or whenever you are feeling congested.

SKIN TYPE
All

WHEN TO USE
Morning and night

**Makes
1 oz (30 mL)**

TIP

This serum may be used underneath a moisturizing cream or on its own. Use twice a day, morning and night.

KNOW THE BENEFITS

Tea tree, frankincense and cajuput essential oils help to decongest the nasal passages. When gently massaged onto the face, they help you breathe and open up congested pores.

- 2 small beakers
- Glass stir stick
- Glass pump or dropper bottle (1 oz/30 mL) sprayed with 70% ethyl alcohol

ESSENTIAL OIL SYNERGY

3 drops	tea tree EO
5 drops (0.25 mL)	frankincense EO
3 drops	cajuput EO

BASE

2 tsp (10 mL)	hempseed oil
4 tsp (20 mL)	sunflower seed oil

1. *Essential Oil Synergy:* In a beaker, combine tea tree, frankincense and cajuput essential oils. Cover with foil or plastic wrap and set aside.
2. *Base:* In second beaker, combine hempseed and sunflower seed oils. Stir well.
3. Add prepared synergy blend and whisk to combine. Transfer to prepared bottle and seal tightly. Properly stored (see page 219), the serum will keep for up to 6 months.

Variations

If you have sensitive skin, reduce the amount of each essential oil by a drop.

LUNG SUPPORT FACIAL MASK: Substituting this serum, follow the mask instructions on page 280.

HOW TO USE

Fill a clean basin with warm water. Add 6 drops serum and agitate. Soak a facecloth in the solution. Drape soaked cloth over your face for 30 seconds, then remove slowly. Repeat 3 to 6 times. Follow by massaging 3 to 4 drops of serum into skin.

Kidney Support Serum

Dark circles and puffiness around the eyes indicate a potential imbalance in the kidneys. Eliminate sugar, caffeine and alcohol; supplement your diet with fresh fruits and vegetables. Increase physical activity and get a good night's sleep on a regular basis. Use this serum when you are experiencing mental fatigue.

SKIN TYPE
All

WHEN TO USE
Morning and night

**Makes
1 oz (30 mL)**

TIP

This serum may be used underneath a moisturizing cream or on its own. Use twice a day, morning and night.

KNOW THE BENEFITS

When the mind and body are exhausted, geranium, juniper berry and rose otto essential oils are restorative and balancing. When gently massaged onto the face, they help to relieve inflammation and calm the nervous system.

- 2 small beakers
- Glass stir stick
- Glass pump or dropper bottle (1 oz/30 mL) sprayed with 70% ethyl alcohol

ESSENTIAL OIL SYNERGY

3 drops	geranium EO
5 drops (0.25 mL)	juniper berry EO
3 drops	rose otto EO

BASE

4 tsp (20 mL)	apricot kernel oil
2 tsp (10 mL)	rosehip seed oil

1. *Essential Oil Synergy:* In a beaker, combine essential oils. Cover and set aside.
2. *Base:* In second beaker, combine apricot kernel and rosehip seed oils. Whisk well.
3. Add prepared synergy blend and whisk to combine. Transfer to prepared bottle and seal tightly. Properly stored (see page 219), the serum will keep for up to 6 months.

Variations

If you have sensitive skin, reduce the amount of each essential oil by a drop.

LUNG SUPPORT FACIAL MASK: Substituting this serum, follow the mask instructions on page 283.

HOW TO USE

Fill a clean basin with warm water. Add 6 drops serum and agitate to disperse. Thoroughly soak a facecloth in the solution. Drape over face for 30 seconds, then remove. Repeat 3 to 6 times. Follow by massaging 3 to 4 drops of serum into skin

Heart Support Serum

Breakouts and redness around the nose indicate a potential imbalance in the cardiovascular system. Eliminate fatty foods, alcohol and cigarettes and let go of sadness, worry and concerns.

SKIN TYPE
All

WHEN TO USE
Morning and night

**Makes
1 oz (30 mL)**

TIP

This serum may be used underneath a moisturizing cream or on its own. Use twice a day, morning and night.

KNOW THE BENEFITS

Neroli, lavender and rose otto essential oils are oils of the heart, creating a sense of being embraced and protected. When gently massaged onto the face, they help to relieve inflammation and calm the nervous system.

- 2 small beakers
- Glass stir stick
- Glass pump or dropper bottle (1 oz/30 mL) sprayed with 70% ethyl alcohol

ESSENTIAL OIL SYNERGY

5 drops (0.25 mL)	lavender EO
3 drops	neroli EO
3 drops	rose otto EO

BASE

4 tsp (20 mL)	apricot kernel oil
2 tsp (10 mL)	rosehip seed oil

1. *Essential Oil Synergy:* In a beaker, combine lavender, neroli and rose otto essential oils. Cover with foil or plastic wrap and set aside.
2. *Base:* In second beaker, combine apricot kernel and rosehip seed oils. Stir well.
3. Add prepared synergy blend and whisk to combine. Transfer to prepared bottle and seal tightly. Properly stored (see page 219), the serum will keep for up to 6 months.

Variation

HEART SUPPORT FACIAL MASK: In a bowl, combine 6 drops serum, 2 tbsp (30 mL) white (kaolin) clay and 3 tbsp (45 mL) water. Mix until a smooth paste forms. Apply to clean face and let dry for 10 to 15 minutes. Rinse off with warm water. Makes 1 application.

HOW TO USE

Fill a clean basin with warm water. Add 6 drops serum and agitate to disperse. Thoroughly soak a facecloth in the solution. Drape over face for 30 seconds. Repeat 3 to 6 times. Follow by massaging 3 to 4 drops of serum into skin.

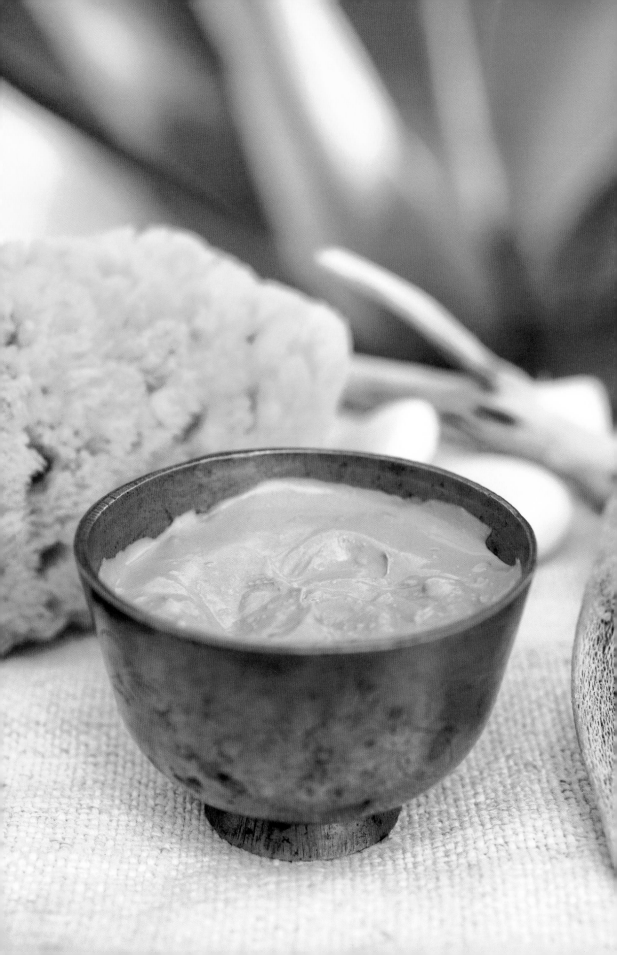

Facial Masks

Facial masks are soothing and nurturing for your skin. They are also an important part of the cleansing process and should be used two or three times a week. Functionally, masks remove impurities, help nutrients penetrate and improve the appearance of your skin. Choosing the right facial mask for your skin type will help keep your skin refreshed and alive, prevent premature aging and help prevent blemishes and breakouts. Taking the time to use a mask also gives you an opportunity to relax and put your mind at ease.

Facial masks should feel calming on your skin and help you to feel relaxed. They should not cause any burning sensation. If you feel more than a gentle tingle when using a mask, your skin is reacting to the product. This can lead to irritation and create sensitivities. If you find that your mask begins to dry out in the jar, add a little water and stir well before using.

Restorative Facial Mask for Dry and Aging Skin

During the autumn and winter months there is much less humidity in the air, which can lead to dry, flaky skin and exacerbate common conditions such as rosacea, eczema and psoriasis. Give your skin some tender loving care with this moisturizing mask.

SKIN TYPE

All, especially dry, chapped skin

WHEN TO USE

Night

Makes 12 oz (360 mL)

TIPS

Adding the antimicrobial synergy and essential oils to your mixture gradually (rather than all at once) prevents clumps from forming.

When you apply any mask to your face, you may feel a tingling sensation. This is caused by its strong astringent properties and the tightening of the mask as it dries; it is a completely normal response. However, if you experience a burning sensation, wash off the mask immediately. Apply jojoba oil to soothe your skin.

- 2 small beakers
- Glass stir stick
- Bowl-style double boiler
- Electric mixer
- Glass or PET wide-mouth jar (14 oz/400 mL) sprayed with 70% ethyl alcohol

ESSENTIAL OIL SYNERGY

5 drops (0.25 mL)	geranium EO
10 drops (0.5 mL)	patchouli EO

BASE

¼ cup (60 mL)	rosehip seed oil
¼ cup (60 mL)	sweet almond oil
2 tbsp (30 mL)	emulsifying wax NF
1 cup (250 mL)	warm (86°F/30°C) filtered water
20 drops (1 mL)	Rose-Scented Antimicrobial Synergy (see page 36)
1 tbsp (15 mL)	kaolin clay

1. *Essential Oil Synergy:* In a beaker, combine geranium and patchouli essential oils. Cover with foil or plastic wrap and set aside.

2. In second beaker, combine rosehip seed and sweet almond oils and whisk to blend. Set aside.

3. *Base:* Set a heatproof glass bowl over a saucepan of hot, not boiling, water (86°F/30°C) and heat until warm to the touch. Add emulsifying wax and let melt completely. Add rosehip and almond oil mixture and stir until evenly combined. Remove pan from heat.

This restorative mask delivers the hydrating benefits of omega-3, -6 and -9 fatty acids, which are abundant in sweet almond and rosehip seed oils. The minerals in the clay help to detoxify and balance skin tone. Patchouli is antimicrobial and helps to repair scar tissue, while its scent is calming and relaxes the mind. Geranium essential oil helps to liven up dull, scaly skin.

4. In a bowl, whisk together warm water, antimicrobial synergy and clay. Using electric mixer at low speed, gradually add to oil-wax solution and beat until mixture is white and fluffy.

5. Gradually add prepared synergy blend and mix until combined. Transfer to prepared jar and seal tightly. Properly stored (see page 219), the mixture will keep for up to 3 months.

Variations

You can substitute an equal amount of hempseed oil for the rosehip seed oil. It also contains an abundance of omega-3, -6 and -9 fatty acids.

RESTORATIVE SERUM: You can easily transform some of the components of this mask into a restorative serum to nurture all types of skin. In a beaker, combine the sweet almond oil, rosehip seed oil and prepared essential oil synergy and whisk well. Transfer to a prepared 5 oz (125 mL) pump bottle. Use nightly as required, following the basic instructions for Emerald Dynasty Serum (page 270). For extra hydration, apply to your face after washing off the mask and leave on overnight.

HOW TO USE

Cleanse face well (exfoliate, if possible). Using your fingers, scoop out 1 to 2 tbsp (15 to 30 mL) and smooth over skin in an even layer. Leave on for 15 to 20 minutes, until completely dry, then gently rinse off with warm water. Ideally, mist your face with rose hydrolat and moisturize with Silky Rose Omega Moisturizing Cream (page 260). Use 2 to 3 times per week, at night.

NUT ALLERGY ALERT

If you are sensitive to nuts, you can use an alternative carrier oil. Substitute an equal amount of grapeseed, fractionated coconut or apricot kernel oil for the sweet almond oil. Using one of these oils will also result in a light-textured base.

Instant Facelift Mask

A natural part of aging is that your skin begins to lose volume and is not as toned as it was when you were younger. Using a facial mask that promotes circulation and softens and smoothes fine lines is a wonderful boost.

SKIN TYPE

Aging

WHEN TO USE

Night

Makes about 3 oz (100 mL)

TIPS

Do not use this mask if you have sensitive or cracked skin.

KNOW THE BENEFITS

Once liquids are added to gum arabic powder, it forms a gel-like base. When applied, it causes the skin to cool and tighten, leaving your face feeling refreshed. Cocoa and caffeine are antioxidants; they also lighten blemishes and tighten skin, smoothing out fine lines. Bergamot balances excessive oiliness and tones the skin while calming the nervous system.

- Small beaker
- Glass stir stick
- Glass or PET jar (4 oz/100 mL) sprayed with 70% ethyl alcohol

10 drops (0.5 mL)	bergamot EO
¼ tsp (1 mL)	sweet almond oil
1 tbsp (15 mL)	gum arabic (acacia) powder
1 tbsp (15 mL)	cocoa powder
¼ cup (60 mL)	warm brewed coffee

1. In beaker, combine bergamot essential oil and sweet almond oil. Cover with foil or plastic wrap and set aside.
2. In a bowl, whisk together gum arabic and cocoa powders. Add oil mixture and stir well. While stirring, gradually add coffee and stir until a gel forms.
3. Transfer to prepared jar and seal tightly. Properly stored (see page 219), the mixture will keep for up to 2 weeks.

Variations

Substitute an equal amount of patchouli essential oil for the bergamot.

If you are sensitive to nuts, use an alternative carrier oil (see Nut Allergy Alert, page 287).

HOW TO USE

Cleanse face well (exfoliate, if possible). Using your fingers, scoop out 1 to 2 tbsp (15 to 30 mL) and smooth over skin in an even layer. Leave on for 15 to 20 minutes, until completely dry, then gently rinse off with warm water (you may need a wet cloth to remove all of it). Follow by misting face with Neroli-Enriched Floral Hydrolat Toner (page 247) and moisturizing with Green Beauty Moisturizing Cream (page 258). Use up to 2 times a week, at night.

Acne Spot-Treatment Mask

There are many reasons for acne breakouts. When they occur, apply this spot treatment before bed.

Oily, acne-prone skin

WHEN TO USE

Night

Makes about 12 oz (375 mL)

TIPS

Adding the witch hazel to your mixture gradually (rather than all at once) prevents clumps from forming.

KNOW THE BENEFITS

French green clay contains minerals that help to detoxify the skin. Witch hazel is an astringent, which helps to close pores. Tea tree and cajuput essential oils are extremely antimicrobial and astringent, which helps prevents infection. Grapefruit essential oil has a fresh citrus scent that will leave you feeling uplifted.

- Small beaker
- Glass stir stick
- Glass or PET wide-mouth jar (14 oz/400 mL) sprayed with 70% ethyl alcohol

ESSENTIAL OIL SYNERGY

5 drops (0.25 mL)	tea tree EO
5 drops (0.25 mL)	cajuput EO
5 drops (0.25 mL)	grapefruit EO (see Sensitivity Alert, page 275)
½ tsp (2 mL)	jojoba oil

BASE

1 cup (250 mL)	French green clay
½ cup (125 mL)	witch hazel hydrolat

1. *Essential Oil Synergy:* In beaker, combine tea tree, cajuput and grapefruit essential oils and jojoba oil. Set aside.
2. *Base:* In a bowl, combine clay and prepared synergy blend. Gradually pour in witch hazel hydrolat and stir until a paste forms.
3. Transfer to prepared jar and seal tightly. Properly stored (see page 219), the mixture will keep for up to 3 weeks.

Variation

For sensitive skin, substitute an equal amount of warm (86°F/30°C) filtered water for the witch hazel hydrolat.

HOW TO USE

Wipe your face with a cloth soaked in warm water. Using your fingers, scoop out ¼ tsp (1 mL) and apply to blemishes. Leave on overnight. In the morning, gently rinse off with warm water. Ideally, mist with witch hazel hydrolat, then apply aloe vera gel. Apply Sensitive Skin Serum (page 276) overtop. Use when needed.

For a longer shelf life (6 to 8 months): Combine all ingredients except the witch hazel hydrolat and store in the jar. When ready to use, scoop up 2 tbsp (30 mL) of the mixture and activate with 1 to 2 tbsp (15 to 30 mL) witch hazel.

Skin-Lightening Face Mask

This formulation is inspired by ancient recipes from North Africa and eastern India, used for their skin-lightening effects. Use at night, once a week.

SKIN TYPE

All, especially dry skin with hyperpigmentation

WHEN TO USE

Night

Makes about 6 oz (200 mL)

TIPS

Look for chickpea flour (also known as garbanzo bean flour) at well-stocked grocers.

KNOW THE BENEFITS

Chickpea flour is rich in amino acids such as lysine, which helps to relieve acne and cold sores; arginine, which helps skin regenerate when applied topically; and glutamic acid, which helps moisturize and lighten skin. Sandalwood essential oil has skin-lightening properties and can help to repair damage caused by the sun. Rose otto essential oil has a calming and balancing effect on the skin and nervous system.

- Small beaker
- Glass stir stick
- Glass or PET wide-mouth jar (7 oz/225 mL) sprayed with 70% ethyl alcohol

ESSENTIAL OIL SYNERGY

5 drops (0.25 mL)	sandalwood EO
5 drops (0.25 mL)	rose otto EO

BASE

1 tsp (5 mL)	organic cane sugar
½ cup (125 mL)	warm (86°F/30°C) filtered water
¼ cup (60 mL)	chickpea flour

1. *Essential Oil Synergy:* In beaker, combine sandalwood and rose otto essential oils. Cover and set aside.
2. In a bowl, combine sugar and warm water and stir well. Set aside for 5 minutes to let the sugar dissolve.
3. Place chickpea flour in another bowl. Add sugar solution and stir to combine. Add essential oil synergy and stir until a paste forms. If the mixture seems too thick, add water, 1 tsp (5 mL) at a time, until desired consistency is reached.
4. Transfer to prepared jar and seal tightly. Properly stored (see page 219), the mixture will keep for up to 2 days.

Variation

SKIN-LIGHTENING FACE OIL: In a beaker, combine the synergy with 6 tbsp + 2 tsp (100 mL) marula oil. Transfer to a 5 oz (125 mL) bottle and seal well. Use nightly, massaging a few drops into the skin after cleansing.

HOW TO USE

Cleanse face well (exfoliate, if possible). Using your fingers, scoop out 1 to 2 tbsp (15 to 30 mL) and smooth over skin in an even layer. Leave on for 15 to 20 minutes, until completely dry, then gently rinse off with warm water or a wet cloth. Ideally, mist face with floral hydrolat and moisturize with Silky Rose Omega Moisturizing Cream or Saffron Night Repair Moisturizing Cream.

Troubled Skin Mask

The minerals in this mask have a soothing effect on oily and acne-prone skin.

(see page 219)

SKIN TYPE
Oily and acne-prone

WHEN TO USE
Night

Makes
4 oz (120 mL)

TIPS
. . . .

To achieve a smoother consistency when blending clays with other ingredients, always add the carrier oil(s) last

KNOW THE BENEFITS
. . . .

Jojoba oil helps the skin retain its natural moisture and balances the astringent properties of the witch hazel and essential oils. Tea tree, sweet marjoram and cajuput essential oils fight bacteria. Green clay helps remove impurities from the skin, while kaolin clay is rich in minerals that relieve inflammation.

- Small beaker
- Glass stir stick
- Glass or PET wide-mouth jar (4 oz/120 mL) sprayed with 70% ethyl alcohol

ESSENTIAL OIL SYNERGY

5 drops (0.25 mL)	tea tree EO
5 drops (0.25 mL)	sweet marjoram EO
5 drops (0.25 mL)	cajuput EO

BASE

¼ cup (60 mL)	French green clay
¼ cup (60 mL)	kaolin clay
¼ cup (60 mL)	witch hazel hydrolat
1 tbsp (15 mL)	jojoba oil

1. *Essential Oil Synergy:* In beaker, combine tea tree, sweet marjoram and cajuput essential oils. Cover with foil or plastic wrap and set aside.
2. *Base:* In a bowl, combine green and kaolin clays. Add prepared essential oil synergy and stir well. While stirring, gradually add witch hazel hydrolat and stir until a smooth paste forms. Gradually stir in jojoba oil, until completely incorporated.
3. Transfer to prepared jar and seal tightly. Properly stored (see page 219), the mixture will keep for up to 4 weeks.

HOW TO USE

Cleanse face well (exfoliate, if possible). Using your fingers, scoop out 1 to 2 tbsp (15 to 30 mL) and smooth over skin in an even layer. Leave on for 15 to 20 minutes, until completely dry, then gently rinse off with warm water or a wet cloth. Mist face with rose hydrolat and a moisturizing cream for sensitive skin. Use at night, 1 or 2 times a week.

For a longer shelf life (6 to 8 months): Combine everything except the witch hazel and jojoba oil and store in the jar. When ready to use, scoop up 2 tbsp (30 mL) of the clay mixture and activate with 1 tbsp (15 mL) witch hazel and ¾ tsp (3 mL) jojoba oil.

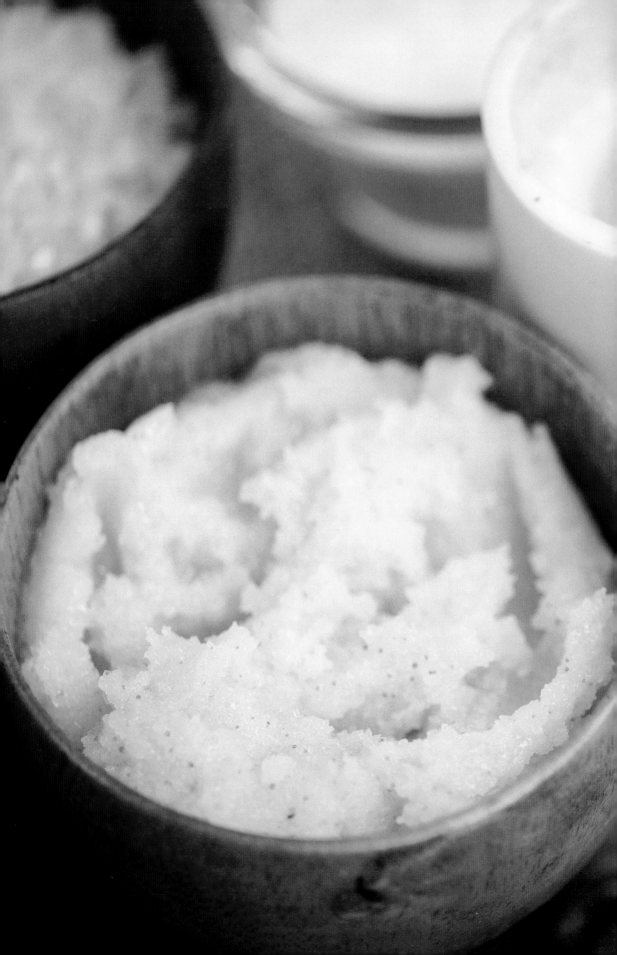

Exfoliants

Exfoliation is an integral part of the cleansing process and can help you achieve healthy, glowing skin. Exfoliation removes dead skin cells and helps uncover new skin while at the same time opening the pores, allowing your skin to absorb the nutrients supplied by natural products. It is important to note that your skin does not need intensive exfoliating to achieve positive results. Gently exfoliate the skin on your face 1 or 2 times a week, preferably in the evening.

Similar to the process used on your face, exfoliating your body helps to remove dead skin cells. The massaging action boosts circulation and helps drain your lymph nodes by increasing blood flow to the skin's surface. The extra bonus is that exfoliation encourages moisturizing products such as body oils and lotions to penetrate more deeply into the skin.

IRRITATION ALERT

Refrain from hair removal 48 hours before and after using an exfoliant, to prevent damage to the skin from the resulting excessive exfoliation.

Facial Exfoliants

Body Exfoliants

Honey-Flow Exfoliant

This exfoliant works quickly to naturally cleanse the skin and remove dead cells, evening overall skin tone.

SKIN TYPE

All

WHEN TO USE

Once or twice a week, in the evening

**Makes
2 oz (60 mL)**

TIPS

If the exfoliant solidifies, place the bottle in a bowl of warm water.

Consider adding dehydrated citrus zest to this and any of the exfoliant formulations in this book. Add 1 to 2 tbsp (15 to 30 mL) to any of the facial exfoliants, and 2 to 4 tbsp (30 to 60 mL) to body exfoliants.

KNOW THE BENEFITS

Honey has antioxidant and antibacterial properties that support the skin's immunity and help to reduce the signs of aging. Pomegranate extract lightens and firms up the skin. Benzoin helps to balance the pH of the skin and relieve dryness and chapping.

- Bowl-style double boiler
- Small beaker
- Glass stir stick
- Glass bottle (2 oz/60 mL) sprayed with 70% ethyl alcohol (see page 219)

2 tbsp (30 mL)	organic raw honey
10 drops (0.5 mL)	pomegranate extract
5 drops (0.25 mL)	benzoin EO
2 tbsp (30 mL)	organic raw cane sugar

1. Set a heatproof glass bowl over a saucepan of hot (not boiling) water (86°F/30°C) and heat until warm to the touch. Add honey and let melt completely. Remove from heat.
2. Add pomegranate extract and benzoin essential oil and stir well. While stirring, gradually add sugar.
3. Transfer to prepared bottle and seal tightly. Properly stored (see page 219), the exfoliant will keep for up to 2 weeks.

Variation

For an anti-inflammatory boost, substitute an equal amount of patchouli essential oil for the benzoin.

HOW TO USE

Wipe your face with a cloth soaked in warm water. Using your fingers, gently massage the exfoliant onto slightly moist skin. Leave on for 1 minute, then gently rinse off with a cloth dampened with warm water. Follow with toner and moisturizer, if needed. Use once or twice a week, in the evening.

Tunisian Marmalade Exfoliant

Hyperpigmentation is a very common problem of aging skin and one of the main reasons why people turn to chemical peels. This lovely blend, which is very rejuvenating, is derived from my mother's recipe for natural hair removal. Freshly squeezed lemon juice, which contains citric acid, lightens the skin and produces a natural glow.

SKIN TYPE
All, especially oily or dry

WHEN TO USE
Evening

Makes 4½ oz (135 mL)

TIP
To dehydrate lemon zest, use a fine-tooth grater to remove the zest from 1 organic (unwaxed) lemon. Spread zest evenly over a nonstick or parchment-lined baking sheet and heat in a 150°F (70°C) oven for 1 hour, until completely dried. If the lemon zest is not dehydrated properly, mold or bacteria may form prematurely in the finished exfoliant.

KNOW THE BENEFITS
Both lemon and sugar are effective skin-lightening and exfoliating agents.

- Glass bottle (5 oz/135 mL) sprayed with 70% ethyl alcohol (see page 219)

½ cup (125 mL)	organic raw cane sugar
½ cup (125 mL)	freshly squeezed organic lemon juice
1 tbsp (15 mL)	dehydrated organic lemon zest (see Tip, left)
10 drops (0.5 mL)	lemon EO

1. In a saucepan over low heat, combine sugar and lemon juice and bring to a simmer. Heat, stirring continuously, until the mixture turns a caramel color. Remove from heat.
2. While stirring, gradually add lemon zest. Add lemon essential oil and stir well.
3. Transfer to prepared bottle and seal tightly. Properly stored (see page 219), the exfoliant will keep for up to 2 weeks.

Variation
You can substitute an equal amount of lime (distilled) or mandarin essential oil for the lemon.

HOW TO USE
Wipe your face with a cloth soaked in warm water. Using your fingers, gently massage ¼ cup (60 mL) exfoliant onto slightly moistened skin. Leave on for 1 minute, then gently remove with a cloth dampened with warm water. Ideally, follow with Saffron Nights Skin-Lightening Toner (page 237) and Saffron Night Repair Moisturizing Cream (page 254), if needed. Use at night, once or twice a week.

Bioactive Exfoliant

This exfoliant is designed especially for sensitive skin, which can be irritated when even slightly coarse products are rubbed on it.

Sensitive

WHEN TO USE
Evening

Makes 4½ oz (135 mL)

TIPS
· · · · · · · · · · · · · · · · · · · ·

Substitute an equal amount of Emulsimulse, an eco-certified wax, for the National Formulary wax.

For a finer and more liquid version, add an additional 3 tbsp (45 mL) warm (86°F/30°C) filtered water.

- Small beaker
- Glass stir stick
- Bowl-style double boiler
- Glass jar (5 oz/135 mL) sprayed with 70% ethyl alcohol

ESSENTIAL OIL SYNERGY

5 drops (0.25 mL)	pine EO
5 drops (0.25 mL)	lavender EO

BASE

1 tbsp (15 mL)	emulsifying wax NF
2 tbsp (30 mL)	jojoba oil
6 tbsp (90 mL)	warm (86°F/30°C) filtered water
10 drops (0.5 mL)	Floral Antimicrobial Synergy (page 37)
1 tbsp (15 mL)	kaolin clay

1. *Essential Oil Synergy:* In beaker, combine pine and lavender essential oils. Cover and set aside.
2. *Base:* Set a heatproof glass bowl over a saucepan of hot (not boiling) water (86°F/30°C); heat until warm to the touch. Add emulsifying wax and let melt completely. Add jojoba oil and stir to combine. Remove from heat.
3. In a small bowl, combine warm water and antimicrobial synergy. While stirring, gradually add to melted wax mixture. Stir until cool, thickened and creamy. Fold in clay until incorporated and paste-like.
4. Add prepared synergy blend and stir until combined. Transfer to prepared jar and seal tightly. Properly stored (see page 219), the exfoliant will keep for up to 3 months.

Kaolin clay is rich in minerals that help to reduce inflammation and calm the skin. Gentle jojoba oil contains eicosanoic acid, which helps treat conditions such as rosacea. Pine essential oil contains pinene, which gently cleanses. In addition to its relaxing scent, lavender essential oil delivers anti-inflammatory, antibacterial and relaxing effects.

Variation

Substitute an equal amount of French green clay for the kaolin.

HOW TO USE

Wipe your face with a cloth soaked in warm water. Using your fingers, gently massage 1 tsp (5 mL) exfoliant onto slightly moist skin. Leave on for 3 to 5 minutes, then gently remove with a cloth dampened with warm water. Ideally, follow with a light lavender hydrolat misting and Orange Blossom Moisturizing Cream (page 264). Use once a week.

Balancing Body Exfoliant

Hot, dry temperatures can lead to dry, scaly, itchy skin. Use this exfoliant when showering to help restore moisture to the skin.

SKIN TYPE

All

WHEN TO USE

2 to 3 times
per week

**Makes about
½ cup (105 mL)**

TIP

If you find the scent of the cocoa butter too strong, use fractionated cocoa butter, which is odor-free.

KNOW THE BENEFITS

Cocoa butter is extremely moisturizing, and it's also an antioxidant. Coconut oil has antibacterial and antifungal properties. Avocado oil contains the fat-soluble vitamins E, D and K and is rich in minerals. Baking soda not only provides the granules needed for exfoliating but is also alkalizing and deodorizing.

- Beaker
- Glass stir stick
- Bowl-style double boiler
- Glass or PET jar (4 oz/125 mL) sprayed with 70% ethyl alcohol (see page 219)

ESSENTIAL OIL SYNERGY

20 drops (1 mL)	lime (distilled) EO
20 drops (1 mL)	pine EO

BASE

2 tbsp (30 mL)	cocoa butter
2 tbsp (30 mL)	extra virgin coconut oil
2 tbsp (30 mL)	avocado oil (crude)
1 tbsp (15 mL)	baking soda

1. *Essential Oil Synergy:* In beaker, combine lime and pine essential oils. Cover with foil or plastic wrap and set aside.
2. *Base:* Set a heatproof glass bowl over a saucepan of hot (not boiling) water (86°F/30°C) and heat until warm to the touch. Add cocoa butter and coconut oil and let melt completely.
3. Add avocado oil and warm until mixture is perfectly clear, 1 to 2 minutes. Stir gently to ensure that the ingredients are dissolved and evenly combined. Add baking soda and stir until well incorporated. Remove bowl from heat and let cool.
4. Cover mixture and refrigerate for about 30 minutes.
5. Remove mixture from fridge and stir until softened. Add prepared essential oil synergy and stir well.
6. Transfer to prepared jar and seal tightly. Properly stored (see page 219), the exfoliant will keep for up to 3 weeks.

HOW TO USE

Wet body with water, then massage a scoopful of exfoliant onto skin, focusing on legs and hips. Rinse with warm water and towel dry. Follow with a misting of rose hydrolat and a body oil or lotion.

Saffron Salt Body Scrub

This body exfoliant has an exotic scent and leaves the skin glowing.

TIPS

If you find that the mixture is a bit dry in Step 3, add another 1 tsp (5 mL) melted coconut oil.

KNOW THE BENEFITS

Himalayan salt is an extremely effective exfoliant that detoxifies and softens skin. Saffron is an ancient spice that moisturizes and gives the skin a smooth appearance. Sandalwood essential oil has a relaxing fragrance and also nurtures the skin. Mandarin essential oil is antiseptic and antibacterial. Jasmine absolute helps to create an overall calming and relaxing fragrance.

- Beaker
- Glass stir stick
- Glass jar (10 oz/300 mL) sprayed with 70% ethyl alcohol (see page 219)

ESSENTIAL OIL SYNERGY

5 drops (0.25 mL)	sandalwood (Australian) EO
5 drops (0.25 mL)	jasmine absolute
10 drops (0.5 mL)	mandarin EO

BASE

1 tbsp (15 mL)	witch hazel hydrolat
10 strands	saffron
2 tbsp (30 mL)	melted coconut oil
1 cup (250 mL)	finely ground Himalayan salt (see Tips, left)

1. In a small bowl, cover saffron with witch hazel hydrolat and set aside for 15 minutes, until liquid turns bright yellow.
2. *Essential Oil Synergy:* Meanwhile, in beaker, combine sandalwood, jasmine and mandarin essential oils. Cover with foil or plastic wrap and set aside.
3. *Base:* In a bowl, combine saffron-infused witch hazel, melted coconut oil and Himalayan salt. Stir until a granular paste forms. Add prepared essential oil synergy and stir well.
4. Transfer to prepared jar and seal tightly. Properly stored (see page 219), the exfoliant will keep for up to 3 weeks.

Variation

Substitute an equal quantity of Dead Sea salt for the Himalayan.

HOW TO USE

Use when showering. Wet body with water, then massage a scoopful of exfoliant onto skin, focusing on legs and hips. Rinse with warm water and towel dry. Ideally, follow with a fine misting of rose hydrolat and moisturize with a body oil or lotion.

Body-Flow Exfoliant

Poor circulation may leave the skin looking dimpled. Exfoliating with this coconut and camellia seed oil blend invigorates the skin, improving circulation and overall tone. It reduces the appearance of cellulite and leaves the skin feeling silky.

SKIN TYPE
All

WHEN TO USE
2 to 3 times
per week

**Makes about
3 cups
(735 mL)**

TIP
If you have sensitive skin, omit the sweet basil essential oil, which can cause irritation in some people.

- Bowl-style double boiler
- Beaker
- Glass stir stick
- Glass jar (26 oz/750 mL) sprayed with 70% ethyl alcohol (see page 219)

BASE

1 cup (250 mL)	extra virgin coconut oil
¼ cup (60 mL)	camellia seed oil
10 drops (0.5 mL)	cocoa extract
1 cup (250 mL)	unsweetened desiccated coconut
¾ cup (175 mL)	sodium laurel sulphate (SLS)–free soap

ESSENTIAL OIL SYNERGY

10 drops (0.5 mL)	benzoin EO
20 drops (1 mL)	mandarin EO
5 drops (0.25 mL)	sweet basil EO

1. *Base:* Set a heatproof glass bowl over a saucepan of hot (not boiling) water (86°F/30°C) and heat until warm to the touch. Add coconut oil and let melt completely. Add camellia seed oil and heat until completely dissolved. Remove from the heat and let cool slightly. Once cooled, cover mixture and refrigerate for 30 minutes, until semi-hardened.
2. *Essential Oil Synergy:* Meanwhile, in beaker, combine benzoin, mandarin and sweet basil essential oils. Cover and set aside.
3. Once carrier oil mixture is semi-hardened, add cocoa extract. Using an electric mixer at low speed, beat until mixture is white and fluffy (see Tips, page 314). Add desiccated coconut and mix well. Add soap and mix well.

Cocoa extract has a toning and stimulating effect on the skin and may help to reduce the appearance of cellulite. Benzoin essential oil has a vanilla-like scent and also tones the skin. Mandarin and sweet basil essential oils improve circulation. Camellia seed oil, rich in oleic acid, is moisturizing.

4. Add prepared synergy blend and mix until combined.
5. Transfer to prepared jar and seal tightly. Properly stored (see page 219), the exfoliant will keep for up to 3 weeks.

Variations

Substitute an equal amount of almond meal for the desiccated coconut.

Substitute an equal amount of apricot kernel oil for the camellia seed oil.

HOW TO USE

Use when showering. Wet body with water, then massage a scoopful of exfoliant onto skin, focusing on legs and hips. Rinse with warm water and towel dry. Ideally, follow with a fine misting of rose hydrolat. For extra benefit, moisturize with White Tea Cellulite Body Lotion (page 322).

Body Cleansers, Oils and Lotions

To keep your skin young and supple, replace traditional body washes with those that are oil based. Oil body cleansers can remove dirt and grime just as well as body washes, but they have the added benefit of hydrating your skin without removing its natural oils.

Body oils are the purest and most potent way to deliver nourishment and moisture to your skin. The best time to use a body oil is after a shower or bath and exfoliation, when the skin is clean and the pores are dilated. Under such conditions, the oil is better able to penetrate and moisturize the skin.

Lotions hydrate and protect the skin; they also transport essential oils and other therapeutic ingredients such as herbs and extracts. They have a higher ratio of liquids to lipids and a lighter viscosity than cream-based moisturizers, which makes them ideal for moisturizing the skin on the body.

SAFETY ALERT

For safety, you may wish to use PET packaging to protect against breakage in the bathroom.

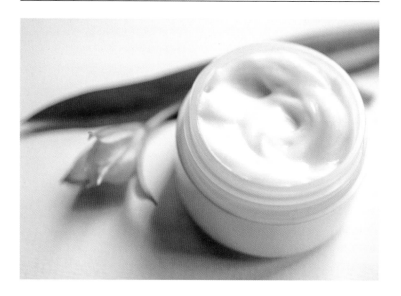

Body Cleansers

Body Oils

Body Lotions

Full-Body Toning Cleanser

Massaging your body for a minute or two while cleansing in the shower can help promote blood circulation and brighten overall skin tone. This gentle but powerful cleanser can be used daily on both the face and body.

SKIN TYPE

All

WHEN TO USE

Morning

**Makes
8 oz (240 mL)**

KNOW THE BENEFITS

Sesame seed oil has antibacterial properties and is beneficial for dry flaky skin.

Hempseed oil contains high levels of omega-3, -6 and -9 fatty acids, which help to nourish and repair damaged skin. Juniper berry essential oil has been used to treat oily skin conditions, congested pores and varicose veins. It is mildly antibacterial and antifungal and has also had good outcomes for managing stress, anxiety and nervous tension. Petitgrain essential oil contributes to a good range of antimicrobial activity. It also has an antispasmodic and calming effect on the whole being.

- 2 beakers
- Glass stir stick
- Glass or PET spray bottle (8 oz/250 mL) sprayed with 70% ethyl alcohol (see Tip, page 309)

ESSENTIAL OIL SYNERGY

5 drops (0.25 mL)	juniper berry EO
10 drops (0.5 mL)	petitgrain EO

BASE

¾ cup (175 mL)	sesame seed oil
¼ cup (60 mL)	hempseed oil

1. *Essential Oil Synergy:* In a beaker, combine juniper berry and petitgrain essential oils. Cover with foil or plastic wrap and set aside.
2. *Base:* In second beaker, whisk together sesame seed and hempseed oils. Add prepared synergy blend and whisk until combined.
3. Transfer to prepared bottle and seal tightly. Properly stored (see page 219), the cleanser will keep for up to 6 months.

Variation

Substitute an equal quantity of camellia seed oil for the hempseed oil.

HOW TO USE

Before showering, use a natural-bristle brush or terry cloth to dry-brush your whole body in a circular motion, working from your calves upward. Then spray the toning cleanser evenly over your entire body. Using your hands, massage the cleanser into your skin for 2 to 3 minutes. Rinse off in a warm shower and towel dry. Follow with a fine misting of Neroli-Enriched Floral Hydrolat Toner (page 247) for an extra-fresh feeling.

Decadent Body Bar

Weather conditions can lead to dry, chapped skin. Using a butter-based body bar can help to relieve these symptoms, especially on the arms and legs.

SKIN TYPE

All, especially dry

WHEN TO USE

Anytime

Makes 12 bars

TIPS

Adding the cider vinegar gradually while stirring helps to avoid clumping. The mixture will resemble thickened milk after blending.

This is a wonderful product to use for shaving legs, to make them look soft and glowing.

KNOW THE BENEFITS

Cocoa butter, shea butter and coconut oil are rich in saturated fats and deeply moisturizing. Calendula helps to relieve chapped and inflamed skin. Kaolin clay acts as an exfoliant and binder. Sandalwood essential oil gives this bar an exotic fragrance and will help ease skin inflammation.

- Bowl-style double boiler
- Glass stir stick
- 12-cup muffin pan, lined with extra-thick paper liners

1 cup (250 mL)	cocoa butter
¼ cup (60 mL)	coconut oil
¼ cup (60 mL)	shea butter
¼ cup (60 mL)	calendula infusion in glycerin
¼ cup (60 mL)	kaolin or French green clay
2 tsp (10 mL)	apple cider vinegar
10 drops (0.5 mL)	sandalwood (Australian) EO

1. Set a heatproof glass bowl over a saucepan of hot (not boiling) water (86°F/30°C) and heat until warm to the touch. Add cocoa butter, coconut oil and shea butter and let melt completely. Add calendula infusion and stir well. Remove from heat.
2. Place clay in a large bowl. Gradually add cider vinegar and stir until a dry paste forms. Add the melted butters and sandalwood essential oil and stir until well combined.
3. Divide mixture evenly among prepared muffin cups. Cover tightly with plastic wrap and refrigerate until hardened, about 24 hours.
4. Transfer bars to an airtight container. Properly stored, unused bars will keep for up to 3 months in the refrigerator.

Variation
Substitute patchouli for the sandalwood EO.

HOW TO USE

Use daily when showering. Wet skin with water, wet body bar and lather over entire body. Leave the creamy emulsion on the skin for 1 to 2 minutes. Rinse thoroughly with warm water and towel dry. Follow with Rose Body Oil (page 308).

Body-Cleanse Massage Oil

Inflammation occurs naturally after all forms of physical activity, a result of stress placed on the body. A bath or gentle massage can help remove accumulated lactic acid. This oil contains warming and anti-inflammatory oils to help prevent soreness after physical exertion.

SKIN TYPE

All

WHEN TO USE

After workout

Makes about 8 oz (250 mL)

KNOW THE BENEFITS

Ginger essential oil is high in zingiberene, which has warming properties. Cardamom essential oil contains eucalyptol, which makes it an effective antispasmodic and decongestant. Sweet basil essential oil has a tonic-like effect on the skin because of its stimulating properties. It has also been found to be a strong antioxidant. Additionally, its eugenol and methyl chavicol constituents make it a leading antimicrobial among the essential oils. Lemongrass essential oil is highly effective in skin-care products that address bacterial and fungal infections.

- 2 beakers
- Glass stir stick
- Glass or PET spray bottle (9 oz/250 mL) sprayed with 70% ethyl alcohol (see Tip, page 309)

15 drops (0.75 mL)	ginger EO
5 drops (0.25 mL)	lemongrass EO
5 drops (0.25 mL)	cardamom EO
5 drops (0.25 mL)	sweet basil EO
1 cup (250 mL)	sesame seed oil

1. In a beaker, combine essential oils. Cover and set aside.
2. Place sesame seed oil in second beaker. Add prepared synergy blend and whisk until combined.
3. Transfer to prepared bottle and seal tightly. Properly stored (see page 219), the oil will keep for up to 6 months. See page 307 for how to use. Ideally, follow with a fine misting of lavender hydrolat (page 246) for a cooling sensation and relaxing scent.

Variation

If you have fair and and/or sensitive skin, reduce the quantity of essential oils by half.

Warming Oils

Warming oils before massaging them onto the skin not only feels delightful but also enhances absorption of the essential oils. You can find oil warmers at suppliers of essential oils (see page 371). Alternatively, place a small amount (2 to 3 tbsp/30 to 45 mL) of the prepared oil in a small bowl, then place that in a bigger bowl filled with hot water. Let stand until the oil is warmer than room temperature.

Patchouli Body Oil

Sesame-based body oils are extremely moisturizing and a wonderful complement to skin-care routines, especially during the winter months, when harsh weather and home heating systems tend to dry out the skin.

SKIN TYPE

Dry

WHEN TO USE

After shower or bath

Makes about 6 oz (190 mL)

KNOW THE BENEFITS

Sesame seed oil is rich in linoleic acid, which protects the skin from dehydration. It is also antibacterial, and provides very mild sun protection (the SPF is 2–3). Caprylic and capric acid (naturally derived from coconut or palm oil fatty acids) provides a stable, silky base. Bamboo extract provide a smooth, non-greasy texture. The deep, warm aroma of patchouli is calming and relaxing; this essential oil is also considered an antioxidant and helps to prevent skin damage caused by UV exposure. In addition to being cooling, peppermint essential oil is antibacterial and analgesic, which means it can help to relieve pain.

- Small beaker
- Large beaker
- Glass stir stick
- Glass or PET flip-top or pump bottle (7 oz/200 mL) sprayed with 70% ethyl alcohol (see Tips, 309)

ESSENTIAL OIL SYNERGY

10 drops (0.5 mL)	patchouli EO
5 drops (0.25 mL)	peppermint EO

BASE

¾ cup (175 mL)	sesame seed oil
1 tbsp (15 mL)	caprylic or capric acid
10 drops (0.5 mL)	bamboo extract

1. *Essential Oil Synergy:* In small beaker, combine patchouli and peppermint essential oils. Cover with foil or plastic wrap and set aside.
2. *Base:* In larger beaker, combine sesame seed oil and caprylic acid. Add bamboo extract and stir well.
3. Add prepared synergy blend and stir until combined.
4. Transfer to prepared bottle and seal tightly. Properly stored (see page 219), the oil will keep for up to 6 months.

Variation

PATCHOULI BODY GEL: In a small bowl, combine 1 tbsp (15 mL) Patchouli Body Oil and 2 tbsp (30 mL) aloe vera gel. Adding this body oil to aloe vera makes a lush moisturizing gel that can be used as a travel-size hand cream (makes about 1 oz/30 mL).

HOW TO USE

Apply to either wet or dry skin after showering. Using your hands, massage 1 to 1½ tbsp (15 to 22 mL) all over body until completely absorbed by the skin.

Rose Body Oil

This body oil feels light and cooling on the skin and has a lovely floral scent.

SKIN TYPE

Dry

WHEN TO USE

After shower or bath

**Makes about
6 oz (190 mL)**

KNOW THE BENEFITS

Sunflower seed oil is high in linoleic acid, which has been found to help dry, chapped skin. Caprylic and capric acid (naturally derived from coconut or palm oil fatty acids) provide a stable, silky base. Bamboo extract provides a smooth, non-greasy texture. Rose essential oil is highly recommended not only for its beautiful fragrance but also for its ability to keep the skin looking supple and toned. Petitgrain lends a green, herbaceous note and is also deodorizing and antibacterial.

- Small beaker
- Large beaker
- Glass stir stick
- Glass or PET flip-top or pump bottle (7 oz/200 mL) sprayed with 70% ethyl alcohol (see Tips, page 309)

ESSENTIAL OIL SYNERGY

10 drops (0.5 mL)	rose otto EO
5 drops (0.25 mL)	petitgrain EO

BASE

¾ cup (175 mL)	sunflower oil
1 tbsp (15 mL)	caprylic or capric acid
10 drops (0.5 mL)	bamboo extract

1. *Essential Oil Synergy:* In small beaker, combine rose otto and petitgrain essential oils. Cover with foil or plastic wrap and set aside.
2. *Base:* In larger beaker, combine sunflower seed oil and caprylic acid. Add bamboo extract and stir well.
3. Add prepared synergy blend and stir until combined.
4. Transfer to prepared bottle and seal tightly. Properly stored (see page 219), the oil will keep for up to 6 months.

Variation

ROSE BODY GEL: In a small bowl, combine 1 tbsp (15 mL) Rose Body Oil and 2 tbsp (30 mL) aloe vera gel. Adding this body oil to aloe vera makes a lush moisturizing gel that can also be used as a travel-size hand cream (makes about 1 oz/30 mL).

HOW TO USE

Apply to either wet or dry skin after showering. Using your hands, massage 1 to 1½ tbsp (15 to 22 mL) all over body until completely absorbed by the skin.

Apricot Kernel Body Oil

This body oil is intensely moisturizing, leaving your skin feeling silky, and has a calming, fresh scent.

Makes about 6 oz (190 mL)

- Small beaker
- Large beaker
- Glass stir stick
- Glass or PET flip-top or pump bottle (7 oz/200 mL) sprayed with 70% ethyl alcohol (see Tip, left)

ESSENTIAL OIL SYNERGY

5 drops (0.25 mL)	neroli EO
5 drops (0.25 mL)	petitgrain EO
5 drops (0.25 mL)	orange EO

BASE

¾ cup (175 mL)	apricot kernel oil
1 tbsp (15 mL)	caprylic or capric acid
10 drops (0.5 mL)	bamboo extract

1. *Essential Oil Synergy:* In small beaker, combine neroli, petitgrain and orange essential oils. Cover with foil or plastic wrap and set aside.
2. *Base:* In larger beaker, combine apricot kernel oil and caprylic acid. Add bamboo extract and stir well.
3. Add prepared synergy blend and stir until combined.
4. Transfer to prepared bottle and seal tightly. Properly stored (see page 219), the oil will keep for up to 6 months.

Variation

APRICOT KERNEL BODY GEL: In a small bowl, combine 1 tbsp (15 mL) Apricot Kernel Body Oil and 2 tbsp (30 mL) aloe vera gel. Adding this body oil to aloe vera makes a lush moisturizing gel that can also be used as a hand cream.

HOW TO USE

Apply to either wet or dry skin after showering. Using your hands, massage 1 to 1½ tbsp (15 to 22 mL) all over body until completely absorbed by the skin.

Jojoba Body Oil

This body oil provides deep moisture and skin repair.

SKIN TYPE

All

WHEN TO USE

After shower or bath

**Makes about
6 oz (190 mL)**

KNOW THE BENEFITS

Jojoba oil is a wonderful emollient for all types of skin, but especially sensitive skin. Both jojoba and evening primrose oil are anti-inflammatory and nurture dry, scaly skin. Bamboo extract provides a smooth, non-greasy texture. German chamomile and helichrysum are also highly beneficial for people who have sensitive, dry, chapped skin.

- Small beaker
- Large beaker
- Glass stir stick
- Glass or PET flip-top or pump bottle (7 oz/200 mL) sprayed with 70% ethyl alcohol (see Tip, page 309)

ESSENTIAL OIL SYNERGY

5 drops (0.25 mL)	German chamomile EO
5 drops (0.25 mL)	helichrysum EO

BASE

¾ cup (175 mL)	jojoba oil
1 tbsp (15 mL)	evening primrose oil
10 drops (0.5 mL)	bamboo extract

1. *Essential Oil Synergy:* In small beaker, combine German chamomile and helichrysum essential oils. Cover with foil or plastic wrap and set aside.
2. *Base:* In larger beaker, combine jojoba and evening primrose oils. Add bamboo extract and stir well.
3. Add prepared synergy blend and stir until combined.
4. Transfer to prepared bottle and seal tightly. Properly stored (see page 219), the oil will keep for up to 6 months.

Variations

JOJOBA BODY GEL: In a small bowl, combine 1 tbsp (15 mL) Jojoba Body Oil and 2 tbsp (30 mL) aloe vera gel. Adding this body oil to aloe vera makes a lush moisturizing gel that can also be used as a hand cream.

Substitute an equal amount of borage essential oil for the evening primrose. Both oils contains a significant amount of GLA.

HOW TO USE

Apply to either wet or dry skin after showering. Using your hands, massage 1 to 1½ tbsp (15 to 22 mL) all over your body until completely absorbed.

After-Sun Repair Body Oil

This body oil contains intensive moisturizers to help repair skin damaged by dehydration and sun exposure.

SKIN TYPE

All

WHEN TO USE

After shower or bath

Makes about 6 oz (190 mL)

TIP

If you have sensitive skin, reduce the quantity of each essential oil to 1 drop.

KNOW THE BENEFITS

This lavish green formula contains an abundance of fatty acids and gamma-linolenic acid (GLA), which will help the skin repair itself, especially after sun exposure. Both hempseed and borage oil rejuvenate dry, chapped skin. Bamboo extract provides a smooth, non-greasy texture. Lavender and peppermint essential oils contribute cooling and anti-inflammatory properties to the blend.

- Small beaker
- Large beaker
- Glass stir stick
- Glass or PET flip-top or pump bottle (7 oz/200 mL) sprayed with 70% ethyl alcohol (see Tip, page 309)

ESSENTIAL OIL SYNERGY

5 drops (0.25 mL)	lavender EO
5 drops (0.25 mL)	peppermint EO

BASE

¾ cup (175 mL)	hempseed oil
1 tbsp (15 mL)	borage or evening primrose oil
10 drops (0.5 mL)	bamboo extract

1. *Essential Oil Synergy:* In small beaker, combine lavender and peppermint essential oils. Cover with foil or plastic wrap and set aside.
2. *Base:* In larger beaker, combine hempseed and borage oils. Add bamboo extract and stir well.
3. Add prepared synergy blend and stir until combined.
4. Transfer to prepared bottle and seal tightly. Properly stored (see page 219), the oil will keep for up to 6 months.

Variation

AFTER-SUN BODY GEL: In a small bowl, combine 1 tbsp (15 mL) prepared After-Sun Repair Body Oil and 2 tbsp (30 mL) aloe vera gel. Adding this oil to aloe vera makes a lush moisturizing gel that is cooling to the skin.

Green Dynasty Body Oil

This deeply moisturizing body oil has an uplifting yet relaxing scent. It contains an abundance of restorative fatty acids that nourish the skin, making it feel naturally silky smooth.

SKIN TYPE
All

WHEN TO USE
After shower or bath

Makes about 5 oz (155 mL)

TIP

If you have sensitive skin, reduce the quantity of each essential oil to 1 drop. Follow the instructions for use on page 313.

KNOW THE BENEFITS

Hempseed and camellia seed oils contain high levels of oleic acid, which has a deep moisturizing effect on skin. Apricot kernel oil is rich in antioxidants, a result of its high levels of vitamin E. Bamboo extract provides a smooth, non-greasy texture. Jasmine and grapefruit essential oils provide a fresh, bright scent.

- 2 beakers
- Glass stir stick
- Glass or PET flip-top or pump bottle (6 oz/200 mL) sprayed with 70% ethyl alcohol (see page 219)

ESSENTIAL OIL SYNERGY

5 drops (0.25 mL)	neroli EO
5 drops (0.25 mL)	grapefruit EO (see Sensitivity Alert, page 275)
5 drops (0.25 mL)	jasmine absolute

BASE

1 tbsp (15 mL)	hempseed oil
1 tbsp (15 mL)	camellia seed oil
½ cup (125 mL)	apricot kernel oil
10 drops (0.5 mL)	bamboo extract

1. *Essential Oil Synergy:* In a beaker, combine neroli, grapefruit and jasmine essential oils. Cover with foil or plastic wrap and set aside.
2. *Base:* In second beaker, combine hempseed, camellia seed and apricot kernel oils. Add bamboo extract and stir well.
3. Add prepared synergy blend and stir until combined.
4. Transfer to prepared bottle and seal tightly. Properly stored (see page 219), the oil will keep for up to 6 months.

Variations

GREEN DYNASTY BODY GEL: In a small bowl, combine 1 tbsp (15 mL) prepared Green Dynasty Body Oil and 2 tbsp (30 mL) aloe vera gel. Adding this oil to aloe vera makes a lush moisturizing gel that can also be used as a hand cream.

Substitute an equal amount of lime (distilled) essential oil for the grapefruit.

Exotic Body Oil

The power of scent plays an important part in personal care products. Jasmine absolute has a deep, exotic floral fragrance that combines with the woody notes of sandalwood to produce a calming and relaxing scent.

SKIN TYPE

All

WHEN TO USE

After shower or bath

Makes about 4½ oz (140 mL)

TIP

If you have sensitive skin, reduce the quantity of jasmine absolute to 5 drops and the sandalwood to 2 drops.

KNOW THE BENEFITS

Jojoba oil leaves the skin feeling soft and moist, without an oily finish. Caprylic and capric acid (naturally derived from coconut or palm oil fatty acids) provide a stable, silky base. The combination of sandalwood and jasmine is a classic feminine fragrance often used in perfumes.

- 2 beakers
- Glass stir stick
- Glass or PET flip-top or pump bottle (5 oz/150 mL) sprayed with 70% ethyl alcohol (see Tips, page 219)

ESSENTIAL OIL SYNERGY

10 drops (0.5 mL)	jasmine absolute
5 drops (0.25 mL)	sandalwood EO

BASE

½ cup (125 mL)	jojoba oil
1 tbsp (15 mL)	caprylic or capric acid

1. *Essential Oil Synergy:* In a beaker, combine jasmine and sandalwood essential oils. Cover with foil or plastic wrap and set aside.
2. *Base:* In second beaker, combine jojoba oil and caprylic acid and stir well.
3. Add prepared synergy blend and stir until combined.
4. Transfer to prepared bottle and seal tightly. Properly stored (see page 219), the oil will keep for up to 6 months.

Variation

EXOTIC BODY GEL: In a small bowl, combine 1 tbsp (15 mL) Exotic Body Oil and 2 tbsp (30 mL) aloe vera gel. Adding this body oil to aloe vera makes a lush moisturizing gel that can also be used as a hand cream.

HOW TO USE

Apply to either wet or dry skin after showering. Using your hands, massage 1 to 1½ tbsp (15 to 22 mL) all over body until absorbed by the skin.

Rich Cream-Based Lotion

This alcohol-free all-purpose lotion can be customized to include any essential oil you prefer (see Variations). It provides all skin types with a lovely protective moisturizing barrier and is particularly good for sensitive or inflamed skin.

SKIN TYPE

All

WHEN TO USE

Morning and night

Makes 2⅔ cups (635 mL)

TIP
....

Always start the mixer at a low speed. Mix patiently, without stopping, so the wax and oils do not cool off before they are emulsified, which can cause the components to separate.

- Glass beaker/measuring cup
- Glass stir stick
- Bowl-style double boiler
- Electric mixer
- Glass or PET jar (22 oz/650 mL) sprayed with 70% ethyl alcohol

1½ cups (375 mL)	warm (86°F/30°C) filtered water
20 drops (1 mL)	antimicrobial synergy of your choice (see page 35)
4 tsp (20 mL)	white or yellow beeswax (cosmetic grade)
¾ cup (175 mL)	extra virgin coconut oil
¼ cup (60 mL)	caprylic or capric triglycerides
20 drops (1 mL)	vitamin E oil
5 drops (0.25 mL)	essential oil of choice (see pages 94 to 203 and Variations)

1. In beaker, combine warm water and antimicrobial synergy. Cover with foil or plastic wrap and set aside (keep warm).
2. Set a heatproof glass bowl over a saucepan of hot (not boiling) water (86°F/30°C) and heat until warm to the touch. Add beeswax and let melt completely. Add coconut oil and stir gently until completely incorporated.
3. Add caprylic triglycerides and stir until completely incorporated. Remove bowl from heat.
4. Using electric mixer at low speed, gradually add prepared synergy blend. Continue to mix until emulsified (thick and creamy), 5 to 10 minutes. Add vitamin E oil and mix until completely incorporated.
5. Add essential oil and mix until completely incorporated.
6. Transfer mixture to prepared jar and seal tightly. Properly stored (see page 219), the lotion will keep for up to 3 months.

The commonly used emulsifying wax contains cetearyl or cetyl alcohol, which may cause sensitivities in some people. Beeswax, the main emulsifying agent in this formulation, provides a neutral base and a protective barrier for the skin. The coconut oil, another neutral ingredient, is rich in lauric acid, an anti-inflammatory. Caprylic and capric triglycerides contribute a silky texture to this lovely cream-based lotion.

Variations

For an everyday lotion, use one of the following essential oil blends:

GROUNDING AND BALANCING: 5 drops patchouli and 3 drops geranium EO

GROUNDING AND RELAXING: 5 drops sandalwood and 3 drops mandarin EO

UPLIFTING AND REFRESHING: 5 drops lavender and 3 drops pine EO

FEMININE AND UPLIFTING: 5 drops rose otto and 3 drops petitgrain EO

FEMININE AND BALANCING: 5 drops neroli and 3 drops rose otto EO

MASCULINE, REFRESHING AND BALANCING: 5 drops juniper berry and 3 drops lavender EO

For inflamed skin, use one of the following essential oil blends:

ANTI-INFLAMMATORY: 5 drops helichrysum and 5 drops lavender EO

ANTI-INFLAMMATORY AND ANTIFUNGAL: 5 drops German chamomile and 5 drops tea tree EO

ANTI-INFLAMMATORY AND CALMING: 5 drops frankincense and 5 drops neroli EO

HOW TO USE

Use after a shower or bath. With your fingertips, massage about 2 tsp (10 mL) all over the body. This lotion can also be used to treat severely dry skin on the face, if needed.

Restore and Repair Body Lotion

This lotion can be used as an all-purpose first-aid treatment to help heal minor injuries such as insect bites, bruises and burns.

SKIN TYPE

All

WHEN TO USE

As needed

**Makes
28 oz (830 mL)**

TIPS

This formulation makes a large quantity. Store extra portions in the fridge for up to 3 months, until ready to use.

Always start the mixer at a low speed. Mix patiently, without stopping, so the wax and oils do not cool off before they are emulsified, which can cause separation of the components.

- Small beaker
- Bowl-style double boiler
- Glass stir stick
- Electric mixer
- 4 glass or PET flip-top or pump bottles (7 oz/200 mL) sprayed with 70% ethyl alcohol (see Tips, left)

ESSENTIAL OIL SYNERGY

5 drops (0.25 mL)	helichrysum EO
5 drops (0.25 mL)	myrrh EO
5 drops (0.25 mL)	benzoin EO

BASE

2 cups (500 mL)	warm (86°F/30°C) filtered water
20 drops (1 mL)	Earthy Antimicrobial Synergy (page 38)
2 tbsp (30 mL)	glycerin
¼ cup (60 mL)	emulsifying wax NF
2 tbsp (30 mL)	shea butter
¼ cup (60 mL)	calendula-infused oil
¼ cup (60 mL)	arnica-infused oil
¼ cup (60 mL)	St. John's wort–infused oil
2 tbsp (30 mL)	aloe vera gel

1. *Essential Oil Synergy:* In beaker, combine helichrysum, myrrh and benzoin essential oils. Cover with foil or plastic wrap and set aside.
2. *Base:* In a bowl, combine warm water, antimicrobial synergy and glycerin.
3. Set a heatproof glass bowl over a saucepan of hot (not boiling) water (86°F/30°C) and heat until warm to the touch. Add emulsifying wax and let melt completely. Add shea butter and let melt completely.

The combination of arnica, St. John's wort and calendula infused oils is recognized as a highly effective first-aid treatment for cuts and sores. When these oils are added to a lotion base, they are a highly beneficial treatment for excessive sun exposure. The combination of helichrysum, myrrh and benzoin essential oils is also known for its wound-healing properties.

4. In a bowl, combine calendula, arnica and St. John's wort infused oils. Add to melted wax mixture and stir until completely incorporated. Remove bowl from heat.

5. Using electric mixer at low speed, gradually add prepared glycerin mixture. Continue to mix until emulsified (thick and creamy), 5 to 10 minutes.

6. Add prepared synergy blend and mix until combined. Add aloe vera gel and mix until well incorporated.

7. Transfer to prepared bottles and seal tightly. Properly stored (see page 219), the lotion will keep for up to 3 months.

Variation

Substitute an equal amount of carrot root–infused oil for the calendula-infused oil.

HOW TO USE

Apply to clean, dry skin after showering or bathing. Massage about 2 tsp (10 mL) into skin all over body, until completely absorbed. Or dab it on minor injuries such as insect bites, bruises and burns.

Troubleshooting Lotions and Creams

Making your own lotions isn't difficult, but you need to follow a few guidelines to achieve consistently good results.

- Work quickly when using an electric mixer to combine melted wax solutions with the remaining ingredients. If the wax cools too soon, your lotion or cream will separate.
- Always set your electric mixture to low speed to prevent the hot wax and oils from splashing. This helps to prevent the ingredients from sticking to the sides of the bowl, which may result in inaccurate measurements. Mixing slowly also helps to prevent air bubbles, which means your lotion or cream will have a much more stable consistency.
- When adding filtered water to a formulation, make sure that it is warm (86°F/30°C) so that the mixture doesn't cool too rapidly.
- Always add the water solution to the wax mixture gradually and while mixing. Otherwise the mixture may cool too quickly and seize, meaning that the oil and water will separate.
- It can take up to 10 minutes of mixing for mixtures to thicken to a creamy consistency. Be patient!
- To remove air bubbles, stir the finished mixture with a clean spatula before transferring to bottles or jars.
- Lotions and creams need to cool at room temperature for about 24 hours to set properly.

Deep Moisture Body Lotion

Climate and environment, especially cold weather or excessive sun exposure, can lead to dry, chapped and scaly skin. Applying moisturizing lotions before and after moderate sun exposure can help maintain healthy skin.

SKIN TYPE

Dry, chapped

WHEN TO USE

As needed

Makes 27 oz (800 mL)

TIPS

This formulation makes a large quantity. Store extra portions in the fridge for up to 3 months, until ready to use.

If you prefer you can divide this and all other formulations in half to make a smaller batch.

Always start the mixer at a low speed. Mix patiently, without stopping, so the wax and oils do not cool off before they are emulsified, which can cause separation of the components.

- Small beaker
- Glass stir stick
- Bowl-style double boiler
- Electric mixer
- 4 glass or PET flip-top or pump bottles (7 oz/200 mL) sprayed with 70% ethyl alcohol (see Tips, left)

ESSENTIAL OIL SYNERGY

5 drops (0.25 mL)	jasmine absolute
5 drops (0.25 mL)	petitgrain EO

BASE

2 cups (500 mL)	warm (86°F/30°C) filtered water
2 tbsp (30 mL)	glycerin
20 drops (1 mL)	Citrus Antimicrobial Synergy (page 36)
3 tbsp (45 mL)	emulsifying wax NF
¼ cup (60 mL)	extra virgin coconut oil
¼ cup (60 mL)	camellia seed oil
¼ cup (60 mL)	avocado oil

1. *Essential Oil Synergy:* In beaker, combine jasmine and petitgrain essential oils. Cover with foil or plastic wrap and set aside.
2. *Base:* In a bowl, combine warm water, glycerin and antimicrobial synergy. Set aside.
3. Set a heatproof glass bowl over a saucepan of hot (not boiling) water (86°F/30°C) and heat until warm to the touch. Add emulsifying wax and let melt completely. Add coconut oil and let melt completely.
4. Meanwhile, in another bowl, combine camellia seed and avocado oils and stir until well combined. Add to melted wax mixture and stir until completely incorporated. Remove bowl from heat.

Camellia seed oil, which is high in oleic acid, is known for its antioxidant properties, as well as it ability to reduce inflammation and help speed recovery from wounds and scrapes. Avocado oil is also very healing, thanks to its high levels of vitamin E and beta-carotene. Coconut oil is both moisturizing and antimicrobial, and it has been shown to resist 20% of UV rays (its SPF is 8).

5. Using electric mixer at low speed, gradually add prepared glycerin blend. Mix until emulsified (thick and creamy), 5 to 10 minutes.
6. Add prepared synergy blend and mix until combined.
7. Transfer to prepared bottles and seal tightly. Properly stored (see page 219), the lotion will keep for up to 3 months.

Variation

Substitute an equal amount of shea butter for the coconut oil.

HOW TO USE

Apply to clean, dry skin after showering or bathing. Massage about 2 tsp (10 mL) into skin, all over body, until completely absorbed.

Sensitive Skin Body Lotion

Some people are born with sensitive skin, while others develop skin conditions because of various factors, including allergies. The health of the nervous system plays a huge role in how the skin responds to circumstances, including inflammation. This lotion is designed to soothe the nervous system while also soothing the skin.

SKIN TYPE

All, especially sensitive

WHEN TO USE

As needed

Makes 27 oz (795 mL)

TIPS

To brew the tea: Use either 1 tbsp (15 mL) loose-leaf organic chamomile tea in an infuser or 1 teabag. Let steep in 2 cups (500 mL) hot water (170°F/80°C) for 10 minutes. (Do not boil the water, as this could damage the herb and reduce its therapeutic properties.)

Always start the mixer at a low speed. Mix patiently, without stopping, so the waxes and oils do not cool off before they are emulsified, which can cause the components to separate.

- Bowl-style double boiler
- Glass stir stick
- Electric mixer
- 4 glass or PET flip-top or pump bottles (7 oz/200 mL) sprayed with 70% ethyl alcohol (see Tip, right)

3 tbsp (45 mL)	emulsifying wax NF
1 tbsp (15 mL)	beeswax
2 cups (500 mL)	brewed organic chamomile tea (see Tips, left)
20 drops (1 mL)	Earthy Antimicrobial Synergy (page 38)
¾ cup (175 mL)	jojoba oil
¼ cup (60 mL)	borage oil
5 drops (0.25 mL)	Roman chamomile EO

1. Set a heatproof glass bowl over a saucepan of hot (not boiling) water (86°F/30°C) and heat until warm to the touch. Add emulsifying wax and let melt completely. Add beeswax and let melt completely.
2. In a bowl, combine chamomile tea and antimicrobial synergy. Set aside.
3. In another bowl, combine jojoba and borage oils and stir until well mixed. Add to melted wax mixture and stir until completely incorporated. Remove bowl from heat.
4. Using electric mixer at low speed, gradually add tea mixture. Continue to mix until emulsified (thick and creamy), 5 to 10 minutes.
5. Add Roman chamomile essential oil and mix until completely incorporated.

. . . .

This formulation makes a large quantity. Store extra portions in the fridge for up to 3 months, until ready to use.

KNOW THE BENEFITS
. . . .

As a herb, chamomile is a calming and soothing tonic; as an essential oil, its fragrance helps to calm the nervous system. Jojoba oil is an effective moisturizer for all skin types, especially skin that is sensitive or affected by rosacea. Borage oil is very healing and reduces inflammation due to skin disorders.

6. Transfer to prepared bottles and seal tightly. Properly stored (see page 219), the lotion will keep for up to 3 months.

Variations

SENSITIVE SKIN BODY OIL: In a beaker, combine jojoba and borage oils and Roman chamomile essential oil. Stir well. Transfer to a glass or PET flip-top or pump bottle (8 oz/250 mL) sprayed with 70% ethyl alcohol.

Substitute an equal amount of evening primrose oil for the borage oil. Both contain a significant amount of gamma-linolenic acid (GLA).

HOW TO USE

Apply on clean, dry skin after showering or bathing. Massage about 2 tsp (10 mL) into skin, all over body, until completely absorbed.

White Tea Cellulite Body Lotion

Cellulite is caused by a number of factors, including lack of exercise, poor diet and genetics. Topical treatments are beneficial only when combined with a lifestyle that includes exercise and healthy eating. When applied to affected areas, this lotion improves blood flow to the surface of the skin, leaving it feeling invigorated and toned.

SKIN TYPE

All

WHEN TO USE

After showering, especially in the morning

Makes 27 oz (795 mL)

TIPS

To brew the tea: Use either 1 tbsp (15 mL) loose-leaf organic white tea in an infuser or 1 teabag. Let steep in 2 cups (500 mL) hot water (170°F/80°C) for 10 minutes. (Do not boil the water, as this could damage the tea and reduce its therapeutic properties.)

Always start the mixer at a low speed. Mix patiently, without stopping, so the waxes and oils do not cool off before they are emulsified, which can cause separation of the components.

- Small beaker
- Glass stir stick
- Bowl-style double boiler
- Electric mixer
- 4 glass or PET flip-top or pump bottles (7 oz/200 mL) sprayed with 70% ethyl alcohol (see Tips, right)

ESSENTIAL OIL SYNERGY

10 drops (0.5 mL)	lime (distilled) EO
5 drops (0.25 mL)	pine EO
5 drops (0.25 mL)	ginger EO

BASE

2 tbsp (30 mL)	emulsifying wax NF
2 tbsp (30 mL)	stearic acid
2 tbsp (30 mL)	shea butter
¾ cup (175 mL)	grapeseed oil
¼ cup (60 mL)	camellia seed oil
2 cups (500 mL)	brewed organic white tea (see Tips, left)
2 tbsp (30 mL)	glycerin
10 drops (0.5 mL)	rosemary extract

1. *Essential Oil Synergy:* In beaker, combine lime, pine and ginger essential oils. Cover with foil or plastic wrap and set aside.
2. *Base:* Set a heatproof glass bowl over a saucepan of hot (not boiling) water (86°F/30°C) and heat until warm to the touch. Add emulsifying wax and stearic acid and let melt completely. Add shea butter and let melt completely.

This formulation makes a large quantity. Store extra portions in the fridge for up to 3 months, until ready to use.

Sometimes it is difficult to find packaging in the exact size that you need. Keep small (¼ to 1 oz/10 to 30 mL) jars on hand to store any extra product that doesn't fit into your packaging. They also make good vessels for testers.

KNOW THE BENEFITS

White tea is high in antioxidants, as are grapeseed and camellia seed oils. Lime, pine and ginger essential oils have a stimulating effect that promotes circulation and tones the appearance of dimpled and sagging skin.

3. Meanwhile, in a bowl, combine grapeseed and camellia seed oils and stir until well mixed. Add to melted wax mixture and stir until completely incorporated. Remove bowl from heat and set aside.

4. In another bowl, combine brewed tea, glycerin and rosemary extract.

5. Using electric mixer at low speed, gradually add tea mixture to melted wax mixture. Continue to mix until emulsified (thick and creamy), 5 to 10 minutes.

6. Add prepared synergy blend and mix until completely incorporated.

7. Transfer to prepared bottles and seal tightly. Properly stored (see page 219), the lotion will keep for up to 3 months.

Variation

If you prefer your lotion to have a gel-like consistency, mix in 2 tbsp (30 mL) aloe vera gel at the end of Step 5.

HOW TO USE

Before showering, use a dry natural-bristle brush or terrycloth to dry-brush your whole body in a circular motion, working from your calves upward. Shower, alternating hot and cold water and ending with cold water. Towel dry. Massage in about 2 tbsp (60 mL) lotion all over the legs and hips with vigorous circular motions, until completely absorbed by skin. Finish by misting entire body with Rejuvenating Toner (page 240).

After-Sun Body Lotion

What is more important than sun protection? After-sun protection. When skin is exposed to excessive sunlight, free radicals start to accumulate. The antioxidants in this lotion provide moisturizing compounds that help to repair skin and prevent degeneration.

SKIN TYPE

All

WHEN TO USE

As needed, especially after sun exposure

Makes about 30 oz (895 mL)

TIPS

Always start the mixer at a low speed. Mix patiently, without stopping, so the wax and oils do not cool off before they are emulsified, which can cause separation of the components.

This formulation makes a large quantity. Store extra portions in the fridge for up to 3 months, until ready to use.

Sometimes it is difficult to find packaging in the exact size you need. Keep small (¼ to 1 oz/10 to 30 mL) jars on hand to store any extra product that doesn't fit into your packaging. They also make good vessels for testers.

- Small beaker
- Glass stir stick
- Bowl-style double boiler
- Electric mixer
- 6 glass or PET flip-top or pump bottles (5 oz/150 mL) sprayed with 70% ethyl alcohol (see Tips, left)

ESSENTIAL OIL SYNERGY

5 drops (0.25 mL)	peppermint EO
5 drops (0.25 mL)	lavender EO
5 drops (0.25 mL)	helichrysum EO

BASE

2 cups (500 mL)	warm (86°F/30°C) filtered water
2 tbsp (30 mL)	glycerin
20 drops (1 mL)	Minted Camphor Antimicrobial Synergy (page 37)
¼ cup (60 mL)	emulsifying wax NF
2 tbsp (30 mL)	extra virgin coconut oil
¼ cup (60 mL)	rosehip seed oil
½ cup (125 mL)	sweet almond oil
¼ cup (60 mL)	evening primrose oil
20 drops (1 mL)	vitamin E oil
2 tbsp (30 mL)	aloe vera gel

1. *Essential Oil Synergy:* In beaker, combine peppermint, lavender and helichrysum essential oils. Cover with foil or plastic wrap and set aside.
2. In a bowl, combine warm water, glycerin and antimicrobial synergy. Set aside.
3. *Base:* Set a heatproof glass bowl over a saucepan of hot (not boiling) water (86°F/30°C) and heat until warm to the touch. Add emulsifying wax and coconut oil and let melt completely.

Rosehip seed and evening primrose oils are both powerhouses when it comes to skin repair, thanks to their fatty acid content. Sweet almond oil contains high levels of vitamin E, which is a powerful antioxidant that also moisturizes the skin. The synergy of peppermint, lavender and helichrysum essential oils has a cooling effect, providing comfort to sunburned skin.

4. Meanwhile, in another bowl, combine rosehip seed, sweet almond, evening primrose and vitamin E oils. Stir until well mixed. Add to melted wax mixture and stir until completely incorporated. Remove bowl from heat.

5. Using electric mixer at low speed, gradually add prepared glycerin mixture. Mix until emulsified (thick and creamy), 5 to 10 minutes.

6. Add prepared synergy blend and mix until completely incorporated. Add aloe vera gel and mix until well incorporated.

7. Transfer to prepared bottles and seal tightly. Properly stored (see page 219), the lotion will keep for up to 1 month.

Variation

AFTER-SUN BODY OIL SPRAY: In a beaker, combine essential oil synergy and rosehip seed, sweet almond, evening primrose and vitamin E oils. Stir well. Transfer to an 8 oz (250 mL) spray bottle. Spray onto cleansed skin for after-sun protection.

HOW TO USE

Apply to clean, dry skin after showering or bathing. Massage about 2 tsp (10 mL) into skin, all over body, until completely absorbed.

NUT ALLERGY ALERT

If you are sensitive to nuts, you can use an alternative carrier oil. Substitute an equal amount of grapeseed, fractionated coconut or apricot kernel oil for the sweet almond oil. These oils will also result in a light-textured base.

Decadent Body Lotion

This lotion is rich in emollients, making it beneficial for very dry skin. It leaves the skin feeling and looking supple and radiant.

- 2 beakers
- Glass stir stick
- Bowl-style double boiler
- Electric mixer
- 4 glass or PET flip-top or pump bottles (7 oz/200 mL) sprayed with 70% ethyl alcohol (see Tips, left)

ESSENTIAL OIL SYNERGY

10 drops (0.5 mL)	patchouli EO
5 drops (0.25 mL)	peppermint EO

BASE

2 cups (500 mL)	warm (86°F/30°C) filtered water
10 drops (0.5 mL)	cornflower extract
20 drops (1 mL)	Earthy Antimicrobial Synergy (page 38)
3 tbsp (45 mL)	emulsifying wax NF
2 tbsp (30 mL)	cocoa butter
¾ cup (175 mL)	sesame seed oil
¼ cup (60 mL)	calendula-infused oil

1. *Essential Oil Synergy:* In beaker, combine patchouli and peppermint essential oils. Cover with foil or plastic wrap and set aside.
2. In another beaker, combine warm water and cornflower extract. Stir in antimicrobial synergy and set aside.
3. Set a heatproof glass bowl over a saucepan of hot (not boiling) water (86°F/30°C) and heat until warm to the touch. Add emulsifying wax and let melt completely. Add cocoa butter and let melt completely.
4. Meanwhile, in a bowl, combine sesame seed and calendula-infused oils and stir until well mixed. Add to melted wax mixture and stir until completely incorporated. Remove bowl from heat.

Cocoa butter is an antioxidant-rich moisturizer. Sesame seed and calendula-infused oils have antimicrobial and anti-inflammatory properties that help to repair and protect the skin. Cornflower extract is also an effective antioxidant. Patchouli and peppermint essential oils lend an exotic scent.

5. Using electric mixer at low speed, gradually add warm cornflower blend. Continue to mix until emulsified (thick and creamy), 5 to 10 minutes.

6. Add prepared synergy blend and mix until completely incorporated.

7. Transfer to prepared bottles and seal tightly. Properly stored (see page 219), the lotion will keep for up to 3 months.

Variation

Substitute an equal amount of carrot root–infused oil for the calendula-infused oil.

HOW TO USE

Apply to clean, dry skin after showering or bathing. Massage about 2 tsp (10 mL) into skin, all over body, until completely absorbed.

Benefits of Sesame Oil

Sesame seed oil has been used for thousands of years to nurture and detoxify the skin. It is antimicrobial and also provides a very slight sun protection factor (SPF of 2–3). It is rich in saturated fats, very moisturizing and easily absorbed into the skin (it's also inexpensive).

Hibiscus Body Lotion

Anti-aging formulations need to contain powerful antioxidants that will effectively protect the skin from damage while gently returning it to a balanced state, without the use of harsh chemicals or other ingredients. When this softly scented lotion is used daily, it will help tone and protect the skin and fight the effects of aging.

SKIN TYPE
All, especially aging

WHEN TO USE
Day and night

Makes 26 oz (765 mL)

TIPS

Always start the mixer at a low speed. Mix patiently, without stopping, so the waxes and oils do not cool off before they are emulsified, which can cause separation of the components.

This formulation makes a large quantity. Store extra portions in the fridge for up to 3 months, until ready to use.

This formulation produces a substantial yield. If you prefer, you can divide it and any other formulations in half.

- 2 beakers
- Glass stir stick
- Bowl-style double boiler
- Electric mixer
- 4 glass or PET flip-top or pump bottles (7 oz/200 mL) sprayed with 70% ethyl alcohol (see Tips, left)

ESSENTIAL OIL SYNERGY

5 drops (0.25 mL)	neroli EO
5 drops (0.25 mL)	petitgrain EO
5 drops (0.25 mL)	orange EO

BASE

2 cups (500 mL)	warm (86°F/30°C) filtered water
2 tbsp (30 mL)	glycerin
10 drops (0.5 mL)	bamboo extract
10 drops (0.5 mL)	hibiscus infusion in glycerin
¼ cup (60 mL)	emulsifying wax NF
2 tbsp (30 mL)	stearic acid
¾ cup (175 mL)	apricot kernel oil

1. *Essential Oil Synergy:* In beaker, combine neroli, petitgrain and orange essential oils. Cover with foil or plastic and set aside.
2. Meanwhile, in another beaker, combine warm water, glycerin, bamboo extract and hibiscus infusion. Stir until well mixed. Set aside.
3. Set a heatproof glass bowl over a saucepan of hot water (86°F/30°C) and heat until warm to the touch. Add emulsifying wax and let melt completely. Add stearic acid and let melt completely. Stir in apricot kernel oil. Remove bowl from heat.

Hibiscus contains quercetin, which has been shown to help repair sun-damaged skin, reduce the degradation of elastin and improve the appearance of skin and scars. Apricot kernel oil is a light moisturizer that is beneficial for all skin types. The soft scents of neroli, petitgrain and orange essential oils are soothing to the mind as well as the body.

4. Using electric mixer at low speed, gradually add glycerin mixture. Continue to mix until emulsified (thick and creamy), 5 to 10 minutes.

5. Add prepared synergy blend and mix until completely incorporated.

6. Transfer to prepared bottles and seal tightly. Properly stored (see page 219), the lotion will keep for up to 3 months.

Variations

For severely dry skin, add 2 tbsp (30 mL) shea butter in Step 3. Allow it to melt completely before continuing with the rest of the recipe.

For a more cost-effective blend, substitute an equal amount of lavender or bergamot FCF essential oil for the neroli. Both these oils deliver similar calming, antiseptic and antibacterial qualities.

HOW TO USE

Apply to clean, dry skin after showering or bathing. Massage about 2 tsp (10 mL) into skin, all over body, until completely absorbed.

Green Dynasty Body Lotion

As the skin ages or is damaged by environmental or health conditions, its natural fatty-acid content is depleted. Applying creams and lotions rich in oleic acid helps to heal and restore dehydrated and chapped skin.

SKIN TYPE

All, especially combination skin and sensitive skin prone to psoriasis and eczema

WHEN TO USE

As needed

Makes about 24 oz (725 mL)

TIPS

Always start the mixer at a low speed. Mix patiently, without stopping, so the wax and oils do not cool off before they are emulsified, which can cause separation of the components.

This formulation makes a large quantity. Store extra portions in the fridge for up to 3 months, until ready to use.

- 2 beakers
- Glass stir stick
- Bowl-style double boiler
- Electric mixer
- 4 glass or PET flip-top or pump bottles (7 oz/200 mL) sprayed with 70% ethyl alcohol (see Tips, left)

ESSENTIAL OIL SYNERGY

5 drops (0.25 mL)	neroli EO
5 drops (0.25 mL)	grapefruit EO
5 drops (0.25 mL)	helichrysum EO

BASE

2 cups (500 mL)	warm (86°F/30°C) filtered water
20 drops (1 mL)	Citrus Antimicrobial Synergy (page 36)
20 drops (1 mL)	green tea infusion in glycerin
10 drops (0.5 mL)	bamboo extract
¼ cup (60 mL)	emulsifying wax NF
2 tbsp (30 mL)	extra virgin coconut oil
1 tsp (5 mL)	hempseed oil
1 tsp (5 mL)	camellia seed oil
½ cup (125 mL)	apricot kernel oil

1. *Essential Oil Synergy:* In a beaker, combine neroli, grapefruit and helichrysum essential oils. Cover with foil or plastic wrap and set aside.

2. In second beaker, combine warm water, antimicrobial synergy, green tea infusion and bamboo extract. Set aside.

3. Set a heatproof glass bowl over a saucepan of hot (not boiling) water (86°F/30°C) and heat until warm to the touch. Add emulsifying wax and let melt completely. Add coconut oil and let melt completely.

. . . .

The combination of hempseed and camellia seed oils, which are both rich in oleic acid, is extremely nourishing to the skin. Oleic acid is a fatty acid found in the epidermis (the top layer of the skin); it is depleted during the normal course of aging. Supplementing the skin with oils that contain high levels of this fatty acid benefits aging and dry skin, and the oils also have antiviral and antifungal properties. Both hempseed and camellia seed oil also contain high levels of chlorophyll, which helps ease symptoms of psoriasis, eczema and severe dryness of the skin. Apricot kernel oil is very moisturizing. Neroli and helichrysum essential oils help to repair scar tissue. Grapefruit essential oil has a light, fresh aroma.

4. Meanwhile, in a bowl, combine hempseed, camellia seed and apricot kernel oils. Stir until well mixed. Add to melted wax mixture and stir to combine.

5. Using electric mixer at low speed, gradually add water mixture. Continue to mix until emulsified (thick and creamy), 5 to 10 minutes.

6. Add prepared synergy blend and mix until completely incorporated.

7. Transfer to prepared bottles and seal tightly. Properly stored (see page 219), the lotion will keep for up to 3 months.

Variations

You can substitute an equal amount of lime (distilled) or bergamot FCF essential oil for the grapefruit.

Substitute an equal amount of grapeseed oil for the apricot.

GREEN DYNASTY BODY OIL: In a beaker, combine hempseed, camellia seed and apricot kernel oils and prepared essential oil synergy. Stir well. Transfer to a glass or PET flip-top or pump bottle (5 oz/150 mL) sprayed with 70% ethyl alcohol.

HOW TO USE

Apply to clean, dry skin after showering or bathing. Massage about 2 tsp (10 mL) into skin, all over body, until completely absorbed.

Emerald Dynasty Body Lotion

This body lotion contains superior hydrating carrier oils and ingredients that will provide long-lasting moisture. It will keep the skin moist and soft for lengthy periods throughout the day and night.

SKIN TYPE

All, especially combination skin and sensitive skin prone to psoriasis and eczema

WHEN TO USE

As needed

Makes about 26 oz (775 mL)

TIPS

Always start the mixer at a low speed. Mix patiently, without stopping, so the wax and oils do not cool off before they are emulsified, which can cause separation of the components.

When cleaning utensils and equipment, always wipe them down with dry paper towels before rinsing. This will prevent clogged drains and scum accumulating in the sink.

- Small beaker
- Glass stir stick
- 4 glass flip-top or pump bottles (7 oz/200 mL) sprayed with 70% ethyl alcohol (see Tips, right)

ESSENTIAL OIL SYNERGY

5 drops (0.25 mL)	lime (distilled) EO
5 drops (0.25 mL)	helichrysum EO
1 drop	peppermint EO
1 drop	myrrh EO

BASE

2 cups (500 mL)	warm (86°F/30°C) filtered water
20 drops (1 mL)	Earthy Antimicrobial Synergy (page 38)
20 drops (1 mL)	green tea infusion in glycerin
10 drops (0.5 mL)	bamboo extract
¼ cup (60 mL)	emulsifying wax NF
2 tbsp (30 mL)	shea butter
¾ cup (175 mL)	camellia seed oil
1 tsp (5 mL)	hempseed oil
1 tsp (5 mL)	avocado oil

1. *Essential Oil Synergy:* In beaker, combine lime, helichrysum, peppermint and myrrh essential oils. Cover with foil or plastic wrap and set aside.
2. In a bowl, combine warm water, antimicrobial synergy, green tea infusion and bamboo extract. Set aside.
3. Set a heatproof glass bowl over a saucepan of hot (not boiling) water (86°F/30°C) and heat until warm to the touch. Add emulsifying wax and let melt completely. Add shea butter and let melt completely.

TIP
. . . .

This formulation makes a large quantity. Store extra portions in the fridge for up to 3 months, until ready to use.

KNOW THE BENEFITS
. . . .

The combination of camellia, hempseed and avocado oils provides a lovely moisturizing base for dry skin. Helichrysum and myrrh essential oils repair scar tissue, while peppermint and lime provide a fresh, clean scent.

4. Meanwhile, in another bowl, combine camellia seed, hempseed and avocado oils. Stir until well mixed. Add to melted wax mixture and stir to combine. Remove bowl from heat.
5. Using electric mixer at low speed, gradually add prepared antimicrobial synergy mixture. Continue to mix until emulsified (thick and creamy), 5 to 10 minutes.
6. Add prepared synergy blend and mix until completely incorporated.
7. Transfer to prepared bottles and seal tightly. Properly stored (see page 219), the lotion will keep for up to 3 months.

Variation
EMERALD DYNASTY BODY OIL: In a beaker, combine camellia seed, hempseed and avocado oils and prepared essential oil synergy. Stir well. Transfer to a glass or PET flip-top or pump bottle (7 oz/200 mL) sprayed with 70% ethyl alcohol.

HOW TO USE
Apply to clean, dry skin after showering or bathing. Massage about 2 tsp (10 mL) into skin, all over body, until completely absorbed.

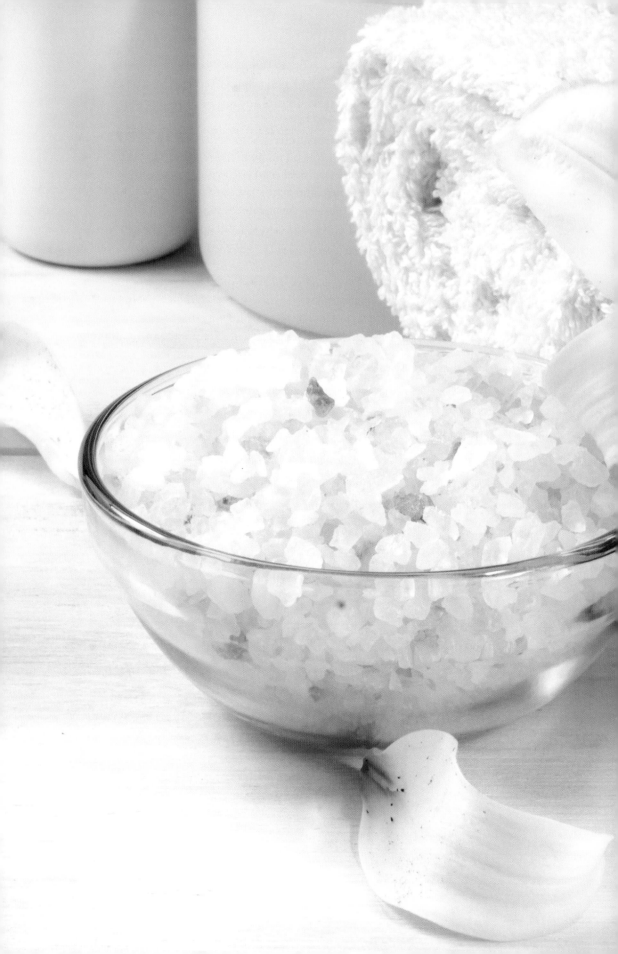

Bath Products and Deodorants

Taking a bath provides the opportunity to enjoy a simple retreat in the comfort of your own home. Bathing is more than a luxurious treatment; it offers wonderful benefits not only for your skin but also for your mind and body. Using essential oils, salts and vinegars in your bath encourages relaxation, healing and rejuvenation for both your body and your mind.

Most commercial antiperspirants and deodorants contain harmful chemicals. Using a natural deodorant helps to prevent toxic ingredients from entering the body.

Bath Products

Deodorants

Himalayan Salt Bath

Bathing is a luxurious way to cleanse. Your body heats up and your skin begins to clean and deodorize through the process of elimination.

SKIN TYPE

All

WHEN TO USE

Evening, or when following a dietary detox program

Makes 3 cups (750 mL)

TIP

See Tips for Taking a Bath, page 337.

KNOW THE BENEFITS

Himalayan salt contains a range of minerals and especially high levels of iron, which is what gives the salt its pink color. The trace minerals found in it are detoxifying and provide penetrating warmth to the skin, opening the pores and relaxing the muscles. Baking soda softens the water, creating a more alkaline medium for bathing. Palmarosa essential oil contributes antifungal and deodorizing properties, and patchouli and juniper berry are both anti-inflammatory.

- Small beaker
- Glass stir stick
- Resealable glass jar (1 quart/1 L) sprayed with 70% ethyl alcohol

ESSENTIAL OIL SYNERGY

5 drops (0.25 mL)	palmarosa EO
10 drops (0.5 mL)	juniper berry EO
10 drops (0.5 mL)	patchouli EO

BASE

1 cup (250 mL)	Himalayan pink salt crystals
2 tbsp (30 mL)	baking soda
2 cups (500 mL)	warm (86°F/30°C) filtered water

1. *Essential Oil Synergy:* In beaker, combine palmarosa, juniper berry and patchouli essential oils. Cover with foil or plastic wrap and set aside.
2. *Base:* In jar, combine Himalayan salt and baking soda.
3. Add prepared synergy blend and stir until combined. Add filtered water and stir well. Cover and set aside for 24 hours before using (the salt will dissolve, creating a deodorizing brine). Properly stored (see page 219), the mixture will keep for up to 3 months.

Variation

FOR SENSITIVE SKIN: Substitute 5 drops (0.25 mL) lavender EO and 10 drops (0.5 mL) juniper berry EO for the essential oil synergy. Omit the baking soda, which may irritate sensitive skin. Prepare as directed.

HOW TO USE BATH FORMULATIONS

Fill tub with warm water, sprinkling in 1 cup (250 mL) bath mixture while water is running. Agitate water to disperse. Soak for at least 20 minutes.

Skin Repair Bath

Bathing is a form of hydrotherapy that helps warm your body and dilate the pores. When your skin is dry, itchy or inflamed, soaking in a warm bath with essential oils and salt provides overall relief and helps to tone the skin.

SKIN TYPE

All, especially acne-prone

WHEN TO USE

Evening, or when following a dietary detox program

Makes 5 cups (1.2 L)

TIP

See "Bathing While Detoxing," page 340.

KNOW THE BENEFITS

Turmeric helps to unclog pores as well as heal wounds; it is an effective treatment for acne and scarring. Helichrysum essential oil has anti-inflammatory properties and helps to repair scar tissue. Lime essential oil has an uplifting scent. Tea tree essential oil is antimicrobial and promotes circulation.

- Small beaker
- Glass stir stick
- 2 resealable glass jars (1 pint/500 mL) sprayed with 70% ethyl alcohol

ESSENTIAL OIL SYNERGY

5 drops (0.25 mL)	helichrysum EO
10 drops (0.5 mL)	lime (distilled) EO
5 drops (0.25 mL)	tea tree EO

BASE

1 cup (250 mL)	Himalayan pink salt crystals
¼ tsp (1 L)	ground turmeric
4 cups (1 L)	filtered water

1. *Essential Oil Synergy:* In beaker, combine helichrysum, lime and tea tree essential oils. Cover with foil or plastic wrap and set aside.
2. *Base:* In a bowl, combine Himalayan salt and turmeric.
3. Complete Step 3 as for Himalayan Salt Bath (page 336).

Variation

STRESS RELIEF BATH: For a soothing bath, replace the essential oils in the recipe with 5 drops (0.25 mL) each of Roman chamomile, jasmine and ylang-ylang essential oils.

Tips for Taking a Bath

- The best time to take a bath is before resting or sleeping. All you need is 30 minutes before sleep.
- Make sure your bathtub is clean.
- Do not bathe on a full stomach.
- Drink plenty of fluids first.
- Prepare your formulations ahead of time.
- Listen to soft music.
- Have your towel and a robe ready.

Mind and Body Detox Bath

Dead Sea salt baths have been used for thousands of years to help relieve the symptoms of many different skin conditions, such as psoriasis and eczema.

SKIN TYPE

Sensitive

WHEN TO USE

As needed

**Makes 6 cups
(1.5 L)**

TIP

Dead Sea salt can be purchased at health food stores or online.

KNOW THE BENEFITS

Dead Sea salt contains the minerals, calcium, potassium, magnesium and bromine, a natural antibiotic. It moisturizes, detoxifies and softens the skin by helping to balance pH levels.

- Glass stir stick
- Resealable glass jar (1½ qt/1.5L) sprayed with 70% ethyl alcohol

5 cups (1.2 L)	hot (170°F/76°C) filtered water
2 tbsp (30 mL)	dried chamomile flowers
1 cup (250 mL)	Dead Sea salt
10 drops (0.5 mL)	Roman chamomile EO

1. In a bowl, combine hot water and dried chamomile. Set tea aside to steep for 10 minutes. Using a fine-mesh strainer, strain into prepared jar; discard solids.
2. Add Dead Sea salt and Roman chamomile essential oil and stir well. Cover and set aside for 24 hours before using (the salt will dissolve, creating a deodorizing brine).

Variation

LAVENDER MIND AND BODY DETOX BATH: To make a soothing lavender bath, substitute 2 tbsp (30 mL) dried lavender for the dried chamomile, and 10 drops (0.5 mL) lavender essential oil for the chamomile essential oil.

HOW TO USE BATH FORMULATIONS

Fill tub with warm water, sprinkling in 1 cup (250 mL) bath mixture while water is running. Agitate water to disperse mixture. Soak for at least 20 minutes.

The Benefits of Bathing

- It's relaxing and restorative. Warm water is calming and cleansing and promotes a good night's sleep.
- It calms the skin. When ingredients such as baking soda, salts and oils are added to water, they help to relieve certain skin conditions such as itchiness and dryness.
- It's detoxifying. Bathing helps the body to get rid of impurities by promoting circulation.
- It's soothing. Bathing in ingredients such as mineral salts can help to ease muscle aches and pains and reduce inflammation.

Deodorizing Vinegar Bath

Vinegar baths are an age-old remedy to relieve the body of impurities and naturally deodorize the skin.

SKIN TYPE

All

WHEN TO USE

As needed

Makes 2 cups (500 mL)

KNOW THE BENEFITS

Apple cider vinegar is high in B-complex vitamins and rich in potassium, calcium and magnesium. It nourishes the skin and balances pH levels and is especially beneficial for dry, sensitive skin. The scent of dried lavender is a nurturing tonic for the nervous system; applied topically, lavender essential oil has antiseptic and antibacterial properties. The two major components of lavender essential oil, linalool and linalyl acetate, calm the nervous system and relax the muscle tissues. Chamomile, both the herb and the essential oil, is relaxing.

- Small beaker
- Glass stir stick
- Resealable glass jar (1 pint/500 mL) sprayed with 70% ethyl alcohol

ESSENTIAL OIL SYNERGY

10 drops (0.5 mL)	lavender EO
5 drops (0.25 mL)	Roman chamomile EO

BASE

1 tbsp (15 mL)	dried lavender flowers
1 tbsp (15 mL)	dried chamomile flowers
1 cup (250 mL)	hot (170°F/76°C) filtered water
1 cup (250 mL)	apple cider vinegar

1. *Essential Oil Synergy:* In beaker, combine lavender and Roman chamomile essential oils. Cover with foil or plastic wrap and set aside.
2. *Base:* In a bowl, combine dried lavender and chamomile. Cover with hot water and set aside to steep for 10 minutes. Using a fine-mesh strainer, strain into prepared jar; discard solids.
3. Add apple cider vinegar and prepared synergy blend. Seal jar and shake to combine. Set aside for 24 hours before using to allow ingredients to synergize. Properly stored (see page 219), the bath tea will keep for up to 6 months.

Variation

Substitute 5 drops (0.25 mL) geranium essential oil for the Roman chamomile, and 1 tbsp (15 mL) dried rose petals for the chamomile flowers.

HOW TO BREW HERBAL TEAS

When brewing herbal teas, always boil the water and then let it stand for 15 minutes before using. To prevent destroying the fragile therapeutic components of herbs, never pour boiling water directly onto them.

Sweet Almond Bath Oil

Indulging in regular baths is calming and comforting.

SKIN TYPE

Dry, chapped skin

WHEN TO USE

As needed

**Makes
1 cup (250 mL)**

TIP

Blending oils at a high speed causes them to emulsify and thicken. To achieve the right consistency, you must use a blender to make this recipe. You may need to scrape down the sides with a spatula to ensure that everything is well incorporated.

- Blender
- Resealable glass jar (8 oz/250 mL) sprayed with 70% ethyl alcohol

1 cup (250 mL)	sweet almond oil
2 tbsp (30 mL)	raw honey, at room temperature
2 drops	rose otto EO

1. In clean blender, combine sweet almond oil and honey. Blend at high speed for 30 seconds, until milky and smooth (see Tip, left).
2. Add rose otto essential oil and pulse to combine.
3. Transfer to prepared jar. Seal and set aside for 24 hours to let oils synergize before using. Properly stored (see page 219), the bath oil will keep for up to 3 months.

Variation

You can also use this bath oil as a facial mask when bathing. Cleanse face and pat dry. Using your fingertips, gently apply oil all over face. Step into warm bath and leave on for 20 minutes. The warmth of the bath helps dilate the pores and allows the honey and oils to penetrate the facial skin. Rinse off with warm water.

Bathing While Detoxing

Bathing is another pathway to help your body eliminate toxins. The external contact with warm water promotes circulation throughout the body, at the same time encouraging it to relax by recruiting the parasympathetic nervous system. This "rest and digest" state allows the involuntary muscles in the digestive tract to relax and permits proper enzymatic functioning, supporting the elimination process.

The skin is the largest organ in the body. In warm bath water it responds through the involuntary nervous system and begins to relax by dilating the pores. It regulates the body's temperature by perspiring, which stimulates detoxification. Adding ingredients such as salts, honey, oils and essential oils amplifies this effect. These additions also help to deodorize the body with subtle scents derived from natural botanicals.

Moisturizing Glycerin Bath

Many people suffer from dry, cracked skin during the winter months. Bathing with humectants such as glycerin helps to keep your skin hydrated.

SKIN TYPE

Severely dry

WHEN TO USE

As needed to treat dry skin, 1 or 2 times a week during winter

Makes about 9 oz (280 mL)

TIP

Sanitization is an important part of making your own skin-care products. Always use dedicated equipment. Wash it with soap and water, then dry with paper towels. Spray with 70% ethyl alcohol, rinse thoroughly and then dry. Use immediately or store in an airtight plastic bin.

KNOW THE BENEFITS

Glycerin is a natural humectant that, when added to bathwater, softens the skin. The combination of rose and jasmine absolute is luxurious and leaves the skin feeling silky smooth.

- Small beaker
- Glass stir stick
- Blender
- Glass flip-top jar (10 oz/300 mL) sprayed with 70% ethyl alcohol

ESSENTIAL OIL SYNERGY

2 drops	rose otto EO
2 drops	jasmine absolute

BASE

1 cup (250 mL)	glycerin
2 tbsp (30 mL)	rose hydrolat

1. *Essential Oil Synergy:* In beaker, combine rose otto essential oil and jasmine absolute. Cover with foil or plastic wrap and set aside.
2. In clean blender, combine glycerin and rose hydrolat. Blend at high speed for 30 seconds, until milky and smooth (see Tip, page 340).
3. Add prepared essential oil synergy and pulse until combined.
4. Transfer to prepared jar and seal tightly. Properly stored (see page 219), the formulation will keep for up to 3 months.

Variation

Jasmine absolute is an expensive oil, as is rose otto. You can substitute 2 drops each of lavender and geranium essential oils for the rose otto and jasmine, if desired.

HOW TO USE BATH OILS

Shake well before using. Fill tub with warm water, sprinkling in ¼ cup (60 mL) of oil while water is running. Agitate water to disperse. Soak for at least 20 minutes.

Basic Deodorant

This is the basic method for making a roll-on deodorant. You can substitute your favorite essential oils to create any scent you like.

**Makes
2½ oz (90 mL)**

TIPS

Use a glass bowl with a spout to make it easier to pour the mixture into the deodorant tube.

To prevent deodorant from staining clothes, be sure to use unscented white beeswax.

When cleaning utensils and equipment, always wipe them down with dry paper towels before rinsing. This will prevent drains from getting clogged and scum from accumulating in the sink.

KNOW THE BENEFITS

Baking soda and potato starch are natural antimicrobial antiperspirants.

- Small beaker
- Glass stir stick
- Bowl-style double boiler
- Deodorant tube (3 oz/90 mL) or glass jar sprayed with 70% ethyl alcohol

ESSENTIAL OIL SYNERGY

10 drops (0.5 mL)	each lavender and geranium EO

BASE

2 tbsp (30 mL)	unscented white beeswax (see Tips, left)
4 tbsp (60 mL)	jojoba oil
2 tbsp (30 mL)	baking soda
2 tbsp (30 mL)	potato starch

1. *Essential Oil Synergy:* In beaker, combine essential oils. Cover and set aside.
2. *Base:* Set a heatproof glass bowl over a saucepan of hot, not boiling, water (86°F/30°C) and heat until warm to the touch. Add beeswax and let melt completely. Add jojoba oil and warm until mixture is perfectly clear, 1 to 2 minutes.
3. Meanwhile, in a small bowl, combine baking soda and potato starch. Add to melted wax mixture and stir well.
4. Add prepared synergy blend and stir until combined.
5. Transfer to prepared container and set aside until completely cool. Once cool, cover with lid and set aside at room temperature for 24 hours to harden. Properly stored (see page 219), the deodorant will keep for up to 1 month.

Variation

To protect sensitive skin, eliminate the baking soda and add 2 tbsp (30 mL) additional potato starch.

HOW TO USE

Apply deodorant to clean armpits after bathing. Let dry before putting on clothing.

Gel Deodorant

This is a simple way to make a refreshing gel-based deodorant. Substitute different essential oils with deodorant properties (see below) to create your preferred scent.

SKIN TYPE

All

WHEN TO USE

After shower or bath

**Makes
3 oz (90 mL)**

TIP

If desired, you can divide these mixtures between two containers. Refrigerate the extra portion until needed.

KNOW THE BENEFITS

Aloe vera is a natural antiseptic that feels light on the skin, and witch hazel is antibacterial. Baking soda and potato starch are natural antimicrobial antiperspirants. Patchouli and geranium essential oils are also antimicrobial.

- 2 beakers
- Glass stir stick
- Glass jar (4 oz/100 mL) or pump bottle sprayed with 70% ethyl alcohol

ESSENTIAL OIL SYNERGY

| 5 drops (0.25 mL) | geranium EO |
| 10 drops (0.5 mL) | patchouli EO |

BASE

¼ cup (60 mL)	aloe vera gel
1 tbsp (15 mL)	witch hazel hydrolat
1 tbsp (15 mL)	baking soda

1. *Essential Oil Synergy:* In a beaker, combine geranium and patchouli essential oils. Cover with foil or plastic wrap and set aside.
2. *Base:* In second beaker, combine aloe vera gel and witch hazel hydrolat. Add baking soda and stir until completely dissolved.
3. Add prepared synergy blend and mix until combined.
4. Transfer to prepared container and set aside until set. Cover with lid and set aside at room temperature for 24 hours to gel. Properly stored (see page 219), the deodorant will keep for up to 3 months.

Variation

Substitute an equal quantity of lavender essential oil for the geranium.

Essential Oils for Deodorants

- geranium
- palmarosa
- petitgrain
- patchouli
- neroli
- lavender
- rose otto

Sensitive Skin Deodorant

This is a simple method for making your own gentle deodorant.

Makes about 3 oz (90 mL)

TIPS

Use a glass bowl with a spout to make it easier to pour the mixture into the deodorant tube.

KNOW THE BENEFITS

Cornstarch and arrowroot powder are natural antiperspirants with a soothing powder feel that absorb moisture. Neroli essential oil is gentle, deodorizing and antimicrobial.

- Bowl-style double boiler
- Glass stir stick
- Deodorant tube (4 oz/100 mL) sprayed with 70% ethyl alcohol

¼ cup (60 mL)	extra virgin coconut oil
1 tbsp (15 mL)	cornstarch
1 tbsp (15 mL)	arrowroot powder
10 drops (0.5 mL)	neroli EO

1. Set a heatproof glass bowl over a saucepan of hot, not boiling, water (86°F/30°C) and heat until warm to the touch. Add coconut oil and let melt completely. Remove from heat and let cool slightly.
2. Meanwhile, in a small bowl, combine cornstarch and arrowroot powder. Add to melted oil mixture and stir until well combined.
3. Add neroli essential oil and stir until combined.
4. Transfer to prepared deodorant bottle and set aside until completely cool. Once cool, cover with lid and set aside at room temperature for 24 hours to firm up. Properly stored (see page 219), the deodorant will keep for up to 3 months.

Variation

To make a powder deodorant: In a bowl, combine 1 tbsp (15 mL) cornstarch, 1 tbsp (15 mL) arrowroot powder and 10 drops (0.5 mL) neroli essential oil. Transfer to a 1 oz (30 mL) glass or PET jar. Close lid and shake well. Dab this powder formulation on clean skin.

Deodorant Packaging

Most people prefer the convenience of a roll-on or stick deodorant. However, if you do not include broad-based preservatives such as parabens — normally used in cosmeceuticals — and you are using a roll-on type applicator, there is a risk that your deodorant will become contaminated, simply through repeated contact with bacteria naturally found on your skin. As an alternative to a roll-on applicator, I recommend decanting the formulation into a glass pump bottle or jar and applying the deodorant with a clean spatula or wooden cosmetic stick.

Gentle Deodorant Body Mist

This gentle deodorant provides a lovely rose scent throughout the day.

TIP
....
If desired, you can divide this mixture between two bottles. Refrigerate extra portions until needed.

KNOW THE BENEFITS
....
Aloe vera is a natural antiseptic that feels light on the skin, and witch hazel is antibacterial. Rose otto essential oil is deodorizing and cooling, with a relaxing scent.

- Small beaker
- Glass stir stick
- Glass spray bottle (4 oz/125 mL) sprayed with 70% ethyl alcohol (see Tip, left)

1 tbsp (15 mL)	aloe vera gel
¼ cup (60 mL)	rose hydrolat
2 tbsp (30 mL)	witch hazel hydrolat
5 drops (0.25 mL)	rose otto EO

1. In beaker, combine aloe vera gel, rose hydrolat and witch hazel hydrolat.
2. Add prepared rose otto essential oil and stir until combined.
3. Transfer to prepared bottle and seal tightly. Properly stored (see page 219), the deodorant will keep for up to 3 months.

Variation
For a lovely rose-scented deodorizing bath, add 2 tbsp (30 mL) of this formula to warm bathwater and agitate to disperse well.

HOW TO USE
Apply to clean armpits. Let dry before putting on clothing.

Preventing Body Odor Naturally

- Shower or bathe daily, using products that contain deodorizing essential oils (see page 343).
- Remove hair from underneath your arms.
- Drink plenty of water: 6 to 8 glasses daily helps the body cleanse itself.

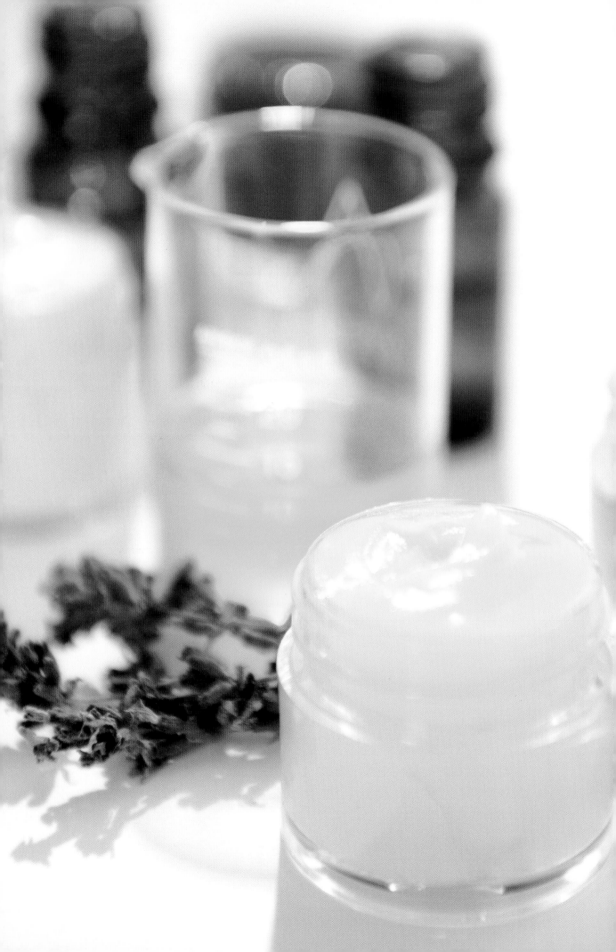

Products for Mothers and Mothers-to-Be

Having a baby is truly one of nature's miracles. During the nine months of gestation your body undergoes substantial hormonal and physiological changes. Some women may experience hyperpigmentation, stretch marks or itchy rashes, which require special care.

Since some topical ingredients, especially essential oils, are absorbed through the skin, women who are pregnant or breastfeeding need to be particularly cautious about the ingredients in their skin-care products. It is important to listen to your body and know what is best for you.

When it comes to pregnancy, it's best to keep the following in mind:

- Eliminate the excess. Reduce your use of products that may contain harmful chemicals and fragrances.
- Less is better. Do not overload your body with too much of a good thing. This is particularly true when it comes to fragrances, as pregnant women often have a heightened sense of smell.
- Let nature take its course. Pregnancy is a natural process. Most pregnancy-related dermatological conditions are temporary and will disappear soon after giving birth.

Citrus Deodorant

During pregnancy and breastfeeding, you not only experience a heightened sense of smell but your body gives off a stronger odor. This is caused by heightened hormone levels and increased weight (which increases body heat and sweating). It's also important to remember that mother and baby bond through touch and smell. Deodorants should be gentle and noninvasive.

SKIN TYPE

All

WHEN TO USE

After bath or shower

**Makes
3 oz (90 mL)**

TIP

See "Deodorant Packaging," page 344.

KNOW THE BENEFITS

Cornstarch and arrowroot powder are scent-free and absorb moisture, making them a wonderful foundation for deodorants. Citrus essential oils are naturally deodorizing.

- Bowl-style double boiler
- Glass stir stick
- 2 deodorant bottles or jars (1 oz/30 mL) sprayed with 70% ethyl alcohol

¼ cup (60 mL)	extra virgin coconut oil
1 tbsp (15 mL)	cornstarch
1 tbsp (15 mL)	arrowroot powder
5 drops (0.25 mL)	mandarin EO

1. Set a heatproof glass bowl over a saucepan of hot, not boiling, water (86°F/30°C) and heat until warm to the touch. Add coconut oil and let melt completely.
2. Meanwhile, in a small bowl, combine cornstarch and arrowroot powder. Add to melted coconut oil and stir until mixture is completely smooth. Remove from heat and let cool slightly.
3. Add mandarin essential oil and stir until combined.
4. Transfer to prepared containers and set aside until completely cool. Once cool, cover with lids and set aside at room temperature for 24 hours to solidify. Properly stored (see page 219), the deodorant will keep for up to 1 month.

Variation

CITRUS DEODORIZING POWDER: Omit the coconut oil. In a 2 oz (50 mL) glass jar, combine cornstarch and arrowroot powder. Add mandarin essential oil, seal and shake well. Use a wooden spoon to scoop the powder onto your fingertips (to avoid cross-contamination) and pat onto clean armpits.

HOW TO USE

Apply to clean armpits after bathing. Let dry before putting on clothing.

Jojoba Body Balm

Stretch marks are a natural occurrence during pregnancy. The body is changing at a fast pace, causing your skin to stretch and leaving marks. Keeping your skin hydrated with oils and balms can help to prevent or lessen stretch marks.

SKIN TYPE

All

WHEN TO USE

After shower or bath

Makes about 7 oz (200 mL)

TIP

Substitute an equal quantity of lemon or mandarin essential oil for the lavender.

KNOW THE BENEFITS

Always use scent-free emulsifiers and butters during pregnancy. Not only do they help offset the effects of a heightened sense of smell, they also result in a gentle, clean fragrance and refreshing product. This lovely body balm is especially emollient, thanks to the beeswax and jojoba oil. Evening primrose oil, vitamin E oil and lavender essential oil all have antioxidant effects.

- Bowl-style double boiler
- Glass stir stick
- Glass or PET jar (7 oz/200 mL) sprayed with 70% ethyl alcohol

2 tbsp (30 mL)	unscented white beeswax
2 tbsp (30 mL)	extra virgin coconut oil
½ cup (125 mL)	jojoba oil
1 tsp (5 mL)	evening primrose oil
10 drops (0.5 mL)	vitamin E oil
5 drops (0.25 mL)	lavender EO

1. Set a heatproof glass bowl over a saucepan of hot (not boiling) water (86°F/30°C) and heat until warm to the touch. Add beeswax and let melt completely. Add coconut oil and heat, stirring occasionally, until melted.
2. Stir in jojoba and evening primrose oils and vitamin E oil. Remove bowl from heat and mix with an electric mixer for 10 minutes.
3. Add lavender essential oil and stir until combined.
4. Transfer to prepared jar and seal tightly. Properly stored (see page 219), the body balm will keep for up to 3 months.

Variation

Substitute an equal amount of natural shea butter for the coconut oil, if desired.

HOW TO USE

After bathing or showering, towel dry. Massage 1 tsp (5 mL) body balm all over skin until completely absorbed.

Neroli Body Oil

Be kind to your skin during pregnancy. Applying emollients to dry, flaky skin can help you feel more comfortable.

SKIN TYPE

All

WHEN TO USE

After showering

**Makes
4 oz (120 mL)**

TIP

When cleaning utensils and equipment, always wipe them down with dry paper towels before rinsing. This will prevent clogged drains and scum accumulating in the sink.

KNOW THE BENEFITS

This gentle serum contains naturally high levels of vitamin E and leaves the skin feeling soft and beautiful. The subtle scent of neroli will calm mother's and baby's nervous systems during breastfeeding.

- Small beaker
- Glass stir stick
- Glass or PET pump bottle (4 oz/120 mL) sprayed with 70% ethyl alcohol

¼ cup (60 mL)	argan oil
¼ cup (60 mL)	apricot kernel oil
10 drops (0.5 mL)	vitamin E oil
2 drops	neroli EO

1. In beaker, combine argan and apricot kernel oils. Add vitamin E oil and stir to combine.
2. Add neroli essential oil and stir until combined.
3. Transfer to prepared bottle and seal tightly. Properly stored (see page 219), the oil will keep for up to 8 months.

Variation

Substitute an equal amount of mandarin essential oil for the neroli.

HOW TO USE

Apply to either wet or dry skin after showering or bathing. Gently massage about 1 tbsp (15 mL) oil all over your body until it is completely absorbed. Avoid the breasts if you are breastfeeding.

Facial Emollient Serum

Keeping things simple is key during pregnancy and breastfeeding. This formulation contains two gentle yet powerful oils, jojoba and argan, to moisturize and nurture the skin.

SKIN TYPE
All

WHEN TO USE
Morning and evening

Makes about 6 oz (190 mL)

TIP

This formulation makes a large quantity. For day-to-day use, decant into a smaller bottle (2 oz/50 mL). Store the remainder in the refrigerator until ready to use.

KNOW THE BENEFITS

Both argan oil and jojoba oil are rich in vitamin E, which has been found to improve the elasticity of skin as well as to moisturize and soften it. Neroli essential oil has a soft, calming and soothing scent and is slightly antibacterial.

- Small beaker
- Glass stir stick
- Glass or PET flip-top or pump bottle (7 oz/200 mL) sprayed with 70% ethyl alcohol (see Tip, left)

¾ cup (175 mL)	jojoba oil
1 tbsp (15 mL)	argan oil
1 drop	neroli EO

1. In beaker, combine jojoba and argan oils.
2. Add neroli essential oil and stir until well combined.
3. Transfer to prepared bottle and seal tightly. Properly stored (see page 219), the serum will keep for up to 8 months.

HOW TO USE

Apply after thoroughly cleansing the skin. Apply 2 to 3 drops of serum to fingertips and gently pat onto forehead, cheeks and chin. Gently massage into skin.

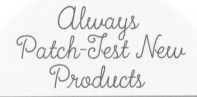

Always Patch-Test New Products

No matter what your normal skin type, your body goes through so many changes during pregnancy that you should always do a patch test before using any product. Apply a bit of the product to the inside of your forearm and wait at least 15 to 20 minutes. If any irritation or redness occurs, do not use the product.

Facial Emollient Gel

This gel helps to balance your skin's pH and prevent it from drying. It will also help minimize blemishes.

SKIN TYPE

All

WHEN TO USE

Morning and evening

Makes about 1 oz (40 mL)

TIP

Overexposure to the sun during pregnancy may cause hyperpigmentation. During the gestation period it is recommended to avoid unnecessary sun exposure.

KNOW THE BENEFITS

Both argan oil and jojoba oil are rich in vitamin E, which has been found to improve the elasticity of skin as well as to moisturize and soften it. Neroli has a soft, calming and soothing scent and is slightly antibacterial.

- Small beaker
- Glass stir stick
- Glass flip-top or pump bottle (2 oz/40 mL) sprayed with 70% ethyl alcohol

2 tbsp (30 mL)	aloe vera gel
1 tsp (5 mL)	jojoba oil
1 tsp (5 mL)	argan oil
1 drop	neroli EO

1. Place aloe vera gel in a small bowl and set aside.
2. In beaker, combine jojoba and argan oils. Add to aloe vera and stir until mixture is emulsified.
3. Add neroli essential oil and stir until well combined.
4. Transfer to prepared bottle and seal tightly. Properly stored (see page 219), the gel will keep for up to 3 months.

Variation

Substitute an equal amount of sunflower oil (page 314) for the argan.

HOW TO USE

After thoroughly cleansing and drying the skin, apply small dollops to forehead, cheeks and chin. Gently massage into skin.

Glowing Mommy Lip Balm

Dry lips are very common during pregnancy and could be an indication that you are not hydrated enough. Dry lips during labor is also very common because of the deep breathing involved. One of the most important items to put in your hospital bag is a lip balm to help moisturize your lips during labor.

SKIN TYPE

All

WHEN TO USE

As needed

Makes 3½ oz (105 mL)

TIP

When cleaning utensils and equipment, always wipe them down with dry paper towels before rinsing. This will prevent clogged drains and scum accumulating in the sink.

KNOW THE BENEFITS

Beeswax and cocoa butter form a protective barrier for the skin while softening and soothing lips.

- Bowl-style double boiler
- Small beaker
- Glass stir stick
- 10 lip balm tubes sprayed with 70% ethyl alcohol

2 tbsp (30 mL)	unscented white beeswax
2 tbsp (30 mL)	cocoa butter
2 tbsp (30 mL)	calendula–infused oil
1 tbsp (15 mL)	jojoba oil
2 drops	lime (distilled) EO

1. Set a heatproof glass measuring cup (with spout) over a saucepan of hot, not boiling water (86°F/30°C) and heat until warm to the touch. Add beeswax and let it melt completely. Add cocoa butter and warm until mixture is perfectly clear, 1 to 2 minutes.
2. Meanwhile, in a bowl, combine calendula–infused and jojoba oils. Add to melted wax mixture and stir until well combined. Remove bowl from heat.
3. Add lime essential oil and stir until combined.
4. Immediately pour into prepared lip balm tubes and set aside until set, about 20 minutes. Once the mixture has set, cap the tubes. Properly stored (see page 219), the balm will keep for up to 6 months.

Variation

In equal amounts, substitute shea butter for the beeswax and mandarin essential oil for the lime.

HOW TO USE

Apply to lips 2 to 3 times a day.

Pure and Simple Acne Mask

Acne is a common problem during pregnancy and is caused by fluctuating hormones. Avoiding harsh chemicals is even more of a priority at this time. White clay is cleansing and draws out impurities; it also helps reduce inflammation.

SKIN TYPE

All

WHEN TO USE

Evening

Makes 3½ oz (105 mL)

TIP

If the mask dries up in its container, stir in water, 1 tbsp (15 mL) at a time, until the desired consistency is reached.

KNOW THE BENEFITS

Kaolin clay is rich in minerals and nourishes the skin, improving its overall appearance. Jojoba oil provides moisture and helps treat inflammation. German chamomile essential oil reduces redness and inflammation, and tea tree essential oil is antibacterial.

- Small beaker
- Glass stir stick
- Glass jar (4 oz/125 mL) sprayed with 70% ethyl alcohol (see page 219)

¼ cup (60 mL)	kaolin clay
¼ cup (60 mL)	warm (86°F/30°C) filtered water
1 tsp (5 mL)	jojoba oil
1 drop	German chamomile EO
1 drop	tea tree EO

1. Place clay in a bowl. While stirring, gradually pour in warm water. Stir until smooth and shiny. If mixture seems too dry, add water, ½ tsp (5 mL) at a time, until desired texture is reached.
2. In beaker, combine jojoba oil and German chamomile and tea tree essential oils. Add to wet clay and stir until well combined.
3. Transfer to prepared jar and seal tightly. Properly stored (see page 219), the mask will keep for up to 2 months.

Variation

Substitute an equal amount of sandalwood for the German chamomile EO.

HOW TO USE

Wash and dry face. Using fingertips, massage about ½ tsp (2 mL) mixture all over face and leave to dry for 10 to 12 minutes. Remove with warm water and a cloth or sponge. Follow with Pure and Simple Acne Gel (page 355).

Alternatively, use the mask as a spot treatment. Apply to spots and leave to dry for 30 minutes. Remove with warm water and a cloth or sponge. Follow with Pure and Simple Acne Gel.

Pure and Simple Acne Gel

Acne is a common problem during pregnancy and is caused by fluctuating hormones. Avoiding harsh chemicals is even more of a priority at this time.

SKIN TYPE

All

WHEN TO USE

As needed

Makes about 4 oz (125 mL)

TIP

When cleaning utensils and equipment, always wipe them down with dry paper towels before rinsing. This will prevent clogged drains and scum accumulating in the sink.

KNOW THE BENEFITS

The combination of German chamomile and tea tree essential oils and jojoba oil reduces inflammation. Aloe vera helps to restore moisture to dry skin.

- Small beaker
- Glass stir stick
- Glass jar (4 oz/125 mL) sprayed with 70% ethyl alcohol (see page 219)

ESSENTIAL OIL SYNERGY

1 drop	German chamomile EO
1 drop	tea tree EO

BASE

2 tbsp (30 mL)	aloe vera gel
1 tsp (5 mL)	jojoba oil

1. *Essential Oil Synergy:* In beaker, combine German chamomile and tea tree essential oils. Cover with foil or plastic wrap and set aside.
2. *Base:* Place aloe vera gel in a bowl. Add jojoba oil and stir until emulsified.
3. Add prepared synergy blend and stir until combined.
4. Transfer to prepared jar and seal tightly. Properly stored (see page 219), the gel will keep for up to 2 months.

Variation

Substitute an equal amount of argan oil for the jojoba.

HOW TO USE

Cleanse skin. Dab gel onto acne spots and let dry. Follow with Facial Emollient Serum (page 351) when needed.

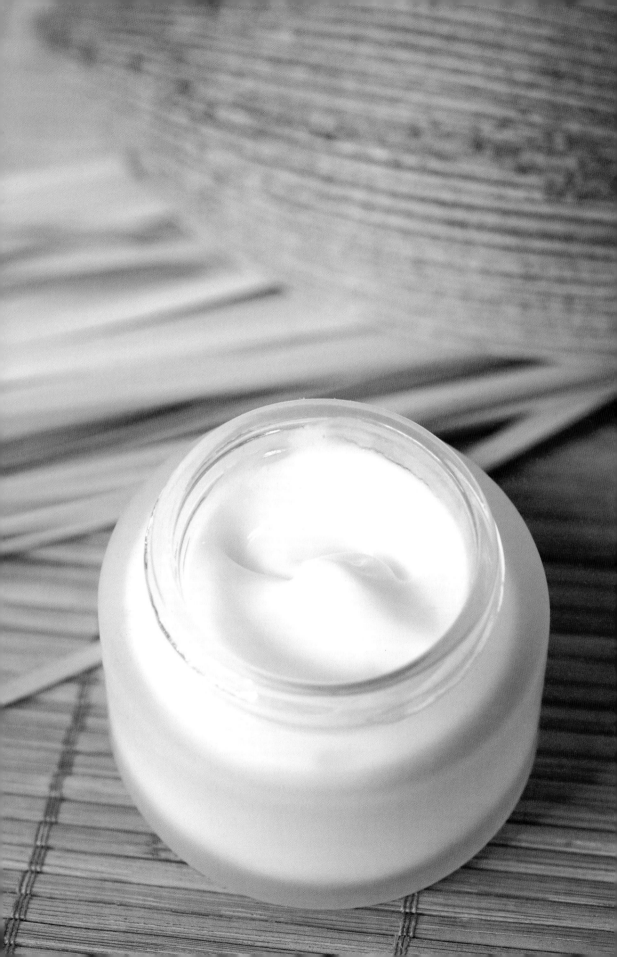

Personal Care
Products for Him

In ancient civilizations, both men and women used scented oils and ointments to cleanse, soften, deodorize and heal the body. But at some point, male grooming became a neglected area of personal care products.

Men do have different skin-care needs. For example, after puberty, their skin produces higher levels of sebum. Men's naturally higher level of androgen hormones (testosterone) results in thicker skin, with a rougher appearance. Men's skin also contains higher levels of collagen, which until the age of 50 delays the appearance of fine lines and wrinkles.

In 2013 the New York State Department of Health and Columbia University's Department of Environmental Health Sciences studied the effects of personal care products on men. They discovered that parabens — known to be harmful to health — were being absorbed through the skin. The World Health Organization has similarly reported that endocrine disruptors in the air and the environment are adversely affecting semen quality. A tailored approach to natural personal care products for men not only supports hygiene but also health and well-being.

Aromatic Sports Bath

Studies conducted by the University of Tokyo in 2014 suggest that post-exercise bathing helps the body repair itself and also improves endurance, especially in older individuals and those who have experienced injuries.

SKIN TYPE

All

WHEN TO USE

1 hour after workout

Makes ⅔ cup (155 mL)

TIPS

This recipe can easily be tripled and stored in a glass jar for up to 3 months.

When cleaning utensils and equipment, always wipe them down with dry paper towels before rinsing. This will prevent clogged drains and scum accumulating in the sink.

KNOW THE BENEFITS

Epsom salts are rich in magnesium. When dissolved in warm water, they help the body to detox and muscles to relax. Rosemary and grapefruit essential oils are warming and uplifting. Lavender essential oil is calming and helps to release tension.

- Small beaker

3 drops	rosemary EO
2 drops	grapefruit EO (see Sensitivity Alert, page 275)
10 drops (0.5 mL)	lavender EO
2 tbsp (30 mL)	hempseed oil
½ cup (125 mL)	Epsom salts

1. In beaker, combine rosemary, grapefruit and lavender essential oils and hempseed oil.
2. Place Epsom salts in a bowl and add prepared blend. Mix well.

Variation

SPORTS MASSAGE OIL: Make the oil blend, transfer to a small bottle (1 oz/30 mL) and seal. Massage into muscles after exercise or other physical activity. Properly stored (see page 219), the mixture will keep for up to 3 months.

HOW TO USE

Fill tub with warm water, sprinkling in bath salts while water is running. Agitate water to dissolve mixture. Soak for at least 20 minutes.

Aroma Dry-Brushing Mist

Dry-brushing stimulates the body, leaving you feeling rejuvenated. It also detoxifies by removing dead skin cells. Lightly spray this mist onto your brush before you begin, enhancing the experience with the refreshing fragrance of the great outdoors.

SKIN TYPE

All

WHEN TO USE

Morning

Makes 4 oz (120 mL)

TIP

This spray can also be used as an aftershave face mist or as a refreshing body spray after a bath or shower.

KNOW THE BENEFITS

Pine essential oil is known for its antiseptic and antibacterial properties. Both basil and geranium essential oils are disinfectants and stimulants that support the body's immune system. Lavender hydrolat is calming and soothing.

- 2 small beakers
- Natural-bristle body brush
- Glass spray bottle (4 oz/120 mL) sprayed with 70% ethyl alcohol (see page 219)

ESSENTIAL OIL SYNERGY

5 drops (0.25 mL)	pine EO
5 drops (0.25 mL)	sweet basil EO
5 drops (0.25 mL)	geranium EO

BASE

¼ cup (60 mL)	lavender hydrolat
¼ cup (60 mL)	warm (86°F/30°C) filtered water

1. *Essential Oil Synergy:* In a beaker, combine pine, sweet basil and geranium essential oils. Cover with foil or plastic wrap and set aside.
2. *Base:* In second beaker, combine lavender hydrolat and water. Stir well.
3. Add prepared synergy blend and stir to combine. Transfer to prepared spray bottle. Properly stored (see page 219), the spray will keep for up to 3 months.

HOW TO USE

Lightly spray dry brush with mist. Brush body in circular movements, starting at the calves and slowly moving upward, for about 5 minutes.

Aroma Shower Oil

This oil works as a decadent moisturizing cleanser, thanks to the power of omega-rich almond and hempseed oils. The essential oil synergy of patchouli, neroli and peppermint will leave you feeling uplifted.

SKIN TYPE

All

WHEN TO USE

Morning or evening

Makes about 9 oz (235 mL)

TIP

You can use this oil as a gentle aftershave. Simply massage 4 to 5 drops all over face until absorbed.

KNOW THE BENEFITS

Almond oil is deeply moisturizing, while hempseed oil is exceptionally rich and high in omega essential fatty acids. The combination of these two oils nourishes dry skin. Patchouli essential oil is anti-inflammatory and helps improve the appearance of scaly skin. Neroli and peppermint essential oils will leave you feeling invigorated.

- Small beaker
- Large beaker
- Glass bottle (9 oz/250 mL) sprayed with 70% ethyl alcohol (see page 219)

ESSENTIAL OIL SYNERGY

10 drops (0.5 mL)	patchouli EO
5 drops (0.25 mL)	neroli EO
5 drops (0.25 mL)	peppermint EO

BASE

¾ cup (175 mL)	sweet almond oil
¼ cup (60 mL)	hempseed oil

1. *Essential Oil Synergy:* In small beaker, combine patchouli, neroli and peppermint essential oils. Cover with foil or plastic wrap and set aside
2. *Base:* In larger beaker, combine sweet almond and hempseed oils. Stir well.
3. Add prepared synergy blend and whisk to combine. Transfer to prepared bottle and seal tightly. Properly stored (see page 219), the oil will keep for up to 6 months.

Variation

Substitute an equal amount of borage oil for the hempseed oil, if desired.

HOW TO USE

Use in the shower. Apply 1 to 2 tbsp (15 to 30 mL) to wet skin and massage all over body. Rinse thoroughly and towel dry.

After-Shower Body Spray

Physical activity and exposure to cold weather can lead to dry, chapped skin. This spray is deeply moisturizing and formulated especially for men.

Makes about 4 oz (125 mL)

KNOW THE BENEFITS

This spray contains a blend of nourishing and soothing oils. Hempseed, arnica-infused and jojoba oils are deeply moisturizing, thanks to their high levels of unique fatty acids. They also have anti-inflammatory properties and can help to relieve muscle tension due to intense physical activity. The combination of mandarin, rosemary, ginger and neroli essential oils has a pleasing masculine aroma and antiseptic and antibacterial properties.

- Small beaker
- Atomizer bottle (4 oz/125 mL) sprayed with 70% ethyl alcohol (see page 219)

ESSENTIAL OIL SYNERGY

20 drops (1 mL)	mandarin EO
5 drops (0.25 mL)	rosemary EO
5 drops (0.25 mL)	ginger EO
5 drops (0.25 mL)	neroli EO

BASE

1/4 cup (60 mL)	hempseed oil
1/4 cup (60 mL)	jojoba oil
1/4 cup (60 mL)	caprylic or capric acid
1/4 cup (60 mL)	arnica-infused oil

1. *Essential Oil Synergy:* In beaker, combine mandarin, rosemary, ginger and neroli essential oils. Cover with foil or plastic wrap and set aside.
2. Pour hempseed, jojoba and caprylic and arnica-infused oils into prepared bottle. Add prepared synergy blend and seal bottle. Gently roll bottle between the palms of your hands to combine the oils.
3. Properly stored (see page 219), the spray will keep for up to 6 months.

Variation

CALMING AFTER-SHOWER BODY SPRAY: Replace the essential oil synergy blend with 20 drops (1 mL) bergamot EO, 5 drops (0.25 mL) Australian sandalwood EO, 5 drops (0.25 mL) sweet marjoram EO and 5 drops (0.25 mL) jasmine absolute.

HOW TO USE

After shower or sauna, spray onto body, focusing on the calves and shoulders. Or massage into skin before a shower or sauna.

Invigorating Liquid Soap and Shampoo

The essential oils in this simple soap/shampoo blend are activated in a hot shower. In conjunction with steam, the essential oil synergy helps to decongest nasal passages and will leave you feeling refreshed.

SKIN TYPE

All

WHEN TO USE

Morning or evening

Makes about 4 oz (125 mL)

TIP

When cleaning utensils and equipment, always wipe them down with dry paper towels before rinsing. This will prevent clogged drains and scum accumulating in the sink.

KNOW THE BENEFITS

Sodium laurel sulfate (SLS)–free soap or shampoo base can be used on its own as a liquid body soap. The essential oil synergy adds benefits. It is antiseptic and antibacterial and, when combined with steam, acts as a decongestant — a great way to start the day during flu season.

- Small beaker
- Electric mixer
- Glass flip-top or pump bottle (5 oz/125 mL) sprayed with 70% ethyl alcohol (see Tips, page 219)

20 drops (1 mL)	mandarin EO
5 drops (0.25 mL)	rosemary EO
5 drops (0.25 mL)	ginger EO
5 drops (0.25 mL)	neroli EO
½ cup (125 mL)	sodium laurel sulfate (SLS)–free soap or shampoo

1. In beaker, combine mandarin, rosemary, ginger and neroli essential oils. Cover with foil or plastic wrap and set aside.
2. Place SLS-free soap in a bowl. Add prepared essential oil synergy and, using electric mixer, mix until well incorporated.
3. Transfer to prepared bottle and seal tightly. Properly stored (see page 219), the soap will keep for up to 12 months.

Variation

CALMING SOAP AND SHAMPOO: Replace the essential oil synergy blend with 20 drops (1 mL) bergamot EO, 5 drops (0.25 mL) Australian sandalwood EO, 5 drops (0.25 mL) sweet marjoram EO and 5 drops (0.25 mL) jasmine absolute.

HOW TO USE

Use in the shower. Apply 1 tbsp (15 mL) to a wet loofah or washcloth and massage all over body. Rinse thoroughly and towel dry. Follow with After-Shower Body Spray (page 361).

Anti-Dandruff Massage Oil

Scalp and facial massage can boost energy levels, ease aches and pains and release tension. Adding antibacterial and invigorating essential oils helps to treat dandruff and also nourishes the scalp, facial skin and hair.

SKIN TYPE

All, especially oily or dry skin

WHEN TO USE

Before washing hair

Makes about 6 oz (185 mL)

TIP

When cleaning utensils and equipment, always wipe them down with dry paper towels before rinsing. This will prevent clogged drains and scum accumulating in the sink.

KNOW THE BENEFITS

When sesame seed oil is combined with jojoba oil, the result is a therapeutic emollient that is perfect for treating dandruff and symptoms related to dry scalp. The essential oil synergy is antibacterial and has a pleasing masculine scent.

- Small beaker
- Atomizer bottle (7 oz/200 mL) sprayed with 70% ethyl alcohol

ESSENTIAL OIL SYNERGY

10 drops (0.5 mL)	sandalwood (Australian) EO
5 drops (0.25 mL)	geranium EO
5 drops (0.25 mL)	patchouli EO
5 drops (0.25 mL)	sweet basil EO

BASE

½ cup (125 mL)	jojoba oil
¼ cup (60 mL)	sesame seed oil

1. *Essential Oil Synergy:* In beaker, combine sandalwood, geranium, patchouli and basil essential oils. Cover with foil or plastic wrap and set aside.
2. Pour jojoba and sesame seed oils into prepared bottle. Add prepared synergy blend and seal bottle. Gently roll bottle between the palms of your hands to combine the oils. Let sit for at least 1 hour before using, to allow oils to meld.
3. Properly stored (see page 219), the oil will keep for up to 6 months.

Variation

DANDRUFF SHAMPOO AND BODY WASH: In a beaker, combine essential oil synergy from Step 1 with ½ cup (125 mL) sodium laurel sulfate (SLS)–free soap or shampoo. Omit remaining ingredients. Transfer to a glass flip-top or pump bottle (5 oz/125 mL) sprayed with 70% ethyl alcohol.

HOW TO USE

Before going to bed, apply 8 or 9 drops of oil to scalp and, using fingers, massage over entire scalp. Leave on overnight. Wash hair in the morning with Invigorating Liquid Soap and Shampoo (page 362).

Beard Serum

Not only does beard serum keep facial hair tidy, it also moisturizes the skin underneath the beard, which can become dry or scaly and even start producing dandruff.

SKIN TYPE

All

WHEN TO USE

After shower or bath

**Makes about
4 oz (125 mL)**

TIP

When cleaning utensils and equipment, always wipe them down with dry paper towels before rinsing. This will prevent clogged drains and scum accumulating in the sink.

KNOW THE BENEFITS

Argan oil conditions and softens facial hair while providing a non-greasy shine. Camellia seed oil provides extra conditioning. Sandalwood and rose otto essential oils have classic fragrances that will ease the mind throughout the day.

- Small beaker
- Atomizer bottle (5 oz/125 mL) sprayed with 70% ethyl alcohol

ESSENTIAL OIL SYNERGY

5 drops (0.25 mL)	sandalwood (Australian) EO
5 drops (0.25 mL)	rose otto EO

BASE

¼ cup (60 mL)	argan oil
¼ cup (60 mL)	camellia seed oil
5 drops (0.25 mL)	bamboo extract

1. *Essential Oil Synergy:* In beaker, combine sandalwood and rose otto essential oils. Cover with foil or plastic wrap and set aside.
2. Pour argan and camellia seed oils and bamboo extract into prepared bottle. Add prepared synergy blend and seal bottle. Gently roll bottle between the palms of your hands to combine the oils. Let sit for at least 1 hour before using, to allow oils to meld.
3. Properly stored (see page 219), the serum will keep for up to 6 months.

Variation

Substitute equal quantities of geranium and patchouli essential oils for the sandalwood and rose.

HOW TO USE

After shower or bath, spray onto beard and comb through.

Aloe Vera Aftershave

This toner acts as an astringent to help close pores after shaving. It also protects the skin from infection caused by razor cuts or scrapes.

All (see Variation, below)

After shaving

Makes 3½ oz (105 mL)

KNOW THE BENEFITS

Aloe vera contains numerous vitamins and minerals, along with saponins that contribute to the cleansing and antiseptic effects of the gel. Witch hazel is astringent, analgesic and anti-inflammatory and reduces erythema (redness of the skin). It has also been found that lotions containing witch hazel can have an antihistamine effect. The essential oil synergy has a grounding, masculine aroma; it is antimicrobial and helps heal sun-damaged skin.

- Small beaker
- Glass jar or pump bottle (4 oz/125 mL) sprayed with 70% ethyl alcohol

ESSENTIAL OIL SYNERGY

5 drops (0.25 mL)	sandalwood (Australian) EO
5 drops (0.25 mL)	patchouli EO
5 drops (0.25 mL)	peppermint EO
5 drops (0.25 mL)	benzoin EO

BASE

¼ cup (60 mL)	green tea infusion in glycerin
2 tbsp (30 mL)	aloe vera gel
1 tbsp (15 mL)	witch hazel hydrolat

1. *Essential Oil Synergy:* In beaker, combine sandalwood, patchouli, peppermint and benzoin essential oils. Cover with foil or plastic wrap and set aside.
2. *Base:* In a bowl, whisk together green tea infusion, aloe vera gel and witch hazel hydrolat. Add prepared synergy blend and mix until combined.
3. Transfer to prepared bottle and seal tightly. Properly stored (see page 219), the gel will keep for up to 3 months.

Variation

ALOE VERA AFTERSHAVE FOR SENSITIVE SKIN: Omit the peppermint and benzoin essential oils. Add 5 drops (0.25 mL) lavender EO.

HOW TO USE

Massage a small amount (less then ¼ tsp/1 mL) all over face after cleansing or shaving.

Aroma Facial

This facial is suitable for all types of skin. However, if your skin is particularly sensitive, reduce the amount of essential oils by half. The best time for a facial is in the evening, when your pores are much more dilated. Follow this process once a week.

SKIN TYPE

All (see Variations)

WHEN TO USE

Evening

Makes 3 cups (750 mL)

TIP

Wash your face with warm water before you begin.

WHEN TO USE

After hot towel treatment

Makes 4 tsp (20 mL)

TIP

If you have sensitive skin, substitute an equal amount of raw honey for the brown sugar.

STEP 1: HOT TOWEL TREATMENT

- Glass or metal bowl
- Small towel

3 cups (750 mL)	warm (86°F/30°C) filtered water
2 drops	essential oil of choice (see Variations, opposite)
1 tsp (5 mL)	glycerin or carrier oil

1. In bowl, combine water, essential oil and glycerin.
2. Place towel in bowl and let it soak up liquid. Wring out and place hot towel on face. Leave on for 7 seconds (count to 7 slowly). Repeat 3 to 6 times.

STEP 2: FACIAL SCRUB

- Glass or metal bowl

1 tbsp (15 mL)	organic brown sugar
½ tsp (5 mL)	argan oil
2 drops	essential oil of choice (see Variations, opposite)

1. In bowl, combine sugar and argan oil.
2. Add essential oil and stir well.
3. Begin by wiping face with a washcloth soaked in warm water (or apply after hot towel treatment, above). Using your fingers, apply ½ to 1 tsp (2 to 5 mL) scrub to slightly moist skin and gently massage face in small circles for 30 seconds. Rinse off with warm water and towel dry. Follow with Moisturizing Facial Massage Serum (opposite).

WHEN TO USE
After Facial Scrub
(page opposite)

**Makes about
⅓ tsp (1.6 mL)**

KNOW THE BENEFITS

Applying a hot, wet towel to your face is warm and comforting hydrotherapy that opens the pores and nasal passages, allowing you to breathe and relax.

Facial scrubs help to thoroughly cleanse your skin, yielding a brighter complexion.

Calming and soothing, this facial massage serum helps skin maintain a healthy balance by preventing clogged pores that can lead to acne and blemishes. It can also be used as an aftershave oil.

- Small beaker

20 drops (1 mL)	argan oil
10 drops (0.5 mL)	rosehip seed oil
3 drops	essential oil of choice (see Variations, below)

1. In beaker, combine argan and rosehip seed oils. Add essential oil and stir well.
2. Begin by wiping face with a washcloth soaked in warm water (or apply after hot towel treatment, opposite). Apply 5 to 8 drops serum to fingertips and gently massage face in small circles for 30 seconds. Rinse off with warm water and towel dry.

Variations

Choose an essential oil to match your skin type from these alternatives:

FOR SENSITIVE SKIN: lavender, neroli, frankincense

FOR OILY SKIN: cajuput, rosemary, grapefruit, petitgrain

FOR DRY SKIN: ylang-ylang, clary sage, Roman chamomile

Pine-Scented Balm

Many men suffer from dry, chapped skin on the hands or feet, especially if they work outdoors. This soothing balm should be used daily.

SKIN TYPE

Dry, chapped

WHEN TO USE

As needed

Makes about 8 oz (235 mL)

TIP

To treat extra-dry and cracked hands or feet, soak them in warm water containing 2 to 3 drops each of pine and lavender essential oils, until water has cooled. Dry completely. Massage with about ½ tsp (2 mL) balm for 3 to 5 minutes, until completely absorbed.

KNOW THE BENEFITS

In addition to being moisturizing and anti-inflammatory, shea butter has wound-healing properties. Calendula-infused oil relieves dry, cracked skin. Borage oil is rich in gamma-linoleic acid, which is also very healing. The essential oil synergy is antiseptic and antibacterial.

- Small beaker
- Bowl-style double boiler
- Electric mixer
- Glass jar (8 oz/250 mL) sprayed with 70% ethyl alcohol (see page 219)

ESSENTIAL OIL SYNERGY

5 drops (0.25 mL)	lavender EO
5 drops (0.25 mL)	pine EO

BASE

1 tbsp (15 mL)	emulsifying wax
2 tbsp (30 mL)	shea butter
¾ cup (175 mL)	calendula-infused oil
1 tbsp (15 mL)	borage oil
10 drops (0.5 mL)	bamboo extract

1. *Essential Oil Synergy:* In beaker, combine lavender and pine essential oils. Cover with foil or plastic wrap and set aside.
2. *Base:* Set a heatproof glass bowl over a saucepan of hot, not boiling, water (86°F/30°C) and heat until warm to the touch. Add emulsifying wax and let melt completely. Add shea butter and warm until clear (1 to 2 minutes).
3. Meanwhile, in a bowl, combine calendula-infused and borage oils.
4. Remove melted wax mixture from heat. Using electric mixer at low speed, beat until cooled, white and fluffy.
5. While mixing, gradually add bamboo extract and mix until thickened. Add prepared synergy blend and mix well.
6. Transfer to prepared jar and seal tightly. Properly stored (see page 219), the balm will keep for up to 6 months.

Variation

For an antifungal effect, substitute equal quantities of tea tree and palmarosa essential oils for the lavender and pine.

HOW TO USE

Massage about ½ tsp (2 mL) balm into clean hands or feet for 3 to 5 minutes, until completely absorbed.

His Deodorant

Natural deodorants can provide long-lasting protection against odor when antimicrobial essential oils and base products are used.

SKIN TYPE

All (see Variation, below)

WHEN TO USE

After shower or bath

Makes 3½ oz (105 mL)

TIP

You can help prevent body odor by drinking plenty of water and eating a diet rich in fruits and vegetables.

KNOW THE BENEFITS

All the essential oils in this synergy blend are naturally deodorizing and antimicrobial. Potato starch, arrowroot powder and baking soda are natural antiperspirants and absorb moisture.

- Small beaker
- Bowl-style double boiler
- 2 deodorant bottles or jars (1 oz/30 mL) sprayed with 70% ethyl alcohol

ESSENTIAL OIL SYNERGY

5 drops (0.25 mL)	petitgrain EO
10 drops (0.5 mL)	patchouli EO
5 drops (0.25 mL)	sweet basil EO

BASE

¼ cup (60 mL)	extra virgin coconut oil
1 tbsp (15 mL)	beeswax
1 tbsp (15 mL)	potato starch
1 tbsp (15 mL)	arrowroot powder
1 tbsp (15 mL)	baking soda

1. *Essential Oil Synergy:* In beaker, combine essential oils. Cover with foil or plastic wrap and set aside.
2. *Base:* Set a heatproof glass bowl over a saucepan of hot, not boiling, water (86°F/30°C) and heat until warm to the touch. Add coconut oil and beeswax and let melt completely. Remove from heat and let cool slightly.
3. Meanwhile, in a small bowl, combine potato starch, arrowroot powder and baking powder. Add to melted oil and stir until well combined. Add prepared synergy blend and mix until combined.
4. Transfer to deodorant bottles, cover with lids and set aside for 24 hours to firm up. Properly stored (see page 219), the deodorant will keep for up to 3 months.

Variation

If you have sensitive skin, omit the baking soda and increase the arrowroot powder to 2 tbsp (30 mL).

HOW TO USE

Apply to clean armpits after bathing. Let dry before putting on clothing.

Shaving Cream

Shaving can take a toll on your skin. Using shaving cream helps the razor glide more smoothly over your skin, reducing the chances of cuts and scrapes.

KNOW THE BENEFITS

Coconut, argan and camellia seed oils are rich in fatty acids, especially lauric acid, which makes them extremely emollient as well as antimicrobial. Argan oil also contains squalane, which helps the skin retain moisture. Camellia seed oil leaves the skin feeling moist and also has antioxidant properties.

- Small beaker
- Bowl-style double boiler
- Electric mixer
- Flip-top or pump bottle (4 oz/125 mL) sprayed with 70% ethyl alcohol

ESSENTIAL OIL SYNERGY

5 drops (0.25 mL)	each cajuput EO and peppermint EO

BASE

¼ cup (60 mL)	extra virgin coconut oil
1 tbsp (15 mL)	shea butter
1 tbsp (15 mL)	argan oil
1 tbsp (15 mL)	camellia seed oil

1. *Essential Oil Synergy:* In beaker, combine essential oils. Cover with foil or plastic wrap and set aside.
2. *Base:* Set a heatproof glass bowl over a saucepan of hot, not boiling, water (86°F/30°C) and heat until warm to the touch. Add coconut oil and let melt completely. Add shea butter and let melt completely. Stir gently until evenly combined. Remove bowl from heat.
3. Add argan and camellia seed oils and stir to combine. Cover and refrigerate for 30 minutes to set.
4. Using electric mixer, whip oil mixture until creamy.
5. Add prepared synergy blend and mix until combined.
6. Transfer to prepared bottle and set aside for 24 hours to set. Properly stored (see page 219), the cream will keep for up to 6 months.

Variation

If you have sensitive skin, replace the essential oil synergy in Step 1 with 2 drops (0.25 mL) each neroli and petitgrain essential oils.

HOW TO USE

Dampen skin. Smooth shaving cream evenly over face before shaving.

Resources

AUSTRALIA

Australian Botanical Products
Essential oils and carrier oils
www.abp.com.au

Native Oils of Australia
Essential oils, carrier oils, herbs
and raw materials
www.nativeoilsaustralia.com.au

New Directions Australia
Essential oils, carrier oils, herbs
and packaging
www.newdirections.com.au

Perfect Potion
Essential oils and aromatherapy
supplies
www.perfectpotion.com

**Sydney Essential Oil
Company**
Essential oils, carrier oils, raw
materials and accessories
www.seoc.com.au

CANADA

Absolute Aromas Canada
Essential oils, carrier oils and
aromatherapy accessories
www.absolute-aromas.ca

Aquatech Skin Care
Base products, raw materials
and packaging
www.aquatech-skincare.com

**Healing Fragrances School
of Aromatherapy**
Educators and distributors of
essential oils and aromatherapy
products
www.healingfragrances.net

New Directions Aromatics
Essential oils and base products
www.newdirectionsaromatics.ca

Rae Dunphy Aromatics Ltd.
Essential oils, carrier oils and
raw ingredients
www.raedunphy.com

Richters Herbs
Plant botanicals and herbs
www.richters.com

Saffire Blue Inc.
Essential oils, carrier oils, raw
materials and accessories
www.saffireblue.ca

Salbro Bottle Inc.
Containers
www.salbrobottle.com

FRANCE

Florihana
Essential oils, carrier oils and
aromatherapy products
www.florihana.com

Pranarōm
Essential oils, carrier oils and
aromatherapy products
www.pranarom.com

ISRAEL

J. D. Schloss Ltd.
Essential oils and carrier oils
www.jd-schloss.com

MEXICO

Shaktili Aromaterapia
Essential oils, carrier oils and
raw materials
www.shaktili.com

UNITED KINGDOM

Absolute Aromas Ltd.
Essential oils, carrier oils, raw
ingredients and aromatherapy
packaging
www.absolute-aromas.com

Gracefruit Ltd.
Essential oils, carrier oils and
raw materials
www.gracefruit.com

**Organic Herb Trading
Company**
Essential oils, carrier oils and
raw materials
www.organicherbtrading.com

Oshadhi Ltd.
Essential oils, carrier oils and
aromatherapy products
www.oshadhi.co.uk

UNITED STATES

Aromatics International
Essential oils, carrier oils and
raw materials
www.aromatics.com

Mountain Rose Herbs
Essential oils, carrier oils and
raw materials
www.mountainroseherbs.com

Nature's Gift Inc.
Essential oils, carrier oils, raw
materials and packaging
www.naturesgift.com

SKS Bottle & Packaging Inc.
Equipment and packaging
www.sks-bottle.com

Specialty Bottle
Packaging
www.specialtybottle.com

Stillpoint Aromatics
Essential oils, carrier oils,
raw materials, packaging and
aromatherapy products
www.stillpointaromatics.com

References

Alcamo, I. Edward, and Barbara Krumhardt. *Anatomy and Physiology the Easy Way.* 1st ed. New York: Barron's, 2004.

Anasari, Shamim A. "Skin pH and Skin Flora." In *Handbook of Cosmetic Science and Technology*, edited by A. Barel, M. Paye and H. Maibach, 163–74. 4th ed. Boca Raton, FL: CRC Press, 2014.

Anitha, T. "Medicinal Plants Used in Skin Protection." *Asian Journal of Pharmaceutical and Clinical Research* 5, suppl. 3 (2012): 40–44.

Asadi-Samani, M., M. Bahmani and M. Rafieian-Kopaei. "The Chemical Composition, Botanical Characteristic and Biological Activities of *Borago officinalis*: A Review." *Asian Pacific Journal of Tropical Medicine* 7 (2014): S22–28. http://dx.doi.org/10.1016/s1995-7645(14)60199-1.

Battaglia, S. *The Complete Guide to Aromatherapy.* 1st ed. Brisbane: International Centre of Holistic Aromatherapy, 2003.

Baumann, Leslie. "The Baumann Skin-Type Indicator: A Novel Approach to Understanding Skin Type." In *Handbook of Cosmetic Science and Technology*, edited by A. Barel, M. Paye and H. Maibach, 29–40. 3rd ed. Boca Raton, FL: CRC Press, 2009.

Bensouda, Y., K. Qiraouani Boucetta, Z. Charrouf, H. Aguenaou and A. Derouiche. "The Effect of Dietary and/or Cosmetic Argan Oil on Postmenopausal Skin Elasticity." *Clinical Interventions in Aging* 10 (2015): 339–49. http://dx.doi.org/10.2147/cia.s71684.

Bergman, Åke, J. Heindel, S. Jobling, K. Kidd and T. Zoeller. "State-of-the-Science of Endocrine Disrupting Chemicals, 2012." *Toxicology Letters* 211, suppl. (2012): S3. doi: 10.1016/j.toxlet.2012.03.020.

Bowles, E. Joy. *The A to Z of Essential Oils.* New York: Barron's, 2003.

Burtenshaw, J.M.L. "The Mechanisms of Self-Disinfection of the Human Skin and Its Appendages." *Journal of Hygiene* 42 (1942), 184–209.

Cabrera-Vique, C., R. Marfil, R. Giménez and O. Martínez-Augustin. "Bioactive Compounds and Nutritional Significance of Virgin Argan Oil: An Edible Oil with Potential as a Functional Food." *Nutrition Reviews* 70, no. 5 (2012): 266–79. http://dx.doi.org/10.1111/j.1753-4887.2012.00478.x.

Campaign for Safe Cosmetics. Parabens. 2016. Accessed June 27, 2016. http://www.safecosmetics.org/get-the-facts/chemicals-of-concern/parabens/.

Catty, S. *Hydrosols.* 1st ed. Rochester, VT: Healing Arts Press, 2001.

Choi, Seo Yeon, Purum Kang, Hui Su Lee and Geun Hee Seol. "Effects of Inhalation of Essential Oil of *Citrus aurantium* L. var. *amara* on Menopausal Symptoms, Stress, and Estrogen in Postmenopausal Women: A Randomized Controlled Trial." *Evidence-Based Complementary and Alternative Medicine* 2014 (2014), 1–7. doi: 10.1155/2014/796518.

Coleman, W.P., III. "*Handbook of Cosmetic Science and Technology*, 3rd Edition" [book review]. *Dermatologic Surgery* 36, no. 3 (2010): 382. http://dx.doi.org/10.1111/j.1524-4725.2009.01444.x.

Couturaud, Virginie. "Biophysical Characteristics of the Skin: Relation to Race, Sex, Age and Site." In *Handbook of Cosmetic Science and Technology*, edited by A. Barel, M. Paye and H. Maibach. 4th ed. Boca Raton, FL: CRC Press, 2014.

Dobrev, H. "Clinical and Instrumental Study of the Efficacy of a New Sebum Control Cream." *Journal of Cosmetic Dermatology* 6, no. 2 (2007): 113–18. http://dx.doi.org/10.1111/j.1473-2165.2007.00306.x.

Dweck, Anthony. "Natural Preservatives." Research paper. http://www.dweckdata.co.uk/Published_papers/Natural_Preservatives_original.pdf.

Eichenfield, L., A. McCollum and P. Msika. "The Benefits of Sunflower Oleodistillate (SOD) in Pediatric Dermatology." *Pediatric Dermatology* 26, no. 6 (2009): 669–75. http://dx.doi.org/10.1111/j.1525-1470.2009.01042.x.

Gabard, B., and J. Ademola. "Lip Sun Protection Factor of a Lipstick Sunscreen." *Dermatology* 203, no. 3 (2001): 244–47. http://dx.doi.org/10.1159/000051758.

Ganceviciene, R., A. Liakou, A. Theodoridis, E. Makrantonaki and C. Zouboulis. "Skin Anti-aging Strategies." *Dermato-Endocrinology* 4, no. 3 (2012): 308–19.

Grotenhermen, F., G. Leson and P. Pless. "Evaluating the Impact of THC in Hemp Foods and Cosmetics on Human Health and Workplace Drug Tests." *Journal of Industrial Hemp* 8, no. 2 (2003): 5–36. http://dx.doi.org/10.1300/j237v08n02_02.

Guillaume, D., and Z. Charrouf. "Argan Oil." *Alternative Medicine Review* 16, no. 3 (2011): 275–77.

Gunstone, F. *The Lipid Handbook.* 1st ed. Hoboken, NJ: CRC Press, 2007.

Gupta, A., P.C. Sharma, B.M.K. Thilakaratne and A.K. Verma. "Studies on Physico-chemical Characteristics and Fatty Acid Composition of Wild Apricot (*Prunus armeniaca* Linn.) Kernel Oil." *Indian Journal of Natural Products and Resources* 3, no. 3 (2012): 366–70.

Harman, A. *Harvest to Hydrosol: Distill Your Own Exquisite Hydrosols at Home.* Washington, DC: botANNicals, 2015.

Health Canada. Safety of Cosmetic Ingredients. 2016. Accessed June 27, 2016. http://hc-sc.gc.ca/cps-spc/cosmet-person/labelling-etiquetage/ingredients-eng.php#a4.1.

Heuberger, Eva, Tapanee Hongratanaworakit and Gerhard Buchbauer. "East Indian Sandalwood and a-Santalol Odor Increase Physiological and Self-Rated Arousal in Humans." *Planta Medica* 72, no. 9 (2006): 792–800. doi: 10.1055/s-2006-941544.

Juhász, Margit Lai Wun, and Ellen S. Marmur. "A Review of Selected Chemical Additives in Cosmetic Products." *Dermatologic Therapy* 27, no. 6 (2014): 317–22. doi: 10.1111/dth.12146.

Khalil, M., J. Marcelletti, L. Katz, D. Katz and L. Pope. "Topical Application of Docosanol- or Stearic Acid-Containing Creams Reduces Severity of Phenol Burn Wounds in Mice." *Contact Dermatitis* 43, no. 2 (2000): 79–81. http://dx.doi.org/10.1034/j.1600-0536.2000.043002079.

Korać, R., and K. Khambholja. "Potential of Herbs in Skin Protection from Ultraviolet Radiation." *Pharmacognosy Reviews* 5, no. 10 (2011): 164–73. http://dx.doi.org/10.4103/0973-7847.91114.

Kristmundsdottir, Thordis, and Skuli Skulason. "Lipids as Active ingredients in Pharmaceuticals, Cosmetics and Health Foods." In *Lipids and Essential Oils as Antimicrobial Agents*, edited by Halldor Thormar, 151–77. Chichester: John Wiley and Sons, 2011.

Kumar, P., S. Singh, D. Mishra and P. Girotra. "Enhancement of Ketorolac Tromethamine Permeability through Rat Skin Using Penetration Enhancers: An Ex-vivo Study." *International Journal of Pharmaceutical Investigation* 5, no. 3 (2015): 142–46. http://dx.doi.org/10.4103/2230-973x.160850.

Kushi, M. *Your Face Never Lies*. 1st ed. Wayne, NJ: Avery, 1983.

Leizer, C., D. Ribnicky, A. Poulev, S. Dushenkov and I. Raskin. "The Composition of Hemp Seed Oil and Its Potential as an Important Source of Nutrition." *Journal of Nutraceuticals, Functional and Medical Foods* 2, no. 4 (2000): 35–53. http://dx.doi.org/10.1300/j133v02n04_04.

Lis-Balchin, Maria. *Aromatherapy Science*. 1st ed. London: Pharmaceutical Press, 2006.

Ma, W., L. Wang, Y. Guo, L. Liu, H. Qi, N. Zhu et al. "Urinary Concentrations of Parabens in Chinese Young Adults: Implications for Human Exposure." *Archives of Environmental Contamination and Toxicology* 65, no. 3 (2013): 611–18. http://dx.doi.org/10.1007/s00244-013-9924-2.

Matsui, M., E. Pelle, K. Dong and N. Pernodet. "Biological Rhythms in the Skin." *International Journal of Molecular Sciences* 17, no. 6 (2016): e801. http://dx.doi.org/10.3390/ijms17060801.

Mehling, A., and J. Fluhr. "Chronobiology: Biological Clocks and Rhythms of the Skin." *Skin Pharmacology and Physiology* 19, no. 4 (2006): 182–89. http://dx.doi.org/10.1159/000093113.

Moreno Gimenez, J.C., J. Bueno, J. Navas and F. Camacho. "Treatment of Skin Ulcer Using Oil of Mosqueta Rose" [article in Spanish]. *Medicina cutánea ibero-latinto-americana* 18, no. 1 (1990): 63–66.

Nayak, B., S. Raju and A. Chalapathi Rao. "Wound Healing Activity of *Persea americana* (Avocado) Fruit: A Preclinical Study on Rats." *Journal of Wound Care* 17, no. 3 (2008): 123–25. http://dx.doi.org/10.12968/jowc.2008.17.3.28670.

Ní Raghallaigh, S., K. Bender, N. Lacey, L. Brennan and F. Powell. "The Fatty Acid Profile of the Skin Surface Lipid Layer in Papulopustular Rosacea." *British Journal of Dermatology* 166, no. 2 (2012): 279–87. http://dx.doi.org/10.1111/j.1365-2133.2011.10662.x.

Pearce, Cedric J. "Review of *Honey in Traditional and Modern Medicine*." *Journal of Natural Products* 78, no. 4 (2015): 967. doi: 10.1021/acs.jnatprod.5b00127.

Prottey, C., P. Hartop and M. Press. "Correction of the Cutaneous Manifestations of Essential Fatty Acid Deficiency in Man by Application of Sunflower-Seed Oil to the Skin." *Journal of Investigative Dermatology* 64, no. 4 (1975): 228–34. http://dx.doi.org/10.1111/1523-1747.ep12510667.

Raghavan, K., A. Pal, F. Khan and A. Singh. "Nutritional, Medicinal and Industrial Uses of Sesame (*Sesamum indicum* L.) Seeds: An Overview." *Agriculturae Conspectus Scientificus* 75, no. 4 (2010): 159–68.

Raichur, P., and M. Cohn. *Absolute Beauty*. 1st ed. New York: HarperCollins, 1997.

Rios Scherrer, Maria Antonieta, and Vanessa Barreto Rocha. "Increasing Trend of Sensitization to Methylchloroisothiazolinone/Methylisothiazolinone (MCI/MI)." *Anais brasileiros de dermatologia* 89, no 3 (2014): 527–28. doi: 10.1590/abd1806-4841.20142852.

Rizer, R.L. "Oily Skin: Claim Support Strategies." In *Cosmetics: Controlled Efficacy Studies and Regulation*, edited by P. Elsner, Howard I. Maibach and Hans F. Merk, 81–91. Berlin: Springer, 1999.

Roosterman, D., T. Goerge, S.W. Schneider, N.W. Bunnett and M. Steinhoff. "Neuronal Control of Skin Function: The Skin as a Neuroimmunoendocrine Organ." *Physiological Reviews* 86, no. 4 (2006): 1309–79. doi: 10.1152/physrev.00026.2005.

Saraf, S., and C. Kaur. "In Vitro Sun Protection Factor Determination of Herbal Oils Used in Cosmetics." *Pharmacognosy Research* 2, no. 1 (2010): 22–25. http://dx.doi.org/10.4103/0974-8490.60586.

Sugawara, Y., C. Hara, K. Tamura et al. "Sedative Effect on Humans of Inhalation of Essential Oil of Linalool." *Analytica Chimica Acta* 365, nos. 1–3 (1998): 293–99. doi: 10.1016/s0003-2670(97)00639-9.

Sultana, Y., K. Kohli, M. Athar, R. Khar and M. Aqil. "Effect of Pre-treatment of Almond Oil on Ultraviolet B–Induced Cutaneous Photoaging in Mice." *Journal of Cosmetic Dermatology* 6, no. 1 (2007): 14–19. http://dx.doi.org/10.1111/j.1473-2165.2007.00293.x.

Thormar, Halldor, ed. *Lipids and Essential Oils as Antimicrobial Agents*. Chichester: Wiley, 2011.

Tisserand, Robert, and Rodney Young. *Essential Oil Safety: A Guide for Health Care Professionals*. 2nd ed. Elsevier Health Sciences, 2013.

Tongnuanchan, Phakawat, and Soottawat Benjakul. "Essential Oils: Extraction, Bioactivities, and Their Uses for Food Preservation." *Journal of Food Science* 79, no. 7 (2014): R1231–49. doi: 10.1111/1750-3841.12492.

Vettor, Manuela, Paola Perugini, Simona Gagliardi et al. "Topical Application of Lignans and Phytosterols in Seborrhoic Skin." *Journal of Applied Cosmetology* 24 (2006): 123–29.

Yates, J., J. Phifer and D. Flake. "Do Nonmedicated Topicals Relieve Childhood Eczema?" *Journal of Family Practice* 58, no. 5 (2009): 280–81.

Library and Archives Canada Cataloguing in Publication

Sade, Danielle, 1957–, author
    The aromatherapy beauty guide : using the science of carrier & essential oils to create natural personal care products / Danielle Sade BSc, CAHP.

Includes index.
ISBN 978-0-7788-0560-1 (softcover)

    1. Aromatherapy. 2. Herbal cosmetics. 3. Natural products.
4. Skin—Care and hygiene. 5. Beauty, Personal. I. Title.

RM666.A68S23 2017   615.3'219   C2017-900377-1

Index